Nursing the Orthopaedic Patient

For Churchill Livingstone

Publisher: Mary Law
Project editor: Dinah Thom
Copy editor: Nairn Reed
Indexer: Nina Boyd
Project manager: Neil Dickson
Sales promotion executive: Hilary Bown

Nursing the Orthopaedic Patient

Edited by

Peter S. Davis MA BEd(Hons) CertEd RGN DN(Lond) ONC

Course Director, Royal National Orthopaedic Hospital (NHS) Trust, Middlesex

Foreword by

Mary Powell OBE SRN MCSP ONC

Formerly Matron, Robert Jones and Agnes Hunt Orthopaedic Hospital, Oswestry, Shropshire

CHURCHILL LIVINGSTONE

EDINBURGH LONDON MADRID MELBOURNE NEW YORK AND TOKYO 1994

CHURCHILL LIVINGSTONE
Medical Division of Longman Group UK Limited

Distributed in the United States of America by Churchill
Livingstone Inc., 650 Avenue of the Americas, New York,
N. Y. 10011, and by associated companies, branches and
representatives throughout the world.

First published 1994

ISBN 0-443-04461-9

British Library Cataloguing in Publication Data
A catalogue record for this book is available from the British
Library.

Library of Congress Cataloging in Publication Data
Nursing the orthopaedic patient / edited by Peter S. Davis; foreword
   by Mary Powell.
        p.   cm.
      Includes index.
      ISBN 0–443–04461–9
      1. Orthopedic nursing.   I. Davis, Peter S., 1953–
      [DNLM: 1. Orthopedic Nursing—methods.   2. Orthopedics—methods.
   3. Patient Care Planning.   WY 157.6 N974 1994]
   RD753.N87   1994
   610.73'677—dc20
   DNLM/DLC
   for Library of Congress   93-43058
                                                                  CIP

The
publisher's
policy is to use
**paper manufactured
from sustainable forests**

Produced by Longman Singapore Publishers (Pte) Ltd
Printed in Singapore

Contents

Contributors

Hilary Addison RGN ONC
Ward Sister in Orthopaedics and
Rheumatology, The Middlesex Hospital,
London

Kathy Balcombe MA DipPDN(Lond) RGN RCNT
Executive Director of Nursing and Quality,
Bromley Hospitals (NHS) Trust, Kent

Peter S. Davis MA BEd(Hons) CertEd RGN DN(Lond)
ONC
Course Director, Royal National Orthopaedic
Hospital (NHS) Trust, Middlesex

Ann F. Gill RGN ONC RCNT FETC
Senior Nurse Manager, Orthopaedic Unit,
Northern General Hospital, Sheffield

Dinah Gould BSc MPhil RGN CertEd
Lecturer in Nursing Studies, London University,
London

Nicholas Hext RGN ENB219
Senior Staff Nurse, Alpington Ward, Norfolk
and Norwich Hospital, Norwich

Carol Horrigan MSc SRN RCNT DN PGCEA RNT
Nurse Tutor (Complementary Therapies and
Oncology), Bloomsbury and Islington College of
Nursing and Midwifery, London; Lecturer
(Complementary Therapies), Institute of
Advanced Nurse Education, Royal College of
Nursing, London

Carol A. Humphreys BSc DPSN FETC RGN OND SEN
Senior Sister, Trauma and Orthopaedics,
Birmingham General Hospital, Birmingham

Ninette Johnson RGN
Clinical Nurse Specialist, The Middlesex
Hospital, London

Jan McCall MSocSci RGN DipN(Lond) ONC FETC
Quality Assurance Adviser, Nuffield
Orthopaedic Centre NHS Trust, Oxford

Amanda Matthew RGN ONC DN
Sister, Trauma / Orthopaedic Directorate, The
Solihull Hospital, West Midlands

Judith Kay Muir MA SRN SCM RNT DipEd(Lond)
Vice-Principal, Bloomsbury and Islington
College of Nursing and Midwifery, London

Elizabeth O'Brien SRN
Ward Sister, The Middlesex Hospital, London

Lorraine Rundell RGN ENB219
Staff Nurse, The Middlesex Hospital, London

Linda C. Russell RGN ONC
Ward Sister, Birmingham Orthopaedic
Oncology Service, Royal Orthopaedic Hospital,
Birmingham

Jacqueline Scott BEd(Hons) RN ONC DN(Lond) RCNT
RNT
Lecturer Practitioner, School of Health Care
Studies, Oxford Brookes University, Nuffield
Orthopaedic Centre, Oxford

Sarah Wallis RGN ONC DN(Lond)
Formerly Nurse Teacher, Bloomsbury and
Islington College of Nursing and Midwifery,
London

Deborah Wheeler BSc(Hons) RGN ONC DN
Senior Nurse/Business Manager, Royal
National Orthopaedic Hospital (NHS) Trust,
Middlesex

Foreword

Orthopaedic nursing in Great Britain can be said to have been 'invented' by Agnes Hunt at the beginning of this century, when the bond between Miss Hunt and Robert Jones united orthopaedic surgery and the appropriate nursing skills for the first time. Later, a course of training was set up and an examination established for the Orthopaedic Nursing Certificate.

Since then, medical, surgical and social changes have overtaken the speciality and it is these changes which are reflected in the pages of this book, including the movement of nursing practice away from the medical model of the past. Nursing diagnosis, primary nursing, the nursing process, nursing models and standards of care are discussed together with the importance of nursing research.

Later chapters deal with the principles of treatment, and the problem of pain is dealt with in Chapter 7. Control of infection is highlighted and there are detailed expositions on osteoarthritis and rheumatoid arthritis. Orthopaedic conditions affecting the spine and limbs are discussed, although paediatric problems and those associated with trauma are not included. In a final chapter the amputee is considered in detail.

The aim of this book is stated to be to 'promote good nursing practice based on present research and understanding and to lay the foundations to enable the orthopaedic nurse to adapt, be innovative and lead the nursing care of clients with problems of mobility in the future'. Peter Davis and his contributors are to be congratulated on the production of this text, which will be required reading not only for the orthopaedic nurse of today but also for her counterpart of tomorrow.

M. P.

Preface

Orthopaedic nursing care is changing at an unprecedented rate and will continue to do so in the future. Almost as soon as pen is put to paper, or fingers to keyboard, the information is out of date. This book does not try to achieve the impossible in containing all the up-to-date information on orthopaedic nursing, but it does provide a solid foundation of current knowledge and understanding of the essence of orthopaedic nursing, and gives direction and guidance to nurses to enable them to identify their own specific needs and achieve their desired objectives.

The book is intended for qualified nurses studying at either diploma or degree level, but pre-registration nurses will find it a useful reference source. The descriptions of nursing care apply mainly to the hospital environment, but the nurse's role within the health care team is referred to in every chapter, and some chapters focus on the interface of hospital and community care provision. A health rather than an illness perspective is adopted in conjunction with models of nursing, and at all times the emphasis is on caring for the patient rather than treating the condition. The care of the child and orthopaedic trauma are not included as they are largely specialty areas in their own right and outside the scope of this book.

The first eight chapters describe and discuss the underlying principles and concepts of orthopaedic nursing, irrespective of the patient/client's medical diagnosis; for example in this section there is a chapter on pain management as it is common to all areas of orthopaedic nursing. This enables the nurse to develop a flexible approach to care based on current research and knowledge and encourages a reflective and critical attitude. In many care situations there is no one right answer but often several, or a number of poor alternatives. The orthopaedic nurse should be able to decide on the most appropriate care for each individual at any particular time.

The second part of the book provides in-depth information on the nursing care of patients with specific conditions and problems. A number of different nursing models are used to describe nursing care, and case studies are included to illustrate and add validity to the discussions.

To avoid confusion, throughout the book the term 'he' is used to refer to patients and clients and 'she' to refer to nurses.

Finally I would like to thank all those nurses from my past who have assisted my learning and development and provided the encouragement and support to enable me to write and edit this book. My fellow contributors and Dinah Thom, my editor at Churchill Livingstone, have worked hard to make my dream a reality. To Lorraine and Holly I give my love for being there and keeping me going when times got hard.

London, 1994   P. S. D.

1

Changing orthopaedic nursing

Peter S. Davis

This chapter looks briefly at some of the changes in society, health care provision and nursing in general that will shape the future of orthopaedic nursing. All aspects of people's lives, including their health, are changing, and predictions suggest that this will continue at an increasing pace. One change that has affected orthopaedic nursing recently is the reduced amount of time that the patient now spends in hospital and the increased amount of nursing that is required in the community. Only two decades ago surgery for scoliosis involved a hospital admission of several months including many weeks of flat bedrest. Today, mobilization may occur in a matter of days and a hospital stay is of a few weeks' duration. Joint replacement surgery for osteoarthritic hips may now involve a preadmission assessment and preparation, a stay of 3 days in hospital and discharge to hotel accommodation.

The role of orthopaedic nurses is changing due to developments within nursing, health care provision and society. As professionals, orthopaedic nurses need to be proactive in adapting their delivery of nursing care to meet the changing needs of society. The Department of Health (1989) warns of a far from stable future: 'If the role of the nursing professions is first and foremost to respond to human needs and if in today's world these needs are continually and rapidly changing then the nursing professions must change with them. Such changes may take many forms.' The orthopaedic nurse must be prepared to care for and support patients in a variety of environments and move between

1

these environments with ease; for example, she may support the patient in his own home, prepare him for hospital and then continue his care whilst he is in hospital. Wherever possible she should seek to promote health, and for this she needs a different set of skills and knowledge base from those required in the past.

Such is the pace of change that often before a particular change has been fully developed or accepted, it is superseded by another; within nursing, the progression from implementing the nursing process to incorporating nursing models and primary nursing is one example. But change tends to be cyclical in nature and few, if any, innovations are totally new. The recent practice of using sugar for cleaning and healing pressure sores is far from original, as honey has been used for such purposes for millenniums.

In the context of change, nurses also need to appreciate the effects of change on others; for instance, patients coming to terms with a change in body image due to the loss of a limb will experience feelings of loss and grief, and colleagues may be reluctant to change their practice for fear of the unknown. By understanding the meaning of change to others, nurses are better able to understand its meaning to themselves (Davis 1991).

ORTHOPAEDIC NURSING

History

The term orthopaedic is derived from the Greek language, *orthos* meaning straight and *paedios* meaning of a child. The original application of the word was the growth or achievement of physically straight children; in the last century, orthopaedics was primarily concerned with children.

Cholmeley (1985) describes how an early London orthopaedic institution appointed its first orthopaedic nurse in 1841 to look after in-patients. The nurse's brief was to visit each patient before she retired to bed between 20 : 00 and 20 : 30, and again at 06 : 00 and at any time during the night if required. In addition to these duties she had to scrub, clean and tidy the wards and lobbies, make beds, be present at all operations, make and prepare bandages and serve the patients' meals. Many of the patients were children with conditions such as club foot and curvature of the spine. By 1871 the Board of Governors had taken steps to improve sanitation and the general conditions in the hospital and had realized the need to appoint a properly qualified person as a superintendent nurse. This nurse had separate sleeping quarters and was paid £5 extra per year. All nurses had their meals off the wards and got an extra pint of beer, a crust of bread or biscuit for their lunch and an extra half day off a fortnight. It must be remembered that at this time Florence Nightingale had only recently returned from the Crimea and that the first preliminary training school was not set up until 1890.

Present practice

Today's orthopaedic nurse owes much to the nursing education and developments achieved in specialist orthopaedic hospitals by such nurses as Dame Agnes Hunt and Mary Powell. Dame Agnes Hunt (1867–1948) with Sir Robert Jones founded what was to become the first orthopaedic hospital at Baschurch, about 7 miles from Oswestry; later she founded the first College for the Disabled in this country. Many of the principles of care adopted by today's orthopaedic nurses were developed at these institutions: the vision and energy of these pioneers has propelled orthopaedic nursing to where it is today.

Powell (1986) suggests that 'alongside her general nursing skills and knowledge the orthopaedic nurse needs expert knowledge of the patient's condition, of his particular needs and, most important, of how these are to be met and how complications are prevented'. This approach to orthopaedic nursing perceives nursing predominantly as a science. Indeed, many significant advances have been made in the science of nursing in the last 20 years. For example, when caring for a patient immediately after surgery, nurses now have the necessary technical skills to manage intravenous infusions, vacuum drainage bottles, positive pressure ventilators and complex traction systems. However, the manner in which nursing care is carried out – the interaction of nurse and patient – owes much to the art of nursing. This includes those aspects of nursing that cannot be analysed scientifically, such as the use of communication skills and in- tuition to decide when and how a nurse should just sit with a patient.

Nursing the orthopaedic patient in the future will be different. During the past 100 years orthopaedic nurses have developed their ideas about nursing, patients, and health and illness. These ideas will be expanded on in Chapter 3 in a proposed model of nursing. Many of them are reflected in the way nurses have developed, ex- panded and changed the existing medical theo- retical frameworks, for example, by moving from:

- A medical model to a nursing model
- An illness belief model to a health belief model
- A health care professional-centred approach to a patient-centred approach
- A perception of the patient as a disease or condition to a holistic perception of the client.

PERSPECTIVES ON PATIENTS/ CLIENTS

Changing role of patients

Orthopaedic nurses should discourage people from taking on the sick role too readily when they seek and receive health care. They should encourage and help patients to understand that they can play an important part in helping to restore their own health and well-being. Nurses can do this by, for example:

- Not using jargon when talking to patients or when talking to colleagues in the presence of a patient
- Using simple language but not treating the patient as simple
- Involving patients in decisions about their health and care
- Not establishing themselves as the all- knowing expert
- Carrying out nursing care *with* the patient and others and not *on* them.

There is now overwhelming evidence through thousands of diverse research studies to show that the person who will not let his illness control him and who takes responsibility for his own health and recovery, recuperates more quickly with fewer complications and with less chance of recurrence. Patients who have a posi- tive attitude and accept more fully their changed situation are more likely to gain a better quality of life ultimately, even if a cure is not possible.

Holism

Many health professionals now view people holistically, i.e. they regard the mind and body as a whole entity which cannot be studied as a collection of discrete parts (Davis 1989). How- ever, Orshan (1988) provides evidence that, although experts believe in this mind–body connection, they are unable to identify exactly what the connection is. The nursing profession is placing increasing emphasis on holistic health care and is in the forefront of its adoption within the Health Service. This is demonstrated in the increasing use, development and evaluation of complementary therapies in pain management, e.g. therapeutic massage, shiatsu, transcutane- ous electrical nerve stimulation, acupuncture, acupressure, reflexology, meditation, relaxation techniques, hypnosis, imagery and music (Rankin-Box 1988).

The changing population

Social and demographic changes have altered dramatically the health needs of the population. Baly (1980) points out that the eradication of the majority of infectious diseases has increased life expectancy and led to a preponderance of the non-infectious diseases. Among these, the degenerative diseases, such as osteoarthritis and osteoporosis, are becoming increasingly preva- lent among the older population. 'It is well known that the British population is rapidly ageing, with an expected doubling of those aged 85 and over between 1971 and 1996. This group makes disproportionately high use of the health services and the need for expansion in the field of care for the elderly will be great' (Royal College of Nursing 1988). As many of the problems suffered by the elderly are orthopaedic in nature, the result of this expansion will be an increase in the demand for orthopaedic nurses and their skills.

The individual's health

The effects of a lifetime of bad habits, such as alcohol and drug abuse, tobacco smoking, dietary excesses and lack of exercise, may become apparent only after a considerable length of time. Many of the diseases due to lifestyle are preventable through health promotion initiatives, which are based on an understanding of why an individual makes certain health or ill health choices. It may at first appear that conditions such as osteoporosis are not susceptible to such health promotion strategies. However, the Office of Health Economics (1990) advocates the use of health promotion interventions to reduce bone loss in women in order to prevent bone fracture due to osteoporosis; there is sufficient evidence to suggest that women who are encouraged to keep up a reasonable level of exercise can prevent bone loss (for example moderate exercise such as 30 minutes walking, jogging or dancing per day). At present one in four women in Britain sustain fractures due to osteoporosis: the development of screening and health education programmes could have a marked impact on these statistics.

The relationship between cause and effect in disease and illness is complex and multifaceted (Boore et al 1987). To be effective health promoters, nurses require a broad understanding of the factors influencing disease and illness, such as genetic predisposition, age, gender, economic, social and psychological conditions, individual response and the immune system.

PERSPECTIVES ON ORTHOPAEDIC NURSES

The recent introduction of clinical nurse specialists and primary nursing into the health service demonstrates the profession's commitment to encouraging nurses to be autonomous, knowledgeable and accountable in their practice. The development of these changes within orthopaedic nursing will be discussed in Chapters 2 and 3.

Clinical nurse specialist

The function of the clinical nurse specialist (CNS) or specialist practice nurse has been widely debated and developed (American Nurses Association 1986, Royal College of Nursing Orthopaedic Nursing Forum 1989). The purpose of this new post is to enable the nurse to focus on nursing issues rather than medical specialities; its introduction has resulted in a fundamental change within nursing. The CNS has the freedom to cross boundaries within defined client groups and is committed to the client rather than the organization. As a practitioner, consultant, educator and researcher the CNS has a significant influence on the nature of the patient's care and therapy, and if necessary acts as the patient's advocate. The orthopaedic nurse specialist is able to provide and advise on the nursing care of patients with orthopaedic problems irrespective of the type of ward the patients or clients are on or whether they are in hospital or in the community. Balcombe (1989) suggests that the component parts of the role of the CNS – practice, education and research – are important in the general maintenance and improvement of standards of care. The development and proliferation of these specialist posts are also a useful way of encouraging nurses, who are expert in caring for orthopaedic patients and who might otherwise move to administrative posts, to maintain close links with patient care: their value is recognized through promotion and remuneration and they increase their job satisfaction.

Primary nursing

The orthopaedic nurse who functions as a primary nurse is responsible and accountable for a patient's nursing throughout his time in hospital and/or the community. Care delivery is based on a care plan agreed with the patient. In the absence of the primary nurse the associate nurse follows the care plan directions.

The orthopaedic nurse's relationship with other health care professionals is of the utmost importance. In the hospital setting the health care team is often led by either a surgeon or a physician. However, only a minority of people with orthopaedic problems are cared for in the hospital environment; the vast majority are outside these carefully controlled, highly organized and expensive institutions. The primary care team is becoming increasingly responsible for the care of these individuals in the community. The composition, number of members, skill mix and leadership of these care teams depend on the environment of care and nature of the person's orthopaedic problem. Nurses may find themselves increasingly leading these teams in future, but only if they can justify the need for their skills and knowledge and accept the professional accountability that is implied. The health care team may consist of a doctor, physiotherapist, occupational therapist, medical social worker, sexual counsellor, dietitian, orthotist, play therapist, disablement resettlement officer and complementary therapist. In addition, the patient's family and friends may be important members of the team, provided that they are given sufficient information and support.

PERSPECTIVES ON ORTHOPAEDIC NURSING

Nursing model vs. medical model

Nursing models are developed from nurses' beliefs, theories, values and concepts (Davis 1988a).

The most successful models evolved from the experience of nurses such as Virginia Henderson and Florence Nightingale who were able to conceptualize clearly their own views on nursing and whose views largely coincided with those of all nurses. Nursing models reflect how nurses comprehend their fellow human beings; the knowledge base for these concepts is taken from the life sciences, i.e. psychology, physiology, anatomy, philosophy and sociology. However, it is the way in which this knowledge is used and prioritized, based on nurses' perceptions of care, that makes a model unique to nursing.

Unfortunately, the rather contorted language used in nursing models often makes them difficult to understand, and nurses are apt to make the simple complex, the understandable incomprehensible and the attainable unreachable, probably in a misguided effort to acquire professional and academic credibility. This can lead to the misuse or rejection of these models.

Nursing models should not be used in a rigid, inflexible way but should be changed and adapted to suit a set of circumstances as well as bring about change through the way they challenge existing understanding, beliefs and attitudes. If an activities of living model is being used (see Roper & Logan 1985) in an orthopaedic nursing setting, then it may be appropriate to prioritize or reorganize the activities so that the main emphasis is placed on the activity of mobilizing (Fig. 1.1). This would be suitable for the rheumatoid patient, for example, who is unable to lift an arm or rotate his wrist and thus

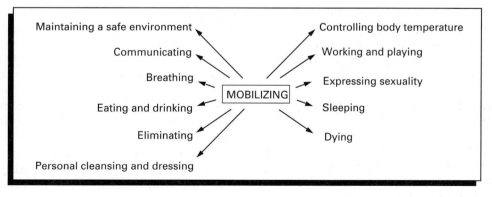

Fig. 1.1   The central position of mobilizing.

has difficulty in eating and drinking. Similarly, other components of the model, such as the dependence–independence continuum, may be reoriented in the same way, as the dependence or independence of the person with orthopaedic problems depends on their degree of mobility.

Prevention vs. cure

Nurses need to take a leading role in illness prevention and reduction. They should increase their understanding of the contexts in which individuals make health choices, rather than persuade people to change their bad behaviour. In promoting health, nurses need to understand the importance of the principles of equity, participation and community development (Gott & O'Brien 1990). For example, back injury is a significant drain on the health and social services. It is essentially preventable, yet nurses, themselves, form one of the largest groups who are affected by it. Resources need to be directed towards providing programmes of instruction in how to lift and handle objects and patients, and the necessary lifting equipment to encourage individuals to take responsibility for their own health.

Research-based care vs. ritualized care

In the past orthopaedic nurses have been content to rely on experience passed on from previous generations. This ensures that nursing knowledge is built on yesterday's experiences, but it can also produce ritualized care, stifle innovation and discourage an enquiring attitude. The lack of good quality nursing research is illustrated in a problem encountered by nurses caring for a person with a skeletal pin as part of a traction system. As Davis (1988b) identifies, there are at present several recommended methods of cleaning and dressing the pin sites with no conclusive research to help the nurse decide. Until research identifies an optimum method, nurses must rely on their own experience and an educated guess.

Despite the above criticisms, there is a considerable body of research-based nursing knowledge which is not being utilized fully. This knowledge needs to be increased and continually evaluated and assessed. Nurses should always be aware, however, that even nursing research can be misused in a ritualized, unquestioning and dogmatic way.

Open vs. closed approach

If orthopaedic nursing is to develop, imaginative and novel approaches to care should be encouraged and nurtured; this may entail looking to unfamiliar disciplines or complementary therapies for ideas. Complementary practices and ideologies are no longer called 'alternative' as this implies the exclusion of traditional methods, whereas 'complementary' implies a process whereby two or more entities mutually make up for each other's deficiencies; that is, they coexist and enhance each other. Complementary practices, such as relaxation techniques based on massage, music and aromatherapy, are now being used increasingly in Western health care in place of medication, which can have unwanted side-effects such as dependency.

The nursing profession's approach to health and nursing is becoming more open: many skills and concepts that had been discarded in the past by Western medicine are now being rediscovered and have been given a prominent place in nursing philosophies – for example, holistic care.

Organizing care

The nursing process

Nursing has developed a systematic approach to care – the nursing process – which many nurses now use. This approach is not unique to nursing. Teachers, for example, use a similar process consisting of the following stages: assessing needs and developing objectives, planning content, implementing methods and carrying out an evaluation. For nurses and teachers, using a systematic approach provides a useful and logical organizational framework; but these frameworks do not contain anything specific to nursing or teaching.

The nursing process is often thought of as

another model of nursing. However, concepts, such as individualizing patient care, are specific to ideas and beliefs about nursing, and form part of a nursing model and not part of the nursing process. The nursing process is a simple organizational tool which is used in many models of nursing but is not a model itself.

The nursing process is usually described as having four phases: assessment, planning, implementation and evaluation. Goals are essential to the process because the evaluative component of nursing cannot take place unless preceded by a statement of expectation (Roper et al 1981). By using the nursing process, nurses should be able to demonstrate accountability for their care and also maintain and improve standards of care.

Quality indicators

The gauging of the quality of nursing care begins and ends with the patient's experience of the service provided (Kitson 1989). A framework for maintaining and improving quality should be based on a patient-centred approach. It should be multidisciplinary in its representation, as nursing care is affected by, and affects, other health care professionals' contribution to the patient's care. It is about setting objectives shared by all members of care groups through developing standards of nursing care. Most patients after hip surgery would want their pain controlled to a level acceptable to them. Therefore, it is the responsibility of the nurse, doctor, physiotherapist and pharmacist, as a team, to assess the patient's pain, provide pain relief, monitor the degree of success and take further action if necessary. A simple standard of no patient having to wait longer than 15 minutes from the time he complains of pain to when he receives a pain relief intervention can make a significant difference to the patient's quality of care.

The setting of standards provides a framework for encouraging nurses at the local level to embrace the objectives and values of the profession at large (Royal College of Nursing Orthopaedic Nursing Forum 1990). Participation in the standard-setting provides an opportunity for nurses to liaise on equal terms with the multidisciplinary team to ensure the best possible service for the patient. Both national and local standards may be used to develop a relevant quality assurance tool in order to measure, improve and maintain the level of service.

The Dynamic Standard-Setting System (DySSSy), developed by Kitson (1989), has been used by orthopaedic nurses in the UK to produce national standards of nursing care. The implementation of the system not only has done much to improve the quality of patient care but has also helped the professional development of orthopaedic nurses. Examples of standards for the organization of care in orthopaedic nursing (Royal College of Nursing Orthopaedic Nursing Forum 1990) are:

1. Standard statement: clients with disorders of the neuromusculoskeletal system will receive competent and individualized care planned by a named nurse according to the concepts of the nursing process.
2. Structure criteria: an agreed philosophy of nursing, reflecting the beliefs of the nursing team, is formulated and held in trust by the ward or unit.
3. Process criteria: all nursing care is based on the ward or unit's agreed philosophy of nursing.
4. Outcome criteria: the client has knowledge of the system of nursing and is able to participate in his care if he so wishes and is able.

In any standard-setting initiatives it is important that nurses, patients and others involved can identify with and believe in the standards set. A system that attempts to enforce standards from above or outside is unlikely to have this level of acceptance and therefore is not likely to succeed.

In, for example, performance indicators (PIs) or financial information projects (FIPs), the gathering and use of objective data are important elements of these quality assurance strategies. (Further information on these strategies is given in Ch. 2.) For instance, it is useful to have data that can indicate whether a new infection control policy has reduced the number of infections in a unit and has thus saved money (by reducing the number of bed days taken up by patients who have delayed discharge dates because of preventable infections). These indicators are, however, only part of the information required to be able to make patient care decisions. The drive for efficiency should be matched by an awareness of the degree of health care that society desires from its health service.

Ballogh and Beattie (1988) argue that the ethical dimension should not be ignored when health service managers use the criteria of efficiency, economy and effectiveness to determine quality of care. The possible scenario of carrying out hip replacements only on under-75-year-olds may be justified on the grounds of efficiency and economy, but may not be ethical in terms of equal health care for all. Commonly, the younger the patient, the fewer the general health problems he has and therefore the shorter is his hospital admission. Statistically, the patient throughput would improve and reduce numbers on the waiting list. However, refusing surgery to over-75-year-olds, whose quality of life would be greatly improved by such surgery, is questionable; and it could be argued that society is prepared to pay for the increased costs of equal health care availability.

CONCLUSION

In future, the orthopaedic nurse will have to become increasingly critical and reflective about the care she provides. Today's important issues will be replaced by equally important but different issues. The aim of this text is to promote good orthopaedic nursing practice based on present research and understanding. In addition, it lays the foundations to enable the nurse to adapt, be innovative and lead the nursing care of clients with problems of mobility in the future.

REFERENCES

American Nurses Association 1986 The role of the clinical nurse specialist. Mercia Publications, Keele University

Balcombe K P 1989 Leading the way. Nursing Standard 16(3): 24

Ballogh R, Beattie A 1988 Performance review. Nursing Times 84(18): 67–69

Baly M E 1980 Nursing and social change, 2nd edn. William Heinemann, London

Boore J R P, Champion R, Ferguson M C 1987 Nursing the physically ill adult. Churchill Livingstone, Edinburgh

Cholmeley J A 1985 History of the Royal National Orthopaedic Hospital. Chapman & Hall, London

Davis P S 1988a Models for orthopaedic nursing. Bare Bones 4 (Spring)

Davis P S 1988b The principles of traction. Nursing 3(34)

Davis P S 1989 Complementary methods in pain management. National study day on the management of pain, 2nd Nov, London

Davis P S 1991 The meaning of change to individuals within a college of nurse education. Journal of Advanced Nursing 16(1): 108–115

Department of Health, Nursing Division 1989 A strategy for nursing. HMSO, London

Gott M, O'Brien M 1990 The role of the nurse in health promotion. Paper presented at Royal College of Nursing research conference, Surrey University

Kitson A L 1989 Standards of care – a framework for quality. Scutari Press, London

Office of Health Economics 1990 Osteoporosis and risk of fracture. Office of Health Economics, London

Orshan S A 1988 Pain and stress management in nursing: controversy and theory. Holistic Nursing Practice 2(3): 9–16

Powell M 1986 Orthopaedic nursing and rehabilitation, 9th edn. Churchill Livingstone, Edinburgh

Rankin-Box D F 1988 Complementary health therapies: a guide for nurses and the caring professions. Croom-Helm, London

Roper N, Logan W W, Tierney A J 1981 Learning to use the process of nursing. Churchill Livingstone, Edinburgh

Roper N, Logan W 1985 The Roper, Logan and Tierney model. Senior Nurse 3(2): 20–26

Royal College of Nursing 1988 The health challenge. Royal College of Nursing, London

Royal College of Nursing, Orthopaedic Nursing Forum 1989 The role of the clinical nurse specialist working in orthopaedics. Bare Bones 9 (Autumn)

Royal College of Nursing, Orthopaedic Nursing Forum 1990 Standards of care in orthopaedic nursing. Royal College of Nursing, London

2

The environment of care

Ann F. Gill

INTRODUCTION

Orthopaedic nursing covers a wide spectrum of conditions affecting all societies throughout the world. Depending on the region and state of the population, these vary from catastrophic congenital deformities and major infection in Third World countries where famine and poor health care provision exist, to problems arising from an affluent lifestyle, culture and social class. Many of these conditions require a wide-ranging team approach to obtain the maximum improvements in quality of life for the patient and family, with the patient and family, or other carers, forming a lynch-pin within the team.

In the United Kingdom the needs identified by the patient or carers will be of a similar nature and pattern. For example, the ability to buy and cook food or to care for oneself will be affected by the immobility which accompanies many orthopaedic conditions, although the environment will vary depending on culture, social class and the level of sophistication of the health care system in which the individual lives. In addition, the nature and pattern of illness or disability and how it affects the patient and family or society at large, has a predictable element the treatment of which, to some extent, may be anticipated. It is known, for example, that in most Western countries, with an increasing number of elderly people in the population, the need for orthopaedic joint restoration will increase and fractured neck of femur in elderly females can be prevented by giving hormone replacement therapy

9

when and if appropriate. The occurrence of these disabilities has implications for nursing practice and the society in which we live. For example, as more is discovered of the treatment and prevention of osteoporosis in older women, the need to care for patients suffering from the effects of this problem will diminish, whereas the increasing demands on the health service by the numbers of patients undergoing joint replacement could change the nature of the service offered.

However, in Third World countries the need for an adequate diet is paramount in maintaining health and minimizing disability within the population. Therefore, the care needs of Third World individuals, although predictable, may be very different from those of the comparatively affluent European.

THE PATIENT AND FAMILY

In order to assess patients' needs and ensure that maximum function is restored, nurses must look at their role within the health care setting in which they work. Meeting the needs of patients has been the stated goal of nurses for many years now. However, often these needs were identified by nurses themselves, with little or no participation from patients or relatives. The concept of the expert deciding what is best for the patient was the commonly used approach until the introduction of holistic care, which occurred at about the same time that nurses were beginning to organize care using the concept of a nursing model, as discussed in Chapter 3.

THE ORTHOPAEDIC NURSE

What is the role of the orthopaedic nurse in present day nursing? Hospitals in the United Kingdom specializing in orthopaedics are rapidly disappearing as conditions requiring long periods of immobilization disappear, and methods of treatment of patients become more home-centred. The trend in today's large general hospitals leans towards the concept of a 'hospital within a hospital', and most areas of specialized nursing may be found within this setting. The orthopaedic nurse now most often works in an orthopaedic unit within a general hospital. She may be a clinical nurse specialist working for a group of wards with only a small number of other orthopaedically qualified nurses employed in the same unit, or she may be the leader of a group of specialist nurses.

Adaptability

The orthopaedic nurse should be able to use her specialist skills in any setting, whether in a hospital or the community, in Western countries or Third World states. The nature of orthopaedic nursing is such that it may be practised with fairly basic amenities, providing the principles of care are followed.

Research

Much knowledge has been gained in recent years as a result of continuing research into, for example:

- Bone growth and healing
- The hormonal influence on growth and repair
- Applying knowledge gained from the space programme, both in the cause and physiology of bone loss
- The use of new materials for prosthetics.

Economics

Nurses in the UK are being increasingly affected by the recent economic evaluation of services that is taking place throughout the health care sector, and are becoming more aware of the financial results of clinical decisions or new clinical practices. This, no doubt, has influenced practices, but not always in a negative way. Option appraisal, in some form or another, has been used for many years in the health service, and the economic aspects of orthopaedic care have been at the forefront of this approach (Drummond 1981).

Change

Many changes are welcomed, and appear to have wholly benefited the patient. For example, who would wish to return to nursing a child on an abduction frame for 2 years in hospital? In addition, the economic results of these changes in patterns of care are quite considerable. The difference in costs at today's budgets between nursing a child in hospital for 2 years or, as at present, approximately 3 weeks (the length of time necessary whilst measuring, making, fitting the splint and providing education and training for the mother or other carer) works out at approximately £150 000 per child, even allowing for the care given in the community. As a member of the health care team, the nurse must be able to, and be prepared to, participate in both the clinical discussions and the wider political debate when changes in health care are being proposed. She is then aware of the effects of decisions made, whether on a clinical basis or as a result of economic pressures, and can maintain her role as patient advocate within the debate and can influence decisions appropriately. (For example, the use of primary nursing has gained acceptance because nurses were prepared to fight for a change which put the patients' interests to the fore and which was also economically sound (see Department of Health and Social Security Orthopaedic Services 1981).)

Nurses should also be more involved in the prevention of health problems and in the health educational and promotional aspects of their role. As orthopaedic nurses, they can contribute significantly to the safe transference of patients into their own homes and can help patients with care needs to maintain their independence within their own environment (Jaffe 1989).

PRIMARY NURSING

Primary nursing as a method of organizing care which acknowledges the essential and unique relationship between the patient and his carer would seem to be a most appropriate solution to the demands for accountability on the one hand and patient advocacy on the other. Moreover, it is a system of care which may be used in any setting. One of its early difficulties of being seen by hospital managers as an economic answer to staffing level problems appears to be disappearing as nurses adapt and modify practice to fit

each setting and become a stronger, professional voice on behalf of and in partnership with patients.

The success of primary nursing is also dependent on an understanding of, and respect for, the work of the whole health care team in order that the patient can receive well-balanced care (Vaughan 1990). As the practice of orthopaedic nursing has also always needed the development of a close, therapeutic relationship between nurse and patient, primary nursing appears to be a natural progression in the orthopaedic care setting.

WRITING STANDARDS

As the role of the orthopaedic nurse changes, it is vital that her involvement in the identification of her standards of care and her commitment to achieve them continues. However, this system of improving the quality of care through the setting of standards (Kitson 1989) is one of many, and it may be necessary to research other methods. For example, there are generic quality assessment instruments which may be bought off the shelf. One of these currently in use in the United Kingdom is Monitor, but there are others available which should be examined before a final choice is made. The establishment of written standards of care involves the nurse in other fields such as the economic effects of setting a standard or the implications for other members of the team. It may alter team relationships and the nurse may be required to gain other skills – e.g. computer training, budget management, assertiveness skills or management skills – for which she will need support, education and training.

The setting of standards offers the nurse the chance to determine and define the standard of care within her area of practice. It is important for nurses to ensure that they themselves set the standards, and not the business or contracts manager whose rationale may be expediency or cost control (Arnold & Wright 1990). However, the need for management to support nurses in the maintenance of standards is essential, and will enhance commitment to quality within the organization.

MONITORING OF STANDARDS

It follows that, if the nurse is involved in setting and writing standards (Arnold & Wright 1990), she must be involved in monitoring standards within her area of work and must be prepared for her own standards of care to be monitored and assessed.

The simplest method of monitoring standards is to use the evaluation of care given in care plans as a simple monitoring tool. However, when standards have been set, nurses need to measure and monitor what they are actually achieving, compare this with the described standards and, if necessary, take action if the quality of care needs to be improved. Again, for this the nurse may require further education and training in order to develop the necessary skills. For example, it is becoming increasingly important that nurses understand the methodology of research so that they can make logical and reasoned arguments to back up their decisions.

Quality assurance

The concept of quality in the provision of health care, although assumed by many to be an integral part of care, is relatively new when expressed as measurable elements which may be defined for any part of the organization, and in all aspects from the physical environment to psychological support. For example, in the 'measurable elements of care' assigned to the physical, as opposed to the emotional elements, quality audit may look at whether nursing procedures are adapted to meet the needs of individual patients, whether a patient's daily hygiene needs for cleanliness and an acceptable appearance are met (Qualpacs, Wandelt & Ager 1974; Pearson 1983).

Workload management systems

A number of quality measurement systems are in use in the UK, many incorporating a manpower planning or assessing system. One such is Monitor, an adaptation of the Rush Medicus Nursing Process Methodology from North America. This was produced in the North West Region of England, following research in hospitals in the UK, and provides the ability to calculate an index of the quality of care delivered to patients, and workload required to support all activities within the ward. This gives an overview of what is being achieved and what can realistically be achieved on the ward with a quality of care element.

Another workload management system which also originates from North America is GRASP (Proprietory to First Consultant Group); again, this incorporates a good quality assurance system. However, further quality criteria were added to fulfil local specifications as, for example, during development of standards of care which were incorporated into the quality of care element for use in Sheffield (Fig. 2.1).

Most ready-made systems are acceptable to non-nurse managers as they have already been tested and offer a less intuitive way of measuring workload, and therefore of assessing staffing level requirements. Other systems in use include:

- Nursing audits
- Qualpacs (Harvey 1990)
- Royal College of Nursing Standards of Care Project
- Dynamic Standard Setting System (DySSSy 1990, Kitson et al 1990)
- Patient satisfaction questionnaires/surveys.

Nurses must be at the forefront in the establishment of quality values (Pearson 1983). A statement of 'philosophy of care' for each area is also an essential part of the initial approach to quality assurance. In her *Therapeutic Nursing Function*, Kitson (1986) gives a clear statement of the philosophy of nursing as 'care which ensured that the patient achieved optimum independence in self-care activities and was treated as an individual, respected and encouraged to make his own decisions'. Questionnaires, or some method of obtaining an understanding of patients' experiences of health care could also be used (Duddy 1990).

The management systems which appear to gain support from nursing staff also incorporate some statement and level of quality assurance. The uptake of quality issues would, therefore,

INSTRUCTIONS: 1. Complete chart by circling activities from patient's care plan
2. Refer to ward operational definitions if in doubt
3. Total the activities circled and divide by ten for final PCH figure

Name:

Week commencing:

Ward: B1/B2/B3

	Mon	Tue	Wed	Thu	Fri	Sat	Sun
Assessment/Evaluation Daily all patients							
E1/E6 Continuous assessment/evaluation	③	③	③	③	③	③	③
Planning Daily all patients							
E5 Update care plan	②	②	②	②	②	②	②
Teaching Circle as applicable							
G10 Knowledge	6	6	6	6	6	6	6
G10 Skills	3	3	3	3	3	3	3
G10 Attiitudes	3	3	3	3	3	3	3
Emotional support As applicable							
F1 Continuous emotional support	1	1	1	1	1	1	1
1334 Care of patient following spinal surgery							
Inc. Pressure area care, hygiene and toileting (Circle as applicable)	77	77	77	77	77	77	77
Elimination Circle one, highest applicable							
205 Toilet on sanichair	9	9	9	9	9	9	9
207 Toilet with supervision/assistance, walking	8	8	8	8	8	8	8
225 Provide/Remove bedpan/commode	18	18	18	18	18	18	18
235 Provide/Remove urinal	7	7	7	7	7	7	7
251 Empty urinary drainage bag Circle as applicable	1	1	1	1	1	1	1
Hygiene Circle as applicable							
608 Partial assistance with hygiene, AM and PM	4	4	4	4	4	4	4
614 Complete assistance with hygiene, AM	6	6	6	6	6	6	6
608 Partial assistance with hygiene, Evening	2	2	2	2	2	2	2
631 Post-Op Wash (2 nurses)	4	4	4	4	4	4	4
657 Wash hair in/out of bed	5	5	5	5	5	5	5
Mobility Circle as applicable							
1335 Turning with Charnley Wedge	16	16	16	16	16	16	16
711 Pressure area care (2 nurses)	4	4	4	4	4	4	4
745 Lifting patient in bed	4	4	4	4	4	4	4
705 Up/return to bed with assistance	2	2	2	2	2	2	2
700 Walk with assistance	5	5	5	5	5	5	5
Diet and fluids Circle as applicable							
115 Feeds self without supervision	2	2	2	2	2	2	2
157 Drink round	1	1	1	1	1	1	1
130 Assist with oral fluids	4	4	4	4	4	4	4
150 Encourage fluids	5	5	5	5	5	5	5
135 Assist with menu completion	1	1	1	1	1	1	1
Drugs Circle as applicable							
904 Ward drug round Daily all patients	②	②	②	②	②	②	②
941 Heparin injection	1	1	1	1	1	1	1
901 Controlled drugs Post-Op	8	8	8	8	8	8	8
Respiratory care Circle as applicable							
415 Continuous oxygen therapy	2	2	2	2	2	2	2

Fig. 2.1 Caption see overleaf.

	Mon	Tue	Wed	Thu	Fri	Sat	Sun
Dressings/suctions Circle as applicable							
525 Wound/suction check	1	1	1	1	1	1	1
530 Empty/change wound suction containers	2	2	2	2	2	2	2
Items may be circled either from this section:							
981 Blood transfusion obs. Post-Op inc. B.P.	15	15	15	15	15	15	15
981 Blood transfusion obs. Top-up inc. B.P.	7	7	7	7	7	7	7
980 Start/change blood transfusion	5	5	5	5	5	5	5
Or this section:							
305 Temp, pulse and B.P. Post-Op	9	9	9	9	9	9	9
305 Temp, pulse and B.P. 4 hourly	4	4	4	4	4	4	4
970 IVI Check	5	5	5	5	5	5	5
976 Change IVI bag/bottle	6	6	6	6	6	6	6
Other direct care Circle as applicable							
971 IV cannula site care	1	1	1	1	1	1	1
974 Discontinue IVI Circle one	1	1	1	1	1	1	1
975 Convert IVI to IV bung only	1	1	1	1	1	1	1
111 Intake and output calculations	1	1	1	1	1	1	1
1205 Pre-operative care/preparation (inc. bath)	4	4	4	4	4	4	4
1150 Receive patient on ward after theatre	2	2	2	2	2	2	2
1220 Apply/Remove anti-embolism stockings	1	1	1	1	1	1	1
1314 Apply Bradford sling	2	2	2	2	2	2	2
1322 Check/maintenance of Bradford sling	1	1	1	1	1	1	1
1216 Apply Flotron Therapy	2	2	2	2	2	2	2
1217 Care of patient receiving Flotron Therapy	6	6	6	6	6	6	6
1300 Plaster check	4	4	4	4	4	4	4
1165 Accompany pt. off ward & stay in attendance	3	3	3	3	3	3	3
1007 Collect any specimen	1	1	1	1	1	1	1
1110 Discharge of instructions	2	2	2	2	2	2	2
Indirect care Daily all patients	㉓	㉓	㉓	㉓	㉓	㉓	㉓
Total							
Total divided by 10 = patient care hours							

(01/01/91)

Fig. 2.1   Sheffield work load management system.

seem to progress in a number of areas – none of which has more or less importance than the others; all will be affected by a good quality assurance programme – from quality awareness, to workload management to resource management, for any unit involved in health care, whether situated in a hospital or the community.

Resource management systems

Resource management now appears to be at the forefront of health care delivery, both in the community and in institutional settings. A large part of this involves the management of the greatest resource within the service – that is, the staff. This includes all members of the caring team and their managers at the highest level, as well as workers such as health care assistants, who are hierarchically lower but no less essential.

Information technology   The use of computers and appropriate programmes is becoming essential to nursing staff at ward and primary care level. Nurses will need to become familiar with and comfortable in handling data to minimize time spent on essential record keeping, which is necessary to maintain good patient care.

Performance review systems

A great deal has been written about performance

review systems. Nurses in the past have been haunted by the appraisal system, which in many cases had become a negative approach to professional performance and one which was open to the most blatant favouritism. Nurses were often assessed not on their competence and ability, but on whether they became socialized to the unit in which they were working. Now nurses are looking for more appropriate ways to assess their own performance or professional competence, usually within a quality of care framework. This allows for the acknowledgement of resource restrictions and most importantly, should include a recognition of professional development needs and the ability and commitment to address those needs, once identified. No nurse should be expected to fulfil her role unless she is given the support and encouragement of her manager to continue her professional development by the ongoing acquisition of expertise and knowledge. Indeed, the professional nurse will not be allowed to re-register unless she has completed a minimum amount of professional development, which at the moment will be 5 days for general nurses.

The orthopaedic nurse may wish to pursue a variety of development opportunities. It would appear that most post-registered nurses now need to acquire a number of additional professional qualifications and skills. The following are examples of courses that can be taken:

1. The Orthopaedic Nurse – ENB Course 219 Orthopaedic Nursing (or its equivalent as modules of a qualification)
2. Teaching and assessing courses
3. Research appreciation and methodology courses
4. Broadened understanding of the chosen fields within orthopaedics
   a. theatre courses
   b. rehabilitation course
   c. advanced nursing courses
   d. degree studies.

The list is endless and varied enough for all nurses to more than fulfil the requirements for re-registering as recommended by the Post-Registration Education and Practice Project (PREPP) 1991 United Kingdom Central Council (UKCC). The nurse may wish to attend study days on subjects as varied as pain control, alternative therapies, word processing and counselling skills. All will enable the nurse to enhance her practice, through meeting and discussing practice and problems with colleagues.

THE HEALTH CARE TEAM

What, precisely, constitutes a health care team? Again, this would depend on the situation in which care is given, but, minimally, it would consist of a doctor and nurse – with or without co-workers.

The patient

The Western world is fortunate in being able to include other professionals in the health care team (Jaffe 1989). However, it is of the utmost importance to remember that the team is acting on behalf of the patient in helping him to return to his maximum potential. As the patient is the focus of the care team's efforts, it is important that his views and those of significant others, if appropriate, are sought when important decisions are made.

Multidisciplinary approach

Although each patient will have specific needs, there is a core team which is more or less common to all orthopaedic patients in hospital. This comprises doctors, nurses, physiotherapists, social workers and occupational therapists. There may also be a need for the services of other professionals, i.e. the orthotist, psychologist, sexual counsellor, dietician, chiropodist, speech therapist, clinical psychologist and pharmacist (Fig. 2.2).

Team leaders

The team is usually headed, at least in the hospital environment, by the doctor, but sometimes the team may be headed by a different member of the multidisciplinary group – for example a

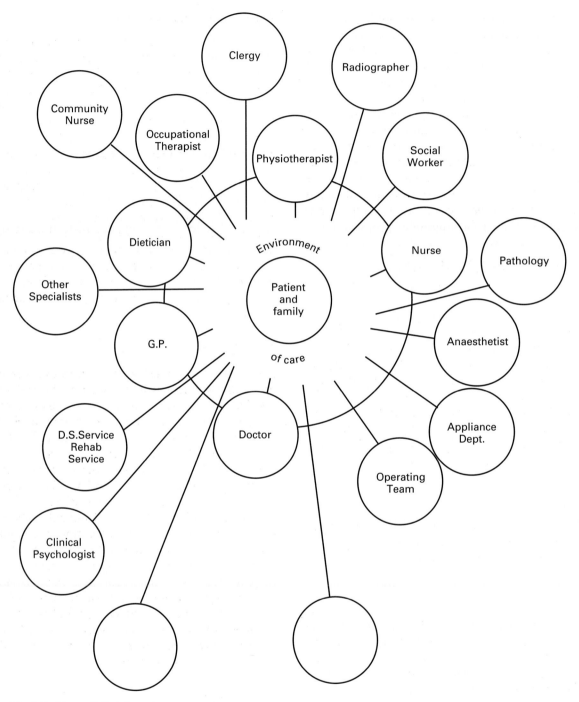

Fig. 2.2 The multidisciplinary team.

nurse or physiotherapist – depending on the needs of the patient, and the phase of care (Turner 1989). The Dulwich Study (Ham et al 1987) suggests that 'within the team, as long as there is at least one experienced person who has the energy and enthusiasm to continue organising the team, and the ability to enable staff training and education to continue, when the team has taken the time and the considerable effort required to formulate agreed policies and standards of care e.g. in discharge procedures, then it can often withstand change within the team', for example, when there is the need to employ agency staff for a short period.

ENVIRONMENT OF CARE

Nurse

The nurse has a key role in promoting a suitable environment of care, both in the hospital and the community. However, no one professional member of the team can work in isolation, and the nurse must be able to work with and use the skills of other members of the team. The orthopaedic nurse must have overlapping skills, for instance in continuing therapeutic programmes of care devised by physiotherapists and occupational therapists.

Advocacy

The nurse can expect to be the advocate for the patient where he does not have the knowledge or skills to act in his own best interests.

Communicating

Effective communication is essential in good patient care. The use of comprehensive, written nursing care plans is useful. The whole nursing team may be involved in the assessment of the patient and his situation, and in an individualized care plan written by the nurse primarily responsible for this care. In some hospitals, each professional member of the team may share and contribute to the written evaluation of the care plan.

Appropriate model of care

It is important that the nurse uses an appropriate model upon which to organize her care; this may be adapted to suit the needs of the patient and the setting in which he is nursed. The model should be capable of being used as a unique source of information for other members of the care team.

Other opportunities for communication are essential in maintaining the adjustment and monitoring of patient care needs. The ward round, case conferences and ward meetings all help to consolidate a consistent, systematic and comprehensive approach to care for each patient.

The nurse may also expect to act in the capacity of 'liaison' person on behalf of the patient. She should know the expectations of the patient, and should have been involved in helping the patient to set realistic goals, or in raising his aims of achievement.

Dependence

Hospitalization almost always produces some degree of dependency in the patient. The patient usually hands over all control of his health care to others, as he needs to derive maximum benefit from the caring situation. He will feel that he must accept the judgement and decisions of others in order to progress. Dependence is often fostered in a hospital setting, and may be continued at home by over-protective relatives or other carers. After all, the dependent patient is more easily nursed or cared for if he is compliant and unquestioning. The patient, therefore, having become dependent will require considerable help to begin working through this phase in order to regain some measure of independence. There will be a period when the patient is not ill, but neither is he better, and nursing attempts to initiate self-care may meet with indignation and frustration from the patient.

Rehabilitation

Rehabilitation of the patient takes place from the time of first contact, which may be at the preoperative assessment, in the patient's own home, at the clinic or on arrival at the hospital.

Wherever this contact takes place, an opportunity is provided for the nurse to begin to assess the patient's needs and potential post-treatment problems. As rehabilitation is provided as part of the continuum of care, it is very useful if the setting can change as part of this process. For example, as soon as the acute surgical phase is over (at approximately the time the drains are removed from the wound), even though mobilization may not be delayed for long, moving the patient physically into a different ward or area of the ward may be a useful tool in the defining of care, both for the care team and for the patient. It allows all concerned to recognize the progression of the patient into another stage of wellness. However, rehabilitation need not necessarily take place in a completely different area (see Department of Health and Social Security, Orthopaedic Services 1981), but may be seen as a progression of the patient into a different type of care with perhaps much greater input from the wider team.

Independence

A return to independence is helped if the patient is cared for in an area different to the acute setting, and many hospitals are recognizing the advantages derived from freeing acute surgical/trauma beds and providing an active rehabilitation setting for patients. Some hospitals also provide a halfway house situation where patients and/or their relatives live within call – usually by intercom or internal telephone system – but are virtually self-caring and self-supporting (Regional Spinal Injuries Unit, Lodge Moor Hospital, Sheffield and Derby Royal Infirmary).

The goals of rehabilitation for a patient should be:

- The prevention of further impairment
- Monitoring of the existing disability
- Restoring function to the maximum attainable degree.

The patient should begin to examine his rehabilitation experience, know his capacity for recovery, and state his needs. The nurse must work with the patient and his family, providing a source of learning, information and support.

Skilled companionship

The nurse must establish what expectations the patient and his family have, and help the patient and his family adapt, acquire new skills, and achieve competence in new functional activities. For example, the change or loss of function of a limb can sometimes have profound effects on the patient; the nurse must be able to offer practical advice and a realistic view of what new skills may eventually be acquired.

The nurse may need to adopt a different care planning concept for this stage of care, and other professionals may need to be included in the care team. A more appropriate model of care may be one which utilizes the self-care continuum, and the nurse may need to make greater use of the liaison nurse as contact with community services are included in care planning.

Nurse-managed preoperative assessment

The Sheffield experiment

One area in which nurses have a very special role to fulfil is preoperative assessment and counselling. An example of the development of this special role was seen in Sheffield in 1986, as a response to a particular problem in bed and theatre management. Patients coming into hospital for major surgery are often totally unprepared. They have, at best, a poor or hazy notion of the implications of their impending surgery, and often are physically and psychologically unfit or unprepared. Delays in discharge are frequent due to poor home facilities or delays in completing adaptations to the home. Patients often have virtually no health education prior to admission; a staggering 48% of cases in a local study carried out by Mrs A. F. Gill and Mr C. Linacre in 1986, needed some health/social intervention before surgery – undetected problems of the circulatory system are common, as are urinary tract infections. An unexpected finding was the number of patients with dependent others who required some support during the absence of the individual from home.

In Sheffield a nurse was diverted from ward

work to assist in addressing some of these problems. The nurse had to have a number of personal qualities:

- Credibility with her peers and other members of the caring team
- Expertise in her field, i.e. orthopaedic nursing
- Excellent interpersonal skills
- Teaching and counselling skills
- Organizational skills!

It was decided that the nurse should visit patients in their own homes initially, as they were more receptive to health education and preoperative information at home and it was also possible for relatives or other carers to be present.

Health screening

A simple basic health screen was possible. Specimens obtained for preoperative screening included:

1. Urine – screened for infection and any other abnormalities
2. Blood – screened for haemoglobin levels; this is frequently low when patients are elderly and have also had long-term anti-inflammatory drugs. A specimen of blood was sent for grouping and retention in a blood bank to enable immediate cross-matching to occur in case the patient was called to fill a cancellation at short notice.

At Sheffield it was possible to establish at short notice (in as little as 4 hours on occasion) a list of patients to fill a theatre roster, but usually longer notice could be given (Fig. 2.3).

When a patient raised other health problems in discussion or as a result of direct questions during the nurse's visit, the nurse could arrange for the patient to attend the outpatient department or make a short day visit to the ward to allow tests such as X-rays or ECGs to take place, or examination by the appropriate anaesthetist or consultant orthopaedic surgeon. The nurse could expedite the treatment of any existing problems by contacting the appropriate consultant and liaising with the general practitioner on the patient's behalf.

Potential discharge problems were identified and dealt with in ample time prior to eventual discharge. Improvements affecting quality of life also were made prior to admission – e.g. simple modifications to the home which called on services already available: the installation of hand rails to stairs, safety rails in bathroom and toilet areas, raised toilet seats. Identified also was the need for support services prior to discharge but which could be commenced before admission. All these measures could be taken prior to admission, to help in the smooth progress of the patient to eventual discharge. Booklets with information on health and the impending operation were left with patients, to be read prior to admission (Williams 1986).

A dramatic, identifiable result of utilizing a preoperative assessment and counselling nurse at Sheffield was a reduction in cancellation or delay in surgery from 48% to 1–2% annually. A less dramatic and not so quantifiable result was a happier, less anxious, better informed, fitter patient attending for surgery, with relatives also happier and better informed. The service provided continuity for the whole caring team, with the patient as the key person. Inpatient time was greatly reduced (Seers 1990) and theatre planning became more logical and controllable (Gill & Fellows 1988).

Doctor

The relationship of the doctor to the other caring team members may be a crucial factor in the effectiveness of multidisciplinary teamwork. If the doctor assumes the role of team leader, he should be seen to take the responsibility of co-ordinating the other professionals' contributions to patient care with serious commitment. He should take time to communicate with other team members, attending ward meetings and case conferences as necessary. This allows for the sharing of ideas and understanding the roles of the various team members. It also allows time for informal teaching and learning to take place. Good multidisciplinary teamwork occurs only through hard work and commitment from all team members, who must be flexible in goal

King Edward VII Orthopaedic Hospital – Pre-operative Health Screening

Home Tel:

Date of Screen: _____

Surgery Planned: _____

Expected Surgery Date: _____

Age: _____

G.P. – Dr. _____ Tel: _____	
Last seen _____ for _____	
Last seen at Orthopaedic Clinic _____ Waiting _____	
Main Orthopaedic Problem	
Other Joints Affected	

Is Joint Painful	Yes/No	
Disturb Sleep	Yes/No	
Limit Mobility	Yes/No –	How far able to walk _____
Cut Toe Nails	Yes/No	Aids to mobility _____
Able to Get Into Bath	Yes/No	_____
Climb Stairs	Yes/No	_____

Home Circumstances: _____

Stairs _____

Toilet _____

Raised toilet seat	Yes	No	N/A	Bath Seat	Yes	No	N/A
High Chair	Yes	No	N/A	Bath Board	Yes	No	N/A

General Health
Heart
Blood Pressure
Chest
Skin
Bladder
Bowels
Digestion
Allergies
Current Medication: _____

Fig. 2.3 Continued on page 21.

Previous Surgery/Illness _____

B/P	Temp.	Pulse	Weight	Urinalysis

Investigations	Specimen obtained	Result	Action
MSU			
Full Blood Count and ESR			
U & E's and LFT's			
Group and save			

Problem	Evaluation

Plan

Nurse's Signature _____ Doctor's Approval _____

Fig. 2.3 Sample of health screen check – nurse-managed preoperative assessment.

planning and must value the contribution from other members of the team. They must be ready to evaluate what is happening and, when possible, participate in research. In the past, there have been spectacularly successful partnerships in orthopaedic nursing, that of Sir Robert Jones and Dame Agnes Hunt being a notable example. Consistent teamwork with good communication from all professionals is in the best interests of the patient.

Coordinator

Of necessity, most orthopaedic wards have more than one consultant attached. As a result, the nurse may be dealing with more than one team leader. In this situation, it may be more appropriate for the nurse to assume the role of head coordinator so that she may facilitate care for all. However, the consultants or senior medical staff are a great source of knowledge, support and commitment to the team they lead.

Anaesthetist

Anaesthetic assessment

The anaesthetist is an often overlooked member of the care team. He is available to examine the patient preoperatively for a number of factors which are potentially life-threatening. The examination may take place at the preoperative assessment clinic or during a ward visit. When elective surgery is planned, it is important that the anaesthetist is involved at an early stage so that the patient, his relatives, if appropriate, and the other members of the care team may make an informed choice with full knowledge of any possible risks, and that appropriate facilities may be made available. This also allows time for the anaesthetist to assess the patient fully and decide upon the method of anaesthesia.

Pain control

The anaesthetist will provide expert advice on pain management for the patient. He could be involved preoperatively with patients suffering

from chronic or acute pain problems, and will be involved postoperatively for most patients. He may also offer support to patients from a wider area at a Pain Control Clinic, when a greater variety of methods are often available for chronic pain sufferers.

Anaesthetists are usually pleased to be involved in care planning for the patient, and can be an ally and source of information for the care team.

Physiotherapist

The physiotherapist is a scarce but valuable member of the health care team, who will contribute greatly to the patient's recovery. She is a professional who often attends the ward to work with the patient, and consequently may be viewed by busy ward staff as just a visitor. It is very important that the effort is made by ward staff, physiotherapists and other team members to communicate freely with each other on problems encountered or progress made by the patient. This is aided if the patient himself is involved in the planned programme of his care and the goals set.

Home visits

Physiotherapists now have a wider remit, visiting patients' homes before their admission for elective surgery; this is a great advantage for both patient and physiotherapist. Much can be gained if the physiotherapist is aware, for example, that the patient has to negotiate very steep stairs with no handrail, to get to the bathroom or bed. This information, if shared with the team, will help them decide what type of prosthesis is to be used and where best to rehabilitate the patient. It will also affect the patient's length of stay in hospital and the degree of safety in mobility the patient must achieve or the number of mobility aids he will require. Additionally, the visit allows the physiotherapist to demonstrate the use of crutches, and to leave a pair to enable the patient to practise before surgery in order to increase his confidence.

Open access

Physiotherapy expertise may also be obtained

at outreach centres and in open access. This may be in the form of direct referral from general practitioners. An outreach centre may be set up in a variety of locations, perhaps as a certain number of sessions per week in suitable accommodation with a general practice surgery, or separate physiotherapy departments may be 'set aside' for the use of general practice patients.

In a study undertaken in 1986 (Fordham 1989), it was found that under a direct referral system, although some additional revenue was required to provide physiotherapy for the open access group of patients, this was offset by the reduction in the number of patients referred to hospital consultants to assess and recommend physiotherapy. The total duration of treatments was also significantly shorter and patients waited for a shorter period of time before obtaining treatment. Using a standardized method of assessing outcome, the majority of patients (70%) obtained, at the very least, some improvement in their condition. However, no statistical difference was found between the improvement rates of directly referred patients and those obtaining physiotherapy via a hospital referral. In this example, despite the similar improvement ratio, costs were reduced for both the hospital and patient.

In the USA (Jaffe 1989), more use is made of physiotherapy in the home, mainly because of the costs of hospitalization and the introduction of Diagnosis Related Group payment. This is a standard assessment for the amount of care paid for by the insurance company or state. However, the patient may opt to have 7 days in hospital or 14 days' physiotherapy at home for the same cost! Perhaps the National Health Service could learn from US practice. In the UK, outreach programmes are running in some health areas. The outcome of these programmes should be examined carefully; there need not necessarily be conflict between economic and clinical goals, provided that patient needs and results are seen as the main priority.

The physiotherapist also contributes to the care of patients in day hospitals or outpatient departments, where their expertise is of great value in the continued support and rehabilita-

tion of spinal-injured patients or chronic back pain sufferers. This practice is a cost-effective way of providing continuing care for patients who have undergone joint replacement surgery and are able to go home or into minimal care accommodation, yet continue to require further physiotherapy.

Occupational therapist

The occupational therapist is an often undervalued member of the caring team when financial restraints make the inclusion of an occupational therapist a low priority. The rehabilitation programme cannot be complete without the services of this professional. However, it would be naive to pretend that occupational therapy has not taken some time to establish its own professional identity, and there has been some confusion within the profession itself as to the parameters it covers. One of the problems this produces is that other professionals tend to view occupational therapists as being 'all things to all men' (Carlisle 1989). On the other hand this very quality provides a unique service which can be utilized by many patients in various specialist areas. For example, a nurse may ask an occupational therapist to offer advice to one of her patients on the types of home aids which are available and to recommend the most appropriate one, whereas a doctor may require an assessment of the patient's ability to care for himself at home. The occupational therapist, in her role of enhancing the quality of life for the chronically sick, for disabled persons and for the elderly population, has the ability to help patients manage change and should be seen as an essential member of the caring team during this time.

The occupational therapist was, perhaps, one of the earliest exponents of the outreach philosophy in patient care. Her ability to assess a patient in his own home is an asset to the whole team, and she may be required in the liaison between hospital and Department of Health and Social Security on behalf of the client. She may be required to carry out a specific functional assessment of several activities incorporating cognitive abilities and orientation; assessment of the patient's diet and nutrition, money management and road safety or domestic abilities may be needed to ascertain his basic safety, nutrition and awareness of kitchen procedures.

Working closely with the patient in deciding and advising on an appropriate aid to daily living in the home, and on home modifications, is an important aspect of occupational therapy. Expert advice can be provided in social service case conferences when extra day support, or even rehousing, is needed for the patient.

More health authorities are adopting the principle of an occupational therapy home service in which patients do not have to spend time in hospital in order to qualify for this life-enhancing professional help. Preadmission visits before elective surgery are other occasions on which occupational therapists can offer help, which may be immediate (e.g. in the supply of toilet hand rails and bath seats) and which improves the patient's quality of life (Katz 1963).

Clinical psychologist

The clinical psychologist may be part of a health care team in specialist units for spinal injuries or for multiple injury patients, as many accidents, particularly road accidents, cause multiple injuries with post-traumatic brain damage. She may take part in pain control clinics, to which patients suffering from such diverse problems as back pain or bone tumours, may be referred. She may also be needed for patients suffering from stress as a result of changes in the patterns of their lives, caused by illness or permanent disability.

The psychologist may offer help to both patients and relatives/carers, and may assist patients through the bereavement process in their loss of function or role. She may help patients to understand, or come to terms with, the reasons for their debilitating problem or disability and in this way enable them to begin to cope. Psychologists may also help parents or partners understand the changes in personality that they may see in the young multiple injury patient, and show them ways of managing their changed lives. They can provide information on effects

of the damage process and how the patient or carers can help themselves, and give advice or suggest strategies to cope with specific problems such as aggressive outbursts or periods of depression. They may also refer the patient or carers to other professionals such as sexual counsellors, and may continue to care for the patient when he returns to his home environment or other care setting, providing him with a lifeline care team member.

Speech therapist

Speech therapists will be members of the health care team when speech problems arise. They are available to patients within the hospital and in the community, and provide expert help for patients and carers. Speech therapists can identify the source of a speech problem, whether it originates in the brain or is a result of functional damage, and may introduce appropriate exercises for brain-damaged patients and those patients who have mechanical problems. They will have a realistic understanding of probable outcomes and can offer sound advice to the patient, relatives and carers, e.g. in teaching and helping the patient. The speech therapist may be the principal care team member for the child with cerebral palsy and for his parents. She can offer hope and support to patients with speech problems, and to their relatives, and should not be overlooked as a further resource for patients.

Social worker

Social workers are invaluable members of the health care team; they fulfil a number of functions within the team for patients, but may also offer a service to staff. Counselling is a major part of their role. The social worker may provide an essential back-up for the team, both in her role as counsellor to individual members of the team and in being able to offer practical advice or help to the patient; she may be the prime counsellor for patients who need help in coming to terms with a life-changing condition, whether this is a sudden change or a more gradual and protracted process. She may offer practical help in the form of advice on benefits available, or may act as a mediator in resolving housing or rehousing problems.

The social worker may offer to accompany the patient if he has to attend a court or tribunal. She would expect to be involved in discharge planning and coordination as she will be aware of the social circumstances of the patient and will be able to refer him to other agencies – i.e. national, local authority or voluntary/charitable agencies.

A placement service for patients can be offered; the social worker acts as expert advisor on other types of care settings available to the patient, enabling the patient, family and team to take part in a full discussion so that an informed choice can be made. She may also be able to initiate the placing of a patient's dependants into respite care, so that the patient can receive the surgery he needs. This service is becoming increasingly necessary, as elderly patients requiring joint replacement are often caring for elderly or infirm relatives and may put off surgery because of these responsibilities. Also, the younger joint replacement patient may have a young family that requires care or supervision while the partner works.

The social worker is one of the few hospital team members to follow the patient through into the community (the patient's home or placement setting) and so provides a bridge between the hospital and community. She may know the appropriate self-help group to which to refer the patient, or an available fund or organization to help provide hospital visits or essential items to enable the patient to continue living at home.

Dietitian

The dietitian can be a great ally and useful source of information to both patient and nurse. She is able to give specific advice tailored to the individual patient's needs, not only within the hospital setting, but also in the community, where her realistic assessment of limited finances will enable her to give sound, practical advice on how the patient can provide himself with a good nutritional base. This may involve a lengthy discussion with the patient to enable the

dietitian to discover his usual diet. An elderly patient with a limited income who is awaiting joint replacement surgery often has to put up with a restricted diet. There is no point in giving such a patient glossy leaflets which show how to lose weight by eating high quality fresh foods. However, a supportive interview with a knowledgeable dietitian is invaluable, both for the patient himself and for his family. The dietitian may liaise directly with nursing staff both prior to the patient's admission to hospital and during his stay there. She can then supply staff with detailed advice on his nutritional needs and how to provide for them. For example, if a patient has food that can be eaten with the fingers at home, she will advise nurses on how to ensure adequate nourishment for him in the vital preoperative and postoperative periods.

The dietitian may advise the parents of children treated for long periods in immobilizing splints on the most appropriate diet to prevent bone loss, or offer advice for patients requiring a high calcium or iron-rich diet or other diets specific to the needs of the individual.

One way of providing support for patients who are trying to achieve a weight loss prior to surgery is by telephone – a weekly telephone call can often supply reassurance and encouragement to the lonely dieter.

Pharmacist

The pharmacist is a member of the caring team whose services are often not adequately used. She is helpful in advising on regimens for patients with special conditions – e.g. rheumatoid patients – and may be a useful source of information for all members of the caring team; for example, in deciding on policies for self-medication within the hospital unit or on strategies for safe-medication in the home.

Disablement resettlement officer

This is a little-known facility provided by the Department of Health and Social Security Unemployment Service. The disablement resettlement officer is a specially trained civil servant who is client-orientated. She is employed to advise and assist any person who has long-term health problems or who is disabled, needs a job and feels able to work. She interviews clients to determine their abilities and special needs, and may advise them to attend an assessment and training centre. These centres, which a client may attend on a regular basis, provide training by experts and assessment for a variety of skills. For example, patients who can no longer continue a job which entails heavy lifting because of back damage, may attend a centre to try other work options and be advised on the opportunities and training available. There is a disablement resettlement officer in every job centre with an employment advisory service, i.e. there is at least one in every major town or city.

These officers can be instrumental in placing disabled clients in employment by building up a knowledge of employers who require the client's skills and would be able to employ him. For example, a spinal-injured young man may be competent at using a word processor or operating a computer and could register with the resettlement officer, who would work with her client to find an appropriate post.

The officer accepts referrals from a variety of sources – general practitioners, social workers, etc. – and provides an additional source of information for patients.

Disablement Advisory Service (DAS)

This service is also based in the local job centre offices but is employer-orientated. It helps employers in firms of all sizes and in all types of industry, commerce, etc. to adopt and implement good policies and practices in the employment of people with disabilities. The service provides advice and practical help in adapting premises. It runs an equipment scheme which gives grants to employers for adaptations for the disabled employee, and will provide special equipment on loan to disabled workers.

The DAS gives disabled workers assistance with their fares to work, and provides many other facilities as a free service; for example, the service may negotiate to pay up to 50% of the employee's salary in a 'sheltered placement' scheme when the disabled person is able to fulfil only half the job requirements.

Wherever encouragement exists to enable our disabled people to achieve greater independence, it enhances their dignity and self-respect.

Hospital resettlement officer

The hospital resettlement officer is an extremely rare member of the health care team. These officers usually work from a hospital, although not necessarily in the hospital: in Yorkshire the officer works from the Regional Limb Fitting Centre and provides a wealth of knowledge and experienced advice for clients within the Centre.

Orthotist/surgical appliance maker

Another important source of help and support for the patient is the hospital or outpatient-based orthotist or surgical appliance maker. Often resourceful and inventive in response to patient needs, these personnel have produced some of the most useful splints and appliances. They may accept the request from one or more members of the health team for an appliance which will hold a limb or part of the body in a particular position, with a number of added restrictions, whilst also working with the patient to make the appliance more comfortable or robust, or satisfying any number of other needs as specified by the patient or carers. One lady had an adaptation fitted which enabled her to wear a moderate heel 'for dancing'; a man with a full limb prosthesis required an easily replaced boot for fell walking.

Orthotists update their knowledge constantly and may initiate or follow closely developmental research. Working with the health care team and parents, they have, for example, made it possible to discard the abduction frame and allow children with Perthes' disease to lead a near-normal life at home and school. Collaboration between medical staff, engineers and orthotists has enabled very effective work to be carried out on new joints for cast-braces, with a more functional result. On a more modest scale orthotists are also expert in producing minor adaptations to plaster of Paris splints or in using modern casting materials to ensure greater comfort and safety for the patient.

ASSOCIATIONS AND PUBLICATIONS

There are a number of useful associations for the disabled and many publications provide further information for members of primary health care teams. One such is *How to Get Equipment for Disability* (Mandelstam 1990) as reviewed by Davis (1990):

Any health care professional requiring in depth or general information about equipment for the disabled is catered for. From nurses, such as orthopaedic ward sisters needing to obtain walking aids for patients, through to community nurses needing to provide pressure relieving beds.

The headquarters of the Royal Association for Disability and Rehabilitation (25 Mortimer Street, London, W1N 8AB) produces a list of publications – e.g. booklets, guides and leaflets – about matters specific to disability. The topics cover rehabilitation, access, mobility allowance and employment. There are branches of this organization in other cities.

Other useful publications include:

1. The King's Fund Directory, King's Fund Publishing Office, 126 Albert Street, London, NEW1 7NF (ISBN 0 900 889 73 X)
2. The Pitman Press, Bath, publisher for Thames Television programme *Help*; Bedford Square Press, NCVO, 26 Bedford Square, London, WC1B 3HU (*Help* – ISBN 07199 1191 5).

REFERENCES

Arnold K, Wright S 1990 Writing and using standards of nursing care. Nursing Practice 4(1)

Carlisle D 1989 More than basket weavers. Nursing Times 85(50)

Davis P S 1990 Bare bones. Royal College of Nursing Society of Orthopaedic Nursing Newsletter (14)

Department of Health and Social Security, Guthrie Report 1981 Orthopaedic services, waiting time for out-patient appointments and in-patient treatment

Drumond M F 1981 Studies in economic appraisal in health care. Oxford University Press, Oxford

Duddy I 1990 The patient's experience. Nursing Standard 5(9)

Fordham R J 1989 Current Orthopaedics. Report of the Health Economics Consortium. University of York, Longman Group UK, vol 3: 33–35

Gill A F, Fellows H 1988 Short reports: home based pre-operative health screening and counselling service. Nursing Times 84(51): 54

Gill A F, Linacre C 1986 Unpublished material

Goldstone L A, Ball J A, Collier M M 1983 Monitor Newcastle upon Tyne Polytechnic Products

Ham R et al, Dulwich Study 1987 Evaluation of introducing the team approach to the care of the amputee. Prosthetics and Orthotics International 11(1): 25–30

Harvey G 1990 Which way to quality? A study of the implementation of four quality assurance tools. A summary report. Royal College of Nursing Standards of Care Project, Oxford

Jaffe K B 1989 The inter-disciplinary team in the health care agency. Nursing Clinics in North America 24(1)

Katz S et al 1963 Quality of life index studies of illness in the aged. Journal of the American Medical Association 185(94–99): 176

Kitson A L 1986 Therapeutic nursing and the hospitalised elderly. Scutari, Harrow

Kitson A L 1989 Standards of care: a framework of quality. Scutari Press, London

Kitson A L, Hyndman S, Harvey G, Yerrell P 1990 Quality patient care: the dynamic standard setting system. Scutari Press, London

Mandelstam M 1990 How to get equipment for disability. Jessica Kingsley Publishers & Kogan Page, London

Pearson A 1983 The clinical nursing unit: quality assurance. Heineman Medical Books, London, ch 7, p 82

Seers K 1990 Early discharge after surgery, its effects on patients and their informal carers. Paper given at the RCN Research Advisory Group Conference 6–8 April 1990, University of Guildford, Surrey

Turner T 1989 Taking the lead. Nursing Times 43(16): 7

UKCC 1991 Post registration education and practice. United Kingdom Central Council, London

Vaughan B 1990 Education for primary nursing. Nursing Practice 4(1)

Wandelt M, Ager J 1974 Quality of patient care scale. Appleton Century Crofts, New York

Williams D 1986 Pre-operative patient education, in the home or in the hospital? American Journal of Orthopaedic Nursing 5(1)

3

Using a nursing model: a model for orthopaedic nursing

Kathy Balcombe

INTRODUCTION

This chapter aims to address the criticism that models are of interest only to theorists, by discussing and examining the elements of a model of nursing as listed in Figure 3.1. These elements will then be related to the concept of mobilization, which is considered to be the core of orthopaedic nursing.

Within nursing, debate continues as to the usefulness of nursing models. Some of the argu-

– The definition of nursing held by the
  nurse and by the society in which
  she is operating

– A description and understanding of the
  society in which the nurse is operating

– The nature of the person requiring
  or seeking nursing care

– The enviroment in which care is to
  be given

– A statement of the knowledge base
  needed by the nurse to make rational
  decisions and reach appropriate conclusions

– The definition of health and illness
  used by society

– The focus of nursing care
  which identifies an assessment
  format, a method of agreeing goals with the
  person receiving nursing, and a
  framework for action

Fig. 3.1   Elements of a model of nursing.

ments against are based on objective reasoning (Roy 1976, Chapman 1990):

1. Their lack of clarity due to the jargon used – e.g. focal, contextual and residual foci in Roy's model
2. The perception that the authors are theoreticians who are distanced from the reality of practical nursing
3. The criticism that the authors have drawn heavily from social sciences.

Other arguments arise out of resistance to change or a reluctance to increase knowledge by further study. For example, the nurse who has not been able to keep up to date with techniques of rapid mobilization or intravenous chemotherapy may refuse to participate in the extension of her role in patient care.

The principal reasons for using a nursing model are as follows:

1. To provide a framework for nursing care that gives a cohesive view of the different aspects of nursing – i.e. physical, social, psychological and spiritual care – and of the art and science of nursing
2. To provide continuity of care from admission to discharge with all nurses involved delivering the same care programme based on a similar philosophy
3. To act as a research tool.

There can be no doubt in the minds of nurses who have analysed and put models into use in hospital and community settings that they have been helpful in planning a consistent approach to patient care. Problems arise when a model is imposed on a nursing team from outside, without sufficient time being allowed for nurses to discuss and assimilate the model and to acquire the knowledge base for its use. This often leads to nurses using the model as an assessment list, as in the activities of living model, rather than adopting its concepts.

Previously, models for nursing have adopted an 'umbrella' approach in that they attempted to provide a way of looking at nursing which could be applied to all specialities. The model described in this chapter can be applied to areas outside orthopaedics; however, it is principally aimed at the orthopaedic nurse and the rest of the orthopaedic multidisciplinary team.

In order to develop an orthopaedic model of nursing it is necessary to consider the differences in the cultural philosophies of North America and the UK, as it is in the former that most nursing models have been formulated.

PHILOSOPHICAL PERSPECTIVES OF NURSING IN THE UK

One of the major criticisms of using models from North America is that the health care system there is different from that in the UK, as is the culture. This may be so. In analysing the philosophical bases of the USA, UK and Europe, Holmes (1981) concludes that the USA has a pragmatic stance, i.e. a practical emphasis, with a concern for the community, whereas society in the UK is more platonic, with a less flexible class structure.

In the USA men are thought to be unequal, but all individuals possess intelligence which enables them collectively to solve their problems. Society is democratic and changing and aims to provide equality before the law and freedom for individuals to compete without destroying the basis of brotherhood. Knowledge is acquired through problem-solving; it is relative, contingent and contextual.

Historically in the UK, men were considered to be unequal by inheriting the conditions which made for inequality. Society was stable and unchanging; men had specific duties to perform, knew their place and were content to occupy it and perform tasks appropriate to their abilities. Knowledge was accessible to a limited number of people who were expected to become leaders. Knowledge consisted of permanent 'ideas', and could be acquired intuitively. In more recent times, British society appears to have adopted many of the features of its US counterpart, but differences in the underlying cultural philosophies are still apparent in the greater reluctance by the British to embrace change.

Nurses share society's beliefs and show the same resistance to change, as demonstrated by their negative reactions toward the introduction of the nursing process and Project 2000 and the changes in the organization of health care in this country.

Changes in UK society resulting from social policy and membership of the European Community (EC), and shifts among countries worldwide toward a market economy are impacting on the profession of nursing, creating conflict. It is important for the orthopaedic nurse to recognize that in part these conflicts arise as a reaction to change, so that she will question more deeply her own response to change. The EC, for example, have already introduced health and safety legislation that will have an effect on lifting and handling procedures within nursing, the Health Service and industry generally.

A MODEL FOR ORTHOPAEDIC NURSING: ESTABLISHING THE UNDERLYING PRINCIPLES

Nursing: the definition of orthopaedic nursing and of the society in which orthopaedic nurses operate

The first step in developing an orthopaedic nursing model is to define orthopaedic nursing. In general, it seems that orthopaedic nurses believe that their aims are either to help the individual to regain mobility and resume his normal occupation, or to assist him to adapt to changes in his life as a result of altered mobility. This does not detract from seeing the person as a whole, as it focuses the aim of nursing on considering how the individual patient's total needs relate to the mobilization/adaptation plan.

The role of the nurse

Neither the public nor nurses themselves have a clear idea of the role of the nurse. The public image of a nurse varies from someone who is dedicated to looking after sick people (an 'angel'), to someone who is available in hospitals and the community to carry out doctors' orders, or to someone who is autonomous and who has special knowledge and skills. In addition a nurse may be

viewed as someone requiring minimal training, not having the authority to make decisions and even as being a sex object (Salvage 1983).

Within the nursing profession there are many who are striving to increase their knowledge so that they can communicate with their medical and paramedical colleagues on an equal basis. These nurses consider that their increased knowledge and skills enable them to provide their patients with improved care and to act as advocates for the patient when necessary.

Other nurses do not value knowledge in the same way; for example, the nurse who proclaims that she has never needed to 'do a course' or read a book since training because she learns all that is necessary on her ward.

Project 2000 courses stress that the role of the nurse is to make autonomous decisions regarding the appropriate assessment, planning, implementation and evaluation of care (UKCC 1986). Until Project 2000 courses and diploma and degree courses become the norm for first level nurses, and it becomes compulsory for qualified nurses to provide evidence that knowledge and expertise are being maintained, it is likely that the nursing profession will be divided on the usefulness of further education.

The nurse of the future will need to be able to work effectively in a changing health care system (Working for patients 1989), whether it is for the National Health Service or within the independent sector. Her role will encompass helping, developing, empowering, caring, counselling, and enabling the patient to work with the health care team to meet his individual needs. She will need to be cognizant of standards of care, be able to negotiate for resources, manage staff and teach.

In order to improve the public's perception of the nurse's role, she will have greater responsibility for communicating the parameters of her job to her patients and to society in general. This may be achieved by contributing to comment and decisions about health care at the national and local level through actions such as lobbying or gaining positions on committees.

In other chapters of this book nursing models have been used to provide a framework for patient care. In all of them, emphasis has been placed on the nurse empowering the patient – for example in his participation in self-care, movement from dependence to independence and adaptation to changes in body image and self-concept.

The roles of the nurse that are identifiable in these chapters are given in Figure 3.2. From this list it is obvious that the nurse is more than a 'skilled doer':

1. She is able to analyse what the patient is 're-ally' telling her by combining her interpretation of his physical symptoms with what he is saying.

2. She empowers the patient by giving him information at a rate and depth with which he can cope.

3. She helps the patient to undertake new roles, skills and techniques to meet his perception of reality for the future.

When the patient cannot cope physically or emotionally with undertaking his own care, or adapt to the changes taking place as a result of his situation, the nurse becomes the helper, carer and knowledgeable practioner; she uses her creative nursing skills to meet the needs of the patient and to assist him in exploring the effect of his present situation on his future aspirations.

The nurse will need to be:

- counsellor – to facilitate the patient's personal exploration and development
- teacher – to help him learn
- agent of change

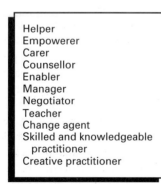

```
Helper
Empowerer
Carer
Counsellor
Enabler
Manager
Negotiator
Teacher
Change agent
Skilled and knowledgeable
  practitioner
Creative practitioner
```

Fig. 3.2   Roles of the nurse.

- negotiator
- manager.

It is acknowledged that the rapid increase in day case surgery and shorter hospitalization will decrease the time for nurse–patient interaction in many instances. Some of the nurse's roles can be fulfilled by the use of patient education booklets, preoperative clinics and creative, informative discharge planning systems that provide patient, family and community nurses with relevant information for continuity of care. A description of the roles of nurses within the community is given in Chapter 2.

The person receiving care

To be able to nurse patients effectively the nurse needs to be aware of how she perceives her patients, and how the patient normally reacts and views life.

Nurses, like doctors, often have identified patients in terms of medical diagnoses, e.g. 'the knee replacement', rather than seeing the patient as a person who has perceptions of life, needs and expectations of care. With encouragement, most nurses are able to identify their ideas and perceptions about the people in their care. It is also possible to determine what the individual nurse uses as a knowledge base and to identify her belief system from these ideas and views. Using a model of nursing reinforces this nursing-focused approach and enables nurses to provide a more comprehensive framework of care than that dictated by medical diagnoses and treatment regimens.

Patients may have obtained a distorted view of available health and medical care from media coverage. Whilst their expectations may be informed, they may also be unrealistic and can influence their behaviour when in contact with the nurse.

Given the decrease in hospital length of stay, it behoves the nurse to help the patient to maintain his individuality and not adopt the sick role too readily (Parsons 1951). Including patients as much as possible in decision-making regarding their own care and encouraging them to wear their own comfortable clothes rather than routinely making them wear nightwear all day, will prevent any tendency to assume the sick role.

Whilst many people entering hospital are sick, some of those who are admitted for surgery or investigations are essentially fit. The young athlete who has a torn meniscus may be fitter than the nurse who is providing his care. This patient's main problem will be achieving maximum muscle tone following surgery. However, if he has hidden fears regarding the effect of surgery on his athletic performance, he may want to continue in his sick role and not participate in physiotherapy. In this instance, his inclusion in decision-making, an exploration of his resistance to treatment, and maintenance of a normal dressing routine will help him to address his negative reactions and empower him to reach his desired health state.

In the community the nurse may be confronted with the person who seems to resist efforts to achieve negotiated goals of care. This may be due to a secondary gain for the patient from adoption of the sick role. For example, the patient who has returned to an empty home following hospitalization for a fractured neck of femur may subconsciously attempt to prolong rehabilitation in order to maintain social contact with the nurse or to increase family visits – in both cases to reduce loneliness.

Society

Analysing different aspects of society can help the orthopaedic nurse to identify her own feelings and prejudices, as well as those of others in the team. It will help her to recognize the beliefs which may be held by her patients and which may affect the way they interact in the care process. For example, the following issues should be explored by the nurse: Does society value nursing and health care? Is there a class system? Are there different levels of health care? What value does society place on preventative medicine/care as opposed to treatment of illness? Is the society multicultural? How does the society value children and the elderly? How does society value education?

In the UK, people's use of health care and their predisposition to disease and accidents is related to their socioeconomic class. Social classes IV and V are more likely to have accidents and diseases related to poor nutrition and living conditions; they are less likely to make their needs known to health care workers or to be understood by them than are people in social classes II and III (Black 1981). The orthopaedic nurse should be aware of these issues when working with patients, in order to provide appropriate access to care and advocacy.

For multifarious reasons, modern society appears to be becoming more violent; orthopaedic nurses find themselves increasingly in situations in which patients or their relatives and friends use physical and verbal violence. The orthopaedic nurse needs to develop sufficient self-awareness and knowledge in these situations to prevent violent conflict.

The increasing number of fit elderly people may result in an expanded role for retired people in society; however, the growing number of frail, elderly individuals will make additional demands on health care provision and will increase its costs. Weighing cost against need is difficult. It is essential that nurses of the future are able to present facts and figures accurately and efficiently if they are to continue their professional and caring role. They will need to be able to analyse, plan, present, discuss and negotiate in order to formulate and monitor nursing and health care standards.

The nurse as a member of society is open to influence and the effects of societal change, and as such has a responsibility to remain abreast of current affairs and to analyse the effects of societal change and policy on the environment in which she operates.

Environment in which care is given

Although many new hospitals, health centres and rehabilitation centres have been built in the past few years, there is still a larger number of old buildings in use which were designed for patients with different expectations or for now outdated systems of health care. For example, the old hospitals had to provide for patients confined to bed for extended periods; little space was made available for privacy, lifting, mobilizing and sanitary care.

Within the community, the nurse may find herself assisting her patient in a warm, well furnished, spacious home, or she may have to work in cramped, overcrowded, damp and insanitary conditions. The increasing number of homeless people is a problem that few nurses have at present confronted in terms of care provision. Wherever nursing care is required, nurses have a duty to respond in a positive manner to the needs of their patients and to respect the United Kingdom Central Council (1992) code of conduct.

Knowledge base for a model for orthopaedic nursing

To use an orthopaedic nursing model effectively, the nurse must have a sound knowledge of anatomy, physiology, psychology and sociology in the context of nursing care. An awareness of social policy, political, economic, demographic, health and medical care/technology trends will become imperative. The nurse will need to be able to understand and use management systems, methods of implementing change and patient education strategies.

The nurse will demonstrate her ability to translate this knowledge base into practice by carrying out appropriate therapeutic care programmes with patients and their families or friends.

The nurse of the future will need to be able to evaluate research and generate questions to participate in the evolution of health care.

Health

The World Health Organization (1948) defined health as 'a state of physical, mental and social well-being and not merely an absence of disease or infirmity'; this suggests a biomedical framework. Parse (1981, 1987) contends that a concept of individual health should include the person's hopes, aspirations and dreams.

This model brings these concepts together and uses the following definition of health developed from Parse (1981): 'a state of physical and mental reality which enables the individual to participate in the achievement of his/her own identified goals. It is more than a wellness of body and mind, in that it enables the individual to incorporate into his/her cultural reality a realistic movement toward his/her dreams of living.'

Using this definition, illness becomes any altered state that leads to an interruption in the person's ability to maintain his own definition of health, temporarily or permanently. The patient's definition of health becomes the reality from which the nurse must plan his care (Fig. 3.3).

As individuals, the patient and nurse may differ in how they define health. The nurse needs to establish the patient's perspective and desires in order to facilitate individualized care planning. She should ask the patient questions to determine his expectations and hopes for the future following his current hospital episode; for example: 'What do you wish could happen in the future?' 'How do you feel this will affect your future hopes for yourself (family, life)?' This will clarify the patient's wishes and identify where health education, counselling or teaching regarding the patient's situation may be required.

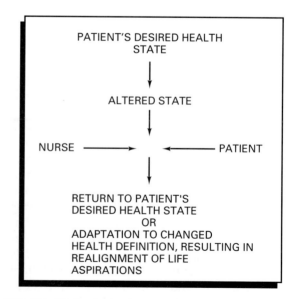

Fig. 3.3 Health construct.

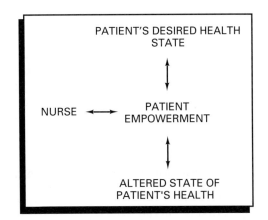

Fig. 3.4 Nurse–patient relationship.

The nurse–patient relationship

To put a model into practice it is necessary to consider the relationship between the nurse and the patient. The principal characteristic of this relationship is empowerment (see Fig. 3.4).

Empowerment of the patient by the nurse commences with the building of trust based on mutual respect, openness, honesty, confidence and acceptance; the nurse avoids being judgemental.

When she first meets the patient, she should let him know that the planning of care will involve him and his family (or significant persons in his life) and will include an understanding of their wishes for his recovery.

The nurse will use verbal and non-verbal communication to imply acceptance of the patient, and show a willingness to listen, understand and give information that will help the patient to make informed choices. In this way the nurse enters into a negotiation of care and avoids adopting an authoritarian mode.

However, if the patient and his family do not trust the nurse, they will not be open and receptive to shared planning and may put up communication barriers, potentially decreasing the nurse's effectiveness in empowering the patient to achieve his own personal aspirations of health.

Each member of the multidisciplinary team must also negotiate a framework of trust and mutual respect in order to have an effective input into the care plan. In this way, conflicts between staff and patients that may be hidden can be explored and confronted, thus removing the potential for misunderstanding and resistance.

THE MODEL FOR ORTHOPAEDIC NURSING

The previous section established the underlying principles for nursing in a modern society, from which a model for orthopaedic nursing could be created which provides a framework for assessment, nursing diagnosis, mutual goal setting, planning and evaluation of care.

Figure 3.5 illustrates the general dynamics of this model: at the centre is the nurse's goal –

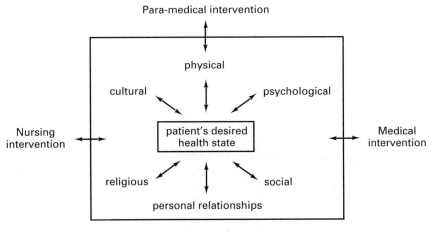

Fig. 3.5 A model for orthopaedic nursing practice.

the attainment of the patient's desired health status – and the linking arrows through the square represent the medical, nursing and paramedical interventions that help bring about this desired health status. Surrounding the goal are the physical, psychological, social, cultural, religious and personal relationships that make the patient a unique person and which will affect the outcome of the interventions.

The orthopaedic model uses empowerment in the nurse–patient relationship to enable the patient to utilize his strengths in his physical, psychological, social, religious and personal relationships with others to help him master the situation which is affecting his ability to mobilize.

Throughout the process of empowerment the nurse uses her roles (Fig. 3.2) as appropriate to the patient's needs; for example, the patient who has received a spinal injury will, at various times, need the nurse as a counsellor to empower him to confront his strengths and weaknesses in all his relationships (see inner circle of Fig. 3.5). He will also need help in exploring the physical and emotional responses which emanate from his loss of control of his physical mobility and the difference between his present and desired health states.

Assessment and nursing diagnosis

Figure 3.6 is the assessment chart for the orthopaedic nursing model which is based on the underlying principles previously discussed, and which makes the model distinctly orthopaedic with its central emphasis on mobility.

During the initial assessment the nurse lays the foundation for her relationship with the patient. Assessment is an ongoing process (see Figs 3.5 and 3.6), but establishment of the priori-

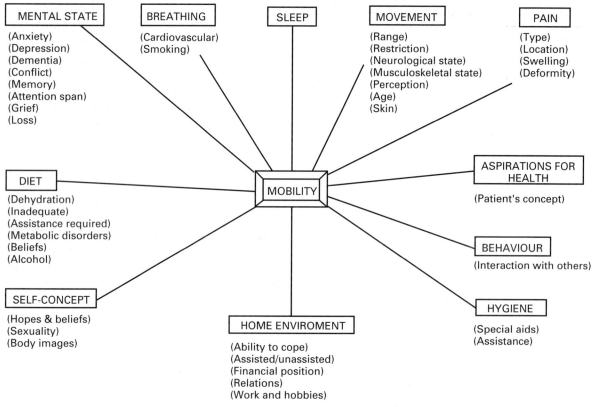

Fig. 3.6 Assessment considerations.

ties is undertaken on admission to facilitate an immediate nursing diagnosis and, where possible, mutual goal setting and planning. In situations in which the patient is unable to communicate directly with the nurse, the nurse should involve the significant others in the patient's life.

Even though there will be limited time available for assessment and care planning if the patient is admitted to hospital for day surgery, it is still imperative that the nurse spends enough time with the patient to give him information to allay his fears, and to enable him to give informed consent to treatment.

The most satisfactory way of carrying this out is to provide a preoperative assessment clinic where the nurse can identify with him any factors which may affect the proposed treatment, including the anaesthetic and discharge (for example, the implications of cigarette smoking for undergoing general anaesthesia). In addition, features in the home environment which could cause difficulties for the patient on discharge can be discussed; for example, stairs and high cupboards can cause problems following hip surgery.

During the assessment, appropriate breathing and mobilization exercises can be taught; this instruction can be reinforced by providing the patient with information leaflets to take home.

Occasions may arise when the nurse feels that the patient is responding to the situation or to her in a manner which indicates that he has been adversely affected by a previous experience. In this situation, it will be important for the nurse to confront the patient with these feelings. For example, a patient admitted for a hip replacement may resist all attempts by the nurse to get him to walk within the first week. He may, when all the indications are to the contrary, insist that he is ill. The nurse should be particularly careful to listen to the patient and to watch non-verbal interactions with other nursing staff and relatives/friends to find clues to explain this behaviour. It may be necessary for the nurse to explore the patient's attitude and behaviour with him by saying, 'Mr . . ., I feel that there is something that has happened to you or somebody that you

know that is making you fearful of walking. Can you think of what this might be?' Or she can directly confront his angry response to her attempts to help him move by saying, 'Mr . . ., whenever we try to help you to walk, as we agreed before your operation, you appear to become angry with us. Can we talk about what is making you angry?' Ignoring the patient's responses will not facilitate his return to health.

The knowledge base that is necessary to carry out the assessment as outlined in Figure 3.6 is contained within this book, and should be enhanced by the nurse gaining a deeper insight into the psychological and social behaviour, cultural reactions and religious beliefs of different sections of the population.

From the assessment will emerge the nursing diagnosis of the patient's care needs. These may fall into one or more of the categories listed in Figure 3.7, each of which relates to alterations in the patient's desired health state.

The diagnoses should encompass the effects of medical intervention and include forward planning with the patient to explore anticipated physical and psychological changes and prepare for discharge (see case study, p. 39).

The emphasis throughout should be on positive progression to assist the patient to view his incapacitation as a temporary episode in his life.

Mutual goal setting

Goals for care should be agreed between the nurse and the patient. It is imperative that the patient explores, with the assistance of the nurse, the potential effects of his orthopaedic condition and the effects of nursing and medical intervention before he agrees on the extent of his participation in his care. For example, a person with osteoarthritis of the hip may be advised to swim every day to improve mobility of the joint, but may decide not to do so. From the information given by the nurse and doctor, he would know that there is a high probability that eventually he will need a joint replacement and would prefer to wait for the surgery and suffer the limited mobility in the meantime.

Potential care needs following surgery or

Pain – locality
      type
      duration

Mobility – reduction of

Diet – dehydration
     inadequate

Hygiene – deficits
      problems in maintaining

Skin – wound
     pressure sore risk/presence

Rest and relaxation – ability/inability to meet

Sexuality – restrictions/adaptations/alterations

Elimination – deficits/alterations

Mood state – current/alterations

Self-concept – positive/negative

Personal relationships – positive/negative resulting
       from orthopaedic condition
Socio-economic – positive/negative resulting from
      orthopaedic condition
Comfort – deficits

Loss – presence of/coping strategy

Body image – alteration in

Fig. 3.7 Categories of nursing diagnosis.

therapy should be used as a basis for patient education and, if necessary, information booklets, group sessions, videos or talking to others with similar experiences, should be built into the programme. Goals for these activities should focus on the patient being able to repeat facts or reproduce behavioural actions related to the information provided.

The mutual goals should state the expected outcome in measurable terms, and dates should be given for evaluation.

Planning care

The care plan will incorporate the goals which have been agreed between patient and nurse (a selection of creative care programmes, based on current and appropriate nursing research, is essential). The plan should also reflect the standards of care identified for the hospital or community environment. These standards should relate to the nursing diagnosis, and state the expectations of care and the criteria to be used in providing the resources (structure), deciding on the action (process), and evaluating the outcome. By having the standards and criteria for care planning in a folder or on computer, the nurse will be able to verify at any time what is available and what is expected. In addition, monitoring the effectiveness of care and the activity of the ward / environment – the nursing audit – can be undertaken more easily.

Evaluation of goal achievement/non-achievement

Perhaps one of the nursing profession's weaknesses is resistance to determine whether a stated goal of care has been achieved. For this model to be effective, it is necessary for the nurse to review the mutual goal with the patient on the date stated, and record the evaluation in a concise, accurate and objective way.

Evaluation is a measurement of the outcome of the patient's care. The most effective method of evaluating a patient's progress is to write and update the care plan at the end of each period spent with the patient rather than at the end of a shift, as this invariably leads to inaccurate recollections and is unlikely to include the patient's views regarding achievement of goals of care. Further planning will depend upon the measured outcome, the changes in the patient's health status and the medical and paramedical intervention. The care plan should be a 'live' document which is used continually and reassessed.

Review of the stated mutual goals provides concurrent audit data, and should be used to identify trends throughout the care setting as well as in the individual patient. For example, examination of goals related to wound healing may reveal an increase in healing time in more than the anticipated number of patients. This should alert the nursing team to analyse potential causes for this trend.

Nursing audit

To evaluate the overall effectiveness of care, it is suggested that each month the nursing records are audited by the nursing team. This would take the form of analysing the outcomes of care and patients' records against the stated standards.

Linking the nursing audit to the medical audit every month would facilitate data collection of health care effectiveness, measured against resources, and enable the nursing team to participate in development planning.

CASE STUDY: THE MODEL IN ACTION

To conclude this chapter and demonstrate the model in action, let us consider the situation of Mr Jones who is to be admitted for a hip replacement in 2 weeks from the date of his preoperative assessment visit.

Assessment

The nurse greets Mr Jones in the assessment clinic and introduces herself by name. Whilst inviting Mr Jones into the clinic the nurse observes the ease/difficulty with which Mr Jones walks and sits in the chair. She notices that Mr Jones uses a walking stick and winces with pain when manoeuvring into the chair.

In order to establish a relationship the nurse gives Mr Jones an outline of the purpose of the visit by explaining why he is going to be asked some questions regarding his life and expectations of his hospitalization. Mr Jones is invited to stop the nurse if he feels that he does not understand or accept what is being said to him. It is emphasized to Mr Jones that the purpose of this clinic is not only to provide the nurse and team who will be looking after him with information, but also for Mr Jones to state his wishes for his care, in order that a plan can be mutually agreed and carried out within the resources available.

At this point the nurse asks Mr Jones to tell her how his hip problem started. He replies that for the past 5 years his right hip has become increasingly painful, to the extent that he has gradually become limited in the distance that he can walk without severe pain, despite pain killers. As Mr Jones seems willing to talk, the nurse does not interrupt but notes that it will be impor-

tant to find out the distance that he can walk before the pain becomes prohibitive.

Mr Jones continues by saying that up until 2 years ago his wife had helped him, but she died suddenly in this hospital from a heart attack. The nurse notes that the hospital may have connotations of death for Mr Jones.

Mr Jones offers the information that when his wife died, nobody in the casualty department told him of her death for some time, and that he felt totally isolated. As he talks he has tears in his eyes. The nurse notes that this may mean that Mr Jones has little trust in the hospital staff, and at this point says, 'Mr Jones, I can see that the death of your wife is still very painful for you and that the experience you had in this hospital might still cause you distress.' Mr Jones affirms that he is frightened that people will not tell him what is happening and will leave him alone.

Rather than stating that this will not happen, the nurse gives Mr Jones the opportunity to express his fears by saying, 'Can you tell me what your real fear is?' In this way Mr Jones is able to confront his fear, instead of being given a meaningless platitude; it is a step forward in his empowerment and the formation of trust between patient and nurse. His fear stems from being alone and not having support.

This statement leads the nurse to ask, 'What do you really wish the outcome of the surgery to be?' In this way the nurse leads Mr Jones into addressing his own expectations of his operation; she can then consider how realistic these expectations are in relation to the planned operation and expected outcomes. The nurse establishes that Mr Jones wants to be able to move easily around his own flat and do his own shopping from the local shops.

The nurse has thus established a relationship with Mr Jones without using a list of questions. She needs to find out the distance that Mr Jones can walk, his previous medical history and his perception of the operation. In order to do this the nurse explains that to plan Mr Jones' postoperative care it is necessary to know how far he can walk now without pain, what usually relieves his pain and his history of illness and health. She then encourages Mr Jones to talk, and discovers that he can walk about 50 metres before pain stops him, that he takes two Brufen tablets 4-hourly to help ease the pain, that he has never been unwell and that health to him is being able to visit his friends, enjoy social gatherings and care for himself. He says that he has felt less like his old social self since his wife died, but that he is now finding it is getting easier to go out.

The nurse checks for environmental factors which could delay discharge and discovers that Mr Jones has a ground floor retirement flat with a high toilet, no steps and a resident warden. From this the nurse concludes that Mr Jones should be able to make an uneventful recovery as he has the motivation of knowing that the operation will relieve the pain in his hip and enable him to reach his desired health state. She further notes that Mr Jones is still passing through the grieving process for his wife.

During a physical examination the nurse discovers that Mr Jones' pulse rate is 68 per minute and regular, blood pressure is 130/90 mmHg, respirations 18 per minute, ECG normal rate and rhythm, blood count normal. The nurse notes that Mr Jones has had his blood taken for grouping and cross-matching, and that X-rays have been taken of his right hip and chest, the latter showing normal lungs and heart.

Nursing diagnosis

The nurse identifies that Mr Jones has pain and limited mobility which will continue in the immediate post-operative period, and that there are still loss feelings associated with the death of his wife. Postoperatively Mr Jones will immediately be at risk from breathing limitations, skin damage, pain and changes in self-concept physiologically and psychologically due to the effects of the surgery and anaesthetic. But Mr Jones' desired health status is achievable.

At this point the nurse checks with Mr Jones that the assumptions of her diagnosis are correct, giving him the opportunity to challenge her.

Mutual goal setting

Having checked that Mr Jones agrees with her diag-nosis, the nurse explains the operation, the immediate postoperative recovery period and the expected mobilization plan. Mr Jones is encouraged to put his wishes for his recovery period into words, and is respected for communicating his fears of pain when mobilization commences. Mutual goals are agreed.

Planning

The nurse shows Mr Jones the proposed programme for pain control, mobilization, postoperative breathing and wound care, allowing him to question and practise the breathing programme, postoperative turning in bed, getting in and out of a chair, and limitations of movement due to the hip replacement.

Before he leaves the clinic the nurse gives Mr Jones information leaflets on the breathing programme for the pre- and postoperative period, mobilization and hip replacement care.

Evaluation

In this context the evaluation takes place first at the assessment meeting, by the nurse checking that Mr Jones has the information to take home, and second on admission to the ward, by checking that Mr Jones is able to relate to the preoperative assessment visit and participate in the expected programme of pre- and postoperative care. The extent of Mr Jones' ability to participate in the latter provides an objective evaluation of the success or failure of the care plan. Evaluation would then be carried out continually during Mr Jones' need for nursing care.

Thus, rather than being purely of theoretical value, the nursing model provides a practical framework on which to base a patient's care. It provides a consistent approach, and ensures continuity and quality of care.

REFERENCES

Chapman P 1990 A critical perspective. In: Salvage J, Kershaw B (eds) Models for nursing: 2. Scutari Press, London
Holmes B 1981 Comparative education. Some considerations of method. Allen & Unwin, London

Inequalities of Health (Report) (Chairman D Black) 1981 HMSO, London
Parse R R 1981 Man – living – health: a theory of nursing. John Wiley & Sons, New York
Parse R R 1987 Nursing science: major paradigms, theories

and critiques. W. B. Saunders, Philadelphia

Parsons T 1951 The social system. The Free Press, New York

Roy C 1976 An introduction to nursing: an adaption model. Prentice Hall, New Jersey

Salvage J 1983 Distorted images. Nursing Times 79(1): 13–15

UKCC for Nursing, Midwifery and Health Visiting 1986

Project 2000. A new preparation for practice. HMSO, London

UKCC for Nursing, Midwifery and Health Visiting 1992 Code of conduct. HMSO, London

Working for patients 1989 HMSO, London

World Health Organization 1948 Constitution. WHO, Geneva

4

Locomotor system

Amanda Matthew   Judith Kay Muir

According to Powell (1986) the nurse must develop an 'orthopaedic eye' – an acute awareness of correct body posture and mechanics – so that she will notice anything that interferes with the patient's treatment. To be able to do this the orthopaedic nurse requires a basic understanding of the underlying anatomy and physiology. This chapter aims to provide a quick reference for the anatomy and physiology of the locomotor system, i.e. the bones, joints, cartilage, muscles and controlling nervous system. These structures combine and influence the way in which people maintain their body posture, form and function. In view of the increasing proportion of elderly people in the population, this chapter also discusses some of the current theories of ageing in relation to the locomotor system.

THE SKELETAL SYSTEM

The skeletal system is the framework of the body. It consists of bone and associated connective tissue, i.e. cartilage and dense fibrous tissue. Bone is a specialized form of connective tissue and is important for its mechanical properties and the maintenance of mineral homeostasis.

Functions of the skeleton

The functions of the skeleton are as follows:

1. Support: the skeleton provides a framework for the body, with surface markings for the attachment and insertion of muscles.

2. Protection: the skeleton maintains body shape, protecting from injury many of the internal organs such as the brain, heart and lungs, and spinal cord.

3. Movement: bones and muscles act as levers producing body movements through joints.

4. Mineral storage: bones store minerals such as calcium and phosphorus.

5. Blood cell formation: red bone marrow produces red blood cells, white blood cells and platelets. This process is called haematopoiesis.

NORMAL BONE STRUCTURE

Bone tissue is highly vascular, combining organic and inorganic material. A system of collagenous fibres forms the organic component, providing resilience and flexibility. The inorganic material consists mainly of mineral salts which form a matrix providing strength and weight-bearing capabilities. Bone is three times stronger than wood and as tensile as cast iron. It is the strength and rigidity of this matrix that gives bone its characteristics.

Bone cells consist of two types of specialized cells:

1. Osteogenic cells
    - are unspecialized cells derived from the mesenchyme
    - are mitotic and differentiate into osteoblasts
    - are found in the periosteum, endosteum, Haversian and Volkmann's canals
   a. osteoblasts
       — do not have mitotic potential
       — are involved in bone formation
       — secrete organic components and mineral salts involved with bone formation
       — are found on the surface of bone
   b. osteocytes
       — are osteoblasts that become trapped within bone
       — do not have mitotic potential
       — maintain bone tissue

2. Osteoclasts
    - develop from the macrophage/monocyte system
    - function in the resorption of bone
    - have a key role in the continuous modelling of bone.

Chemical composition

Bone is normally made up of organic (30–35%) and inorganic (65–70%) material. The organic component consists of protein fibres which are mainly collagen. These collagen fibres make up 90–95% of the organic matrix.

Mineral salts, such as those of calcium and phosphorus, predominate in the inorganic component. These complex crystals combine to produce rod-shaped hydroxyapatite crystals (see Fig. 4.1) which are uniform in shape. The ratio of calcium content to phosphorus content varies depending on the nutritional state of the individual. Their levels are controlled by the parathyroid hormone and calcitonin which are produced in the parathyroid glands.

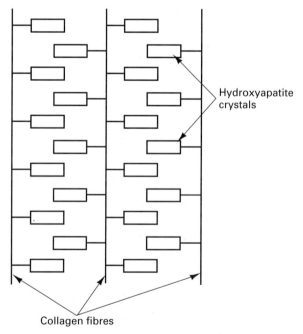

Hydroxyapatite crystals

Collagen fibres

Fig. 4.1 Hydroxyapatite crystals.

Other substances are present, attached in the form of ions:

- Magnesium
- Sodium
- Potassium
- Carbonate.

The chemical composition of bone makes it susceptible to damage. For example, radioactive chemicals attach strongly to the hydroxyapatite crystals. These include emissions from nuclear power stations such as uranium, plutonium and strontium. These destructive chemicals are ionically similar to calcium and phosphorus and do not pass out of the body but accumulate and irradiate bone marrow.

Types of bone

The density of bone varies. There are two major types of bone with differences in weight, strength and function:

- Compact (dense) bone
- Cancellous (spongy) bone.

Compact bone is denser bone tissue with few spaces, whereas cancellous bone has larger spaces filled with red bone marrow. The distribution of compact and cancellous bone is illustrated in Figure 4.2.

Compact bone

Cancellous bone is surrounded by a layer of compact bone. This layer is thicker in the diaphysis than the epiphysis, and in addition to providing support and protection it resists any weight directed through the long bone.

Compact bone is dense with a concentric ring structure. Blood vessels and nerves enter the bone substance from its outer covering, the periosteum, through the Volkmann's canals. Central haversian canals run longitudinally and contain blood vessels and nerves which have merged with vessels from the Volkmann's canals and the medullary cavity.

The central (haversian) canals are surrounded

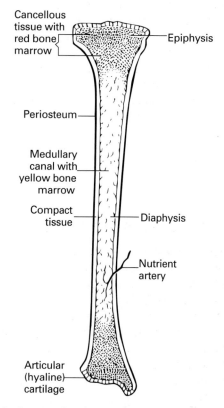

Fig. 4.2 A mature long bone – longitudinal section. (From Wilson 1990, with permission.)

by rings of a hard calcified bone, known as concentric lamellae. In between the lamellae are spaces called lacunae which contain osteocytes. Small canals called canaliculi radiate from these osteocytes. Circumferential lamellae form flat plates and surround the outer surface of the compact bone.

In cross-section (see Fig. 4.3) a haversian system (osteon) consists of a single haversian canal, associated concentric lamellae and osteocytes.

Compact bone is made up of an intricate network allowing the passage of nutrients from the periosteum and endosteum to the osteocytes, with the removal of waste products passing in the opposite direction.

Cancellous bone

Cancellous bone consists of a lattice-work of thin plates of compact bone called trabeculae. Each

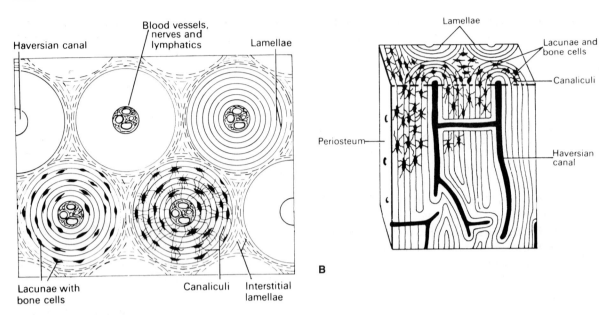

A

Fig. 4.3 Microscopic structure of bone. A. Cross-section; B. Longitudinal section. (From Wilson 1990, with permission.)

trabecula comprises several lamellae containing layers of lacunae that are filled with osteocytes. These osteocytes are associated with other osteocytes through canaliculi, where they obtain their nutrients from the circulating blood.

Trabeculae are laid down along lines of stress.

Structure of a long bone

A typical long bone (see Fig. 4.4) consists of the following components:

1. Diaphysis: the diaphysis is the shaft of a long bone.
2. Epiphysis: the epiphyses are at the ends of a long bone.
3. Epiphyseal plate: the epiphyseal plate consists of cartilage, and joins the diaphysis to the epiphysis in mature bone. It may also be referred to as the 'metaphysis'. This is the area where most growth in length takes place. Growth stops when all of the epiphyseal plate is fully ossified, usually in the late teens to early 20s.
4. Periosteum: the periosteum is essential for bone growth, repair and nutrition. It covers the outer surface of the bone. The periosteum has a

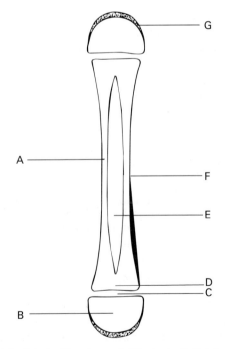

Fig. 4.4 A typical long bone. A. Diaphysis; B. Epiphysis; C. Epiphyseal plate; D. Metaphysis; E. Medullary cavity; F. Periosteum; G. Articular hyaline cartilage. (From Gunn 1992, with permission.)

dense outer fibrous layer composed of connective tissue, containing blood vessels, nerves and lymphatic vessels. The inner layer contains elastic fibres, a few osteoclasts, a single layer of osteoblasts, osteoprogenitor cells and blood vessels. Where ligaments and tendons attach, the periosteal fibres become continuous with the fibres of the tendon or ligament. Perforating fibres called Sharpey's fibres allow the attachment of ligaments and fibres to the bone by penetrating the periosteum.

5. Endosteum: the endosteum lines the medullary cavity of the bone. It consists of a single layer of osteoprogenitor cells and osteoblasts, and some osteoclasts.

6. Medullary cavity: this is found within the diaphysis of long bones and in smaller cavities in the epiphysis. The medullary cavity contains yellow marrow or red marrow.

Bone formation

Embryonic development of bone involves the migration of mesenchymal tissue into the area where bone formation is to begin. The mesenchymal cells increase in size and number and differentiate into osteogenic cells. Then the osteogenic cells differentiate into osteoblasts or chondroblasts. In the embryo, fibrous membranes and cartilage are shaped like bone. Ossification begins around the 6th or 7th week of embryonic life.

Ossification or osteogenesis is the formation of bone by osteoblasts. This process involves the synthesis of an organic matrix and the addition of mineral salts such as hydroxyapatite. Intramembranous ossification refers to the formation of bone within connective tissue membranes. Endochondral ossification is the formation of bone associated with cartilage.

Intramembranous ossification

Osteoblasts formed from osteoprogenitor cells colonize connective tissue membranes. These secrete intercellular substances and form a bony matrix in centres of ossification. Trabeculae radiate out from each centre of ossification into a lattice-work of collagen fibres where inorganic

salts are deposited. The original connective tissue becomes the periosteum and the ossified area becomes spongy bone with a covering layer of compact bone. Blood vessels and unspecialized cells form the bone marrow.

The bones of the skull and the clavicle develop in this manner. In the newborn the bones of the skull are incomplete with membranous gaps called fontanelles between them. The bones eventually grow together and close the gaps.

Endochondral ossification

Most of the bones of the body and the base of the skull are formed by this method. Bone develops from a hyaline cartilage prototype through a process of endochondral ossification (see Fig. 4.5). The cartilage is covered by a membrane called the perichondrium and this is invaded by numerous blood capillaries which stimulate osteoprogenitor cells to form osteoblasts. This layer of osteoblasts forms compact bone around the diaphysis, and is called the periosteum.

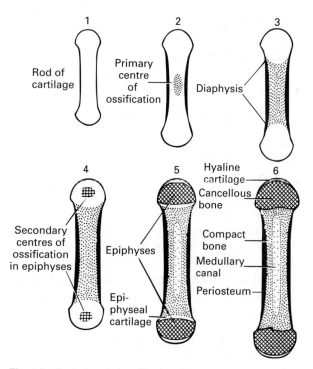

Fig. 4.5 Endochondral ossification. (From Wilson 1990, with permission.)

Changes occur to the cartilage cells, the chondrocytes, within the diaphysis. This area is known as the primary ossification centre. These cells hypertrophy, and the matrix becomes mineralized as the intercellular substance calcifies. The chondrocytes eventually die, leaving large lacunae for blood vessels to grow into. The spaces in the shaft of the long bone join together forming the medullary cavity which becomes filled with bone marrow.

In the long bone, secondary centres of ossification appear in the epiphyses and lay down cancellous bone. Ossification continues until all the cartilage is replaced, except that covering the articular surfaces and in the epiphyseal plate. The articulating cartilage and the epiphyseal plate are directly formed from original embryonic tissue.

Bone growth

Bone grows by appositional growth or endochondral growth.

Appositional growth

This is the formation of new bone on the surface of existing bone. Most bones increase in diameter through this means. Appositional growth occurs along with growth in the length of a bone. Bone lining the marrow cavity is destroyed by osteoclasts, enabling the cavity to increase in size. Simultaneously, osteoblasts from the periosteum produce new compact bone which covers the outer surface of the bone.

Endochondral growth

This is the growth of cartilage in the epiphyseal plate and its eventual ossification and fusion with the diaphysis between 12 and 25 years of age. This process of growth involves interstitial cartilage growth followed by calcification and replacement bone.

Repair and maintenance

Repair and maintenance of bone occurs as a result of several different stimuli:

- Remodelling during bone growth: this involves the replacement of old bone by new bone tissue.
- Exercise and mechanical stress: additional bone is deposited in response to mechanical stress.
- Fracture repair: the time taken for a fracture to repair will depend on the type of fracture; it will also take longer in the elderly because of decreased blood supply and general inefficiency of the repair processes.

Remodelling

Remodelling takes place:

- in bone growth
- during an alteration in shape
- in response to mechanical stress
- in repair.

Bone constantly remodels its matrix. The process allows worn or injured bone to be replaced and helps to regulate the storage of calcium for the rest of the body, as calcium is essential for the normal functioning of many of the body's tissues.

Normal bone replacement relies on sufficient dietary intake or production of:

- calcium and phosphorus
- manganese and boron
- vitamin D, which aids the absorption of calcium from the gastrointestinal tract into the blood, removes calcium from bone and reabsorbs calcium from the kidney tubules
- vitamin C, which maintains the intercellular substance of bone and other connective tissue
- vitamin A, which controls the activity, distribution, and coordination of osteoblasts and osteoclasts
- hormones.

Process of resorption

Osteoclasts are believed to be responsible for resorption. In the normal adult, homeostasis is maintained between the removal and deposition of calcium and collagen. During this process it is thought that osteoclasts develop projections that secrete enzymes as well as lactic acid and citric acid. The acids cause bone to dissolve and the enzymes digest collagen and other organic substances.

Hormones

Human growth hormone, secreted by the anterior pituitary gland, is responsible for bone tissue growth. Under- or over-secretion during childhood may result in dwarfism or gigantism, respectively. Growth hormone stimulates interstitial cartilage growth and appositional bone growth. The thyroid gland produces calcitonin which is also essential for normal growth. Calcitonin inhibits osteoclast activity and accelerates the absorption of calcium by bone.

Parathormone, which is produced in the parathyroid glands, increases osteoclast activity, releasing calcium and phosphate ions from the bones into the circulation.

Sex hormones stimulate bone growth. Oestrogen and testosterone increase the activity of osteoblasts and promote new bone formation. The burst of growth during puberty is due to a release of male/female sex hormones. These hormones also stimulate ossification of the epiphyseal plate as skeletal growth is completed. Females usually stop growing earlier than males.

Exercise

Bone is capable of altering its strength in response to mechanical stress. Mechanical stress increases the deposition of mineral salts and the production of collagen fibres. An absence of this type of stress promotes the removal of mineral salts and collagen fibres.

Athletes whose bones are subjected to a high degree of stress have thicker bones than non-athletes. The effect of regular exercise is to stimulate bone growth and increase the production of calcitonin, thus inhibiting bone resorption.

Fracture repair

Bones vary considerably in the length of time they require to heal. As a rule, in adults upper limb fractures take 6–8 weeks to heal and lower limb fractures require 8–12 weeks.

The following stages occur in the repair of a fracture (see Fig. 4.6):

1. Stage 1 Inflammatory phase. As a result of a fracture, the bone ends and surrounding tissue bleed and a haematoma is formed. The bone ends are subsequently sealed by the fracture haematoma, where osteocyte and periosteal cell death occurs. This results in an inflammatory response with vasodilation and the gathering of polymorphonucleocytes and histiocytes.

2. Stage 2 Reparative phase. This stage is characterized by the formation of callus. External callus is produced by osteoblasts from the periosteum forming a bridge between the bone ends. At this stage the callus is visible on X-ray.

3. Stage 3 Remodelling phase. Remodelling of the original structure takes place over a period of time. Any fragments or dead bone are resorbed by the osteoclasts and compact bone replaces spongy bone around the fracture. On X-ray the surface of the bone will usually retain some evidence of the fracture site.

Axial and appendicular skeleton

The adult skeleton (Fig. 4.7) consists of 206 bones, which can be divided into two categories. The axial skeleton consists of 80 bones and the appendicular skeleton 126 bones.

The exact number of individual bones varies from person to person and may decrease with age owing to the fusion of some bones. The axial skeleton consists of the skull, hyoid bone, vertebral column, ribs and sternum. The appendicular skeleton consists of bones of the upper limbs and pectoral girdle, and the lower limbs and pelvic girdle.

CARTILAGE

Cartilage is made up of cartilage cells called chondrocytes. Cartilage consists of a dense network of collagenous fibres and elastic fibres within an extensive and fairly rigid matrix. The matrix, secreted by the chondrocytes, consists of

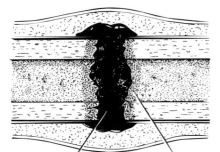

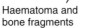

Haematoma and   Inflamed area
bone fragments

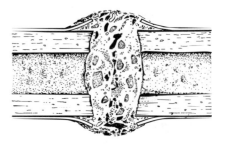

Phagocytosis of clot and debris. Growth of
granulation tissue begins

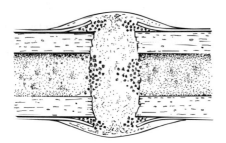

Osteoblasts begin to form new bone

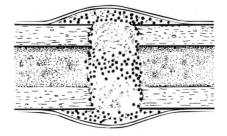

Gradual spread of new bone to bridge gap

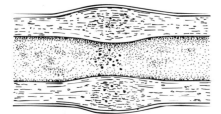

Bone healed. Osteoblasts reshape and
canalise new bone

Fig. 4.6 Stages of fracture repair. (From
Wilson 1990, with permission.)

protein fibres, a ground substance consisting of
non-fibrous protein such as proteoglycans, and
fluid. The proteoglycans are capable of trapping
large quantities of water like a sponge, enabling
the cartilage to spring back after it has been
compressed; the collagen fibres give cartilage its
considerable strength.

Growth of cartilage

Cartilage grows in two ways:

1. Interstitial growth: this is a rapid increase in
size through the division of existing chondrocytes and the continual deposition of increasing
amounts of intercellular matrix by the chondro-

cytes. This growth pattern occurs during childhood and young adolescence.

2. Appositional growth: this occurs as a result
of activity within the inner chondrogenic layer of
the perichondrium. Fibroblasts divide and differentiate into chondroblasts and chondrocytes.
The matrix is deposited beneath the perichondrium on the surface of the cartilage. Appositional growth takes over from interstitial growth
and continues throughout life.

Types of cartilage

There are three types of cartilage:

1. Hyaline cartilage. Hyaline cartilage covers
the surface of bones where they articulate within

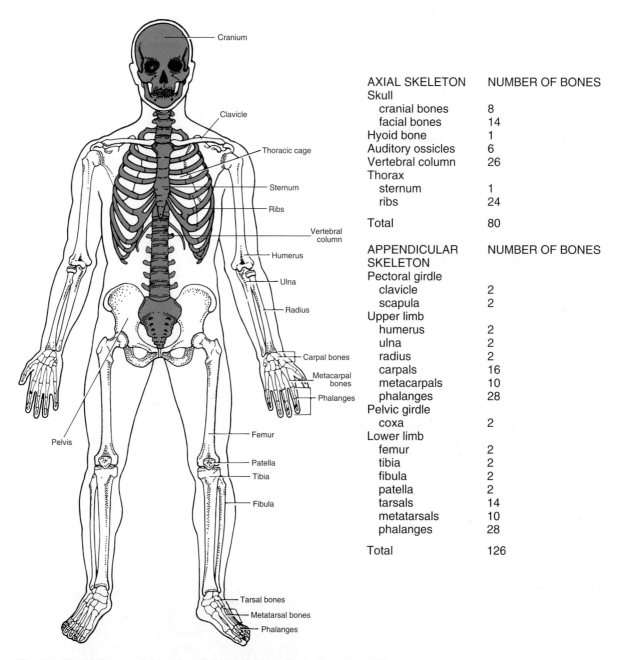

AXIAL SKELETON	NUMBER OF BONES
Skull	
cranial bones	8
facial bones	14
Hyoid bone	1
Auditory ossicles	6
Vertebral column	26
Thorax	
sternum	1
ribs	24
Total	80

APPENDICULAR SKELETON	NUMBER OF BONES
Pectoral girdle	
clavicle	2
scapula	2
Upper limb	
humerus	2
ulna	2
radius	2
carpals	16
metacarpals	10
phalanges	28
Pelvic girdle	
coxa	2
Lower limb	
femur	2
tibia	2
fibula	2
patella	2
tarsals	14
metatarsals	10
phalanges	28
Total	126

Fig. 4.7   The skeleton – anterior view. Axial skeleton – dark shading. (From Wilson 1990, with permission.)

a joint (see Fig. 4.8). It is also found at the ends of the ribs, nasal septum, larynx, trachea, bronchi and bronchial tubes. It appears as a smooth bluish-white shiny substance; the cells are grouped together and the matrix is solid (see Fig. 4.9).

2. Fibrocartilage. Fibrocartilage is flexible and capable of withstanding considerable pressure. Thick dense collagen fibres are arranged in layers; the matrix is similar to that of hyaline cartilage (see Fig. 4.10). Fibrocartilage is found in

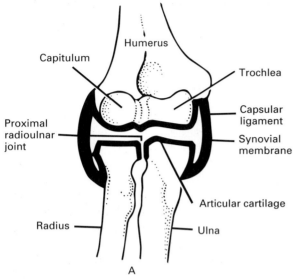

Fig. 4.8 The elbow joint. (From Wilson 1990, with permission.)

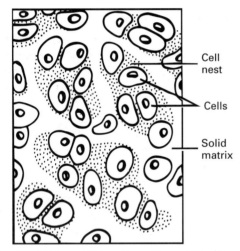

Fig. 4.9 Hyaline cartilage. (From Wilson 1990, with permission.)

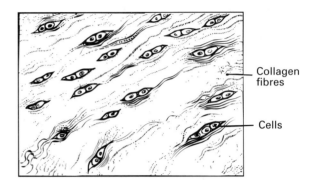

Fig. 4.10 Fibrocartilage. (From Wilson 1990, with permission.)

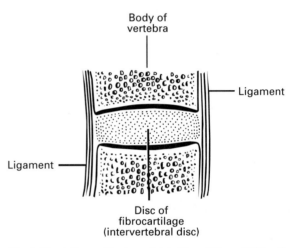

Fig. 4.11 A fibrocartilaginous joint. (From Wilson 1990, with permission.)

the symphysis pubis, in the knee joint as menisci and between the vertebrae as intervertebral discs (see Fig. 4.11).

3. Elastic Cartilage. Elastic cartilage is found in the epiglottis, the larynx, the pinna of the ear and the eustachian tubes. The elastic fibres form a thread-like network which provides strength and flexibility while maintaining the shape of organs (see Fig. 4.12). Otherwise the structure is similar to that of hyaline cartilage.

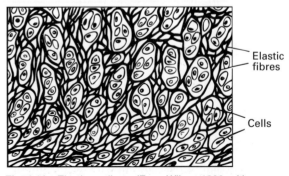

Fig. 4.12 Elastic cartilage. (From Wilson 1990, with permission.)

SKELETAL MUSCLE TISSUE

Muscle tissue consists of highly specialized fibres for the active generation of force from contraction. This characteristic in muscles is responsible for movement, maintenance of posture and heat production.

Muscle tissue can be classified according to its structural and functional characteristics into three types:

1. Skeletal or striated voluntary muscle
2. Cardiac or striated involuntary muscle
3. Smooth or non-striated involuntary muscle.

In this chapter only skeletal muscle tissue is described in detail.

Characteristics

Muscle tissue has four principal characteristics:

1. Contractility; muscle contractions are responsible for the body's movements. Contractility is the ability of muscle tissue to actively generate force by shortening and thickening as a result of a stimulus.
2. Excitability; muscle is termed excitable when it responds to stimuli from nerves, hormones and injury. A stimulus is a change in the internal or external environment which is strong enough to initiate an impulse.
3. Extensibility; this is the ability of muscle to be stretched. Muscles work in opposing groups: while one is contracting and shortening, the other is relaxing and undergoing extension.
4. Elasticity; muscles are elastic and recoil to their original shape if they are stretched.

Functions

Skeletal muscle comprises approximately 40% of body weight. In conjunction with the skeleton, muscle performs three functions:

- Motion (reflex and voluntary); movement relies on a partnership between the bones, joints and skeletal muscles attached to the bones.
- Maintenance of posture; the contraction of skeletal muscles holds the body in stationary positions.
- Heat production; skeletal muscle contractions produce most of the body's heat and therefore assist in the maintenance of normal body temperature.

Embryonic development

All muscles are derived from the mesoderm. During the development of the mesoderm a portion becomes arranged in columns on either side of the developing nervous system. These columns segment into a series of blocks of cells known as somites. Except for the head and extremities which develop from the general mesoderm, skeletal muscles develop from the mesoderm of somites.

The cells of a somite differentiate into three: myotome, dermatome and sclerotome. Skeletal muscle develops from a myotome of a somite.

Skeletal muscle structure

Skeletal muscles are composed of muscle fibres and some connective tissue such as blood vessels and nerves. Muscle fibres develop from multinucleated cells called myoblasts. The myoblasts are converted into muscle fibres as contractile proteins accumulate within their cytoplasm. As the myoblasts form, nerves grow into the area and innervate the developing muscle fibres.

Muscle cells remain constant in number following birth. The enlargement of muscles is then dependent on an increase in the size of muscle fibres rather than their number. Skeletal muscle fibres have a striated appearance due to the arrangement of the myofilaments.

Surrounding each muscle fibre is an external lamina comprising reticular fibres which are indistinguishable from the muscle fibre's cell membrane, the sarcolemma. Outside the lamina is a delicate network of fibres called the endomysium. Each bundle of muscle fibres is surrounded by a heavier layer, the perimysium, and is called a fasciculus. A muscle consists of several fasciculi surrounded by a third layer, the epimysium, covering the entire surface of the muscle. Individual muscles are separated by fascia, a layer of fibrous connective tissue.

Structure of muscle fibres

Each muscle fibre is comprised of several layers (see Fig. 4.13). Skeletal muscle fibres are composed of cylindrical structures called myofibrils. These are thread-like structures running from one end of the muscle to the other. Myofibrils consist of two kinds of smaller structures:

- Actin or thin myofilaments, which contain two additional proteins – tropomysin and troponin – which are involved in the regulation of muscle contractions
- Myosin or thick myofilaments, composed of the protein, myosin.

The actin and myosin myofilaments are arranged in compartments called sarcomeres. Certain areas within a sarcomere can be distinguished. A dense area called the anisotropic (dense band) or A band represents the length of the thick myofilaments. Each isotropic (light band) or I band is composed of thin myofilaments only.

Physiology of skeletal muscle

Skeletal muscle contracts in response to electro-chemical stimuli. Through the central nervous system, nerve cells control and coordinate this muscle contraction.

The neuromuscular junction

The axons of motor neurons, motor nerve cells, enter skeletal muscle along the same pathway as arteries and veins. The axon to a muscle may be as long as 3 feet or more. At the level of the perimysium the axon branches towards a muscle fibre, forming a neuromuscular junction or synapse (see Fig. 4.14). Each axon innervates more than one muscle fibre. The area adjacent to the axon in the muscle cell membrane or sarcolemma is called the end-plate or postsynaptic terminal. The neuromuscular junction refers to the space between the axon terminal of the motor neuron and the end-plate.

The axon terminal is enlarged and forms the presynaptic terminal; the space between this and the muscle fibre is the synaptic cleft. The presynaptic terminal contains sacs, the synaptic vesicles, which store chemicals called neurotransmitters that stimulate or inhibit an action potential.

The neurotransmitter released in skeletal muscle is acetylcholine. Acetylcholine diffuses across the synaptic cleft combining with the receptor sites of the sarcolemma of the muscle fibre. At this point the permeability of the sarcolemma to sodium (Na) and potassium (K) ions is increased. When two acetylcholine molecules bind to the receptor it opens channels. As a result there is an inward movement of sodium (Na) ions which depolarize the membrane to below threshold level causing the muscle fibre to contract.

Acetylcholinesterase or cholinesterase inactivates acetylcholine by breaking it down into its components, acetate and chlorine. In this way it allows time for repolarization of the membrane of the muscle fibre so that another impulse may be transmitted.

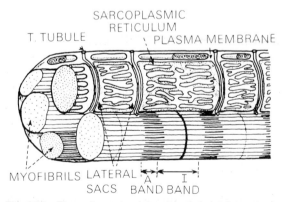

Fig. 4.13 Three-dimensional drawing of skeletal muscle fibre. (From Mackenna & Callander 1990, with permission.)

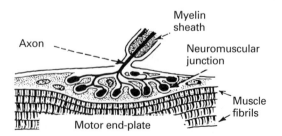

Fig. 4.14 Neuromuscular junction. (From Mackenna & Callander 1990 with permission.)

Energy source

Muscle contraction and relaxation require energy. Adenosine triphosphate (ATP) is the immediate source of energy for contraction. Skeletal muscle fibres contain a high-energy molecule called phosphocreatine. Phosphocreatine and ATP constitute the phosphagen system. The phosphagen system provides enough ATP for bursts of activity, of approximately 15 seconds. If activity is to be sustained for longer, the body's supply of phosphagen becomes depleted. Glucose then becomes the source of energy, derived from the breakdown of glycogen. Glycogen is stored in the muscles and the liver. The breakdown of glycogen is known as glycolysis. This may occur with or without the continued presence of oxygen. Once the immediate oxygen stores have been used for aerobic respiration then anaerobic respiration occurs and lactic acid is produced. This glycogen–lactic acid system will provide sufficient ATP for 30–40 seconds of vigorous muscular activity. After this the muscles will need to rest or drastically reduce their activity in order to repay the oxygen debt they have built up.

In prolonged, less vigorous activity the metabolic process of cellular respiration must take place in the continuous presence of oxygen. This aerobic system combined with glycolysis will continue as long as nutrients and adequate oxygen are available.

Type of muscle contraction

Skeletal muscle contractions are either isometric or isotonic. Isometric contractions occur when the muscle length does not change, but the amount of tension increases during the contraction, for example the contractions of postural muscles. Isotonic contractions occur when the muscle length becomes shorter, but the amount of tension produced by the muscle is constant during the contraction. Most muscle contractions tend to combine isometric and isotonic contractions.

Skeletal muscles and body movement

Body movement is produced by the coordinated action of the muscles, bone, nerves and joints. As a muscle contracts in response to a nerve impulse, a force is applied to a tendon which pulls on a bone. In body movement bones act as levers and joints function as the fulcrum or pivot points. This process allows a force to be transferred along a lever to some other point on that lever. Muscles provide the force to move the lever.

Levers

Levers may be categorized into three types:

1. First class levers: the fulcrum is located between the force (effort) and the weight (resistance), for example, a seesaw or the head resting on the atlas; the atlanto-occipital joint is the fulcrum, the skull is the weight and the muscles at the back of the neck the force.
2. Second class levers: the weight (resistance) is between the force (effort) and the fulcrum; an example is a wheelbarrow or standing on one's toes: the body is the weight, the ball of the foot is the fulcrum and the contracted calf muscle is the force.
3. Third class levers: the weight and the fulcrum are at opposite ends and the force is in between. This is the most common form of leverage in the body. An example is someone carrying a weight with the forearm flexed at the elbow: the hand holds the weight, the elbow is the fulcrum and the biceps muscle acts as the force pulling on the forearm as the lever.

Origin and insertion of muscles

The origin of a muscle or proximal attachment is normally the end of the muscle that is attached to the more stationary of two bones (see Fig. 4.15). The distal attachment is where the muscle inserts into the bone undergoing the greatest movement. Some muscles have multiple origins.

Group actions

Most skeletal muscles work in opposing groups, such as abductors and adductors, flexors and

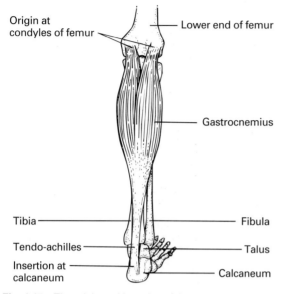

Origin at condyles of femur

Lower end of femur

Gastrocnemius

Tibia

Fibula

Tendo-achilles

Talus

Insertion at calcaneum

Calcaneum

Fig. 4.15 The origin and insertion of the gastrocnemius muscle.

extensors. Muscles, or groups of muscles, that work together to cause movement are known as synergists or agonists, and opposing muscles, or groups of muscles, are called antagonists. A muscle is termed a 'prime mover' if it is predominant in causing a movement. Occasionally prime movers and antagonists act together as fixators or stabilizers to provide a fixed position from which other prime movers can function. For example, the shoulder blade is often fixed in position by its muscles to enable movement of the shoulder joint. For muscle actions, see Table 4.1.

Table 4.1 Principal actions of muscles

Action	Movement
Flexion	decreases angle at a joint
Extension	increases angle at a joint
Abduction	away from the midline
Adduction	towards the midline
Levator	upward movement
Depressor	downward movement
Supinator	turns palm (or sole) upwards
Pronator	turns palm (or sole) downwards
Sphincter	decreases the size of an opening
Tensor	tightens the body part
Rotator	movement around the long axis

JOINTS

Joints are found where two or more bones meet. A joint arises between adjacent bones or areas of ossification. Areas of ossification would include the sutures of the skull where, after ossification, no movement is possible.

Classification of joints

The classification of joints is based upon the presence or absence of a synovial cavity and the type of connective tissue that binds the bones together. There are three main classes:

1. Synovial
2. Fibrous
3. Cartilaginous.

Examples of synovial joints may be found in Table 4.2. Fibrous joints have no joint cavity; they are united by fibrous tissue and have little movement (see Fig. 4.16). There are three types of fibrous joints (see Table 4.3). Cartilaginous joints have no joint cavity; the articulating bones are united by hyaline cartilage or fibrocartilage. There are two types (see Table 4.4).

THE NERVOUS SYSTEM

The function of the nervous system is to co-ordinate and control all parts of the body; it works in close cooperation with the endocrine system to harmonize many complex body functions. Structurally it can be divided into:

1. The central nervous system (CNS) comprising the brain and spinal cord
2. The peripheral nervous system comprising spinal and cranial nerves.

Functionally the nervous system can be divided into:

1. The somatic or voluntary nervous system which transmits impulses to and from non-visceral parts of the body, i.e. skeletal muscles, bones, joints, ligaments, skin, eyes and ears. Impulses carried in this way lead to activities which are conscious and willed.

Table 4.2 Types of synovial joint

Type of joint	Examples	Movements possible
Ball and socket	hip, shoulder	flexion extension abduction adduction rotation circumduction
Condylar (uniaxial)	knee, temporomandibular joint	flexion extension rotation
Ellipsoid (biaxial)	wrist, atlanto-occipital joint	flexion extension abduction adduction
Hinge (uniaxial)	elbow, ankle	flexion extension
Pivot (uniaxial)	median atlanto-axial joint, odontoid process	rotation
Plane	sacroiliac, costovertebral, cubonavicular, sternoclavicular joints	gliding

2. The autonomic or involuntary nervous system which transmits impulses concerned with activities of visceral organs, e.g. muscles in organs, blood vessels and glands.

Neurones

The functional unit of the nervous system is the neurone or nerve cell and its processes. It is composed of a nucleated cell body and cytoplasmic processes which include an axon and one or more dendrites (see Fig. 4.17). The axon conducts nerve impulses from the cell body out towards the dendrites of other neurones or to muscles and glands. Large axons, and especially those of peripheral nerves, are covered by a white lipid protein sheath called myelin which assists the speedy passage of nerve impulses. Dendrites receive stimuli and carry impulses from the axons of other neurones towards the nerve cell body.

Table 4.3 Types of fibrous joints

Example of joint	Structures involved	Movement
Sutures of skull		
coronal	frontal and parietal bones	fixed from
squamosal	parietal and temporal bones	age 2 years
Syndesmosis		
tibiofibular	tibia and fibula	variable
Gomphoses		
dentoalveolar	teeth and alveolar process of maxilla and mandible	minimal

Table 4.4 Types of cartilaginous joints

Example of joint	Structures involved	Movement
Synchondroses		
sternocostal	rib and sternum	minimal
epiphyseal	diaphysis and epiphysis of a long bone	none
Symphyses		
symphysis pubis	the two coxae	variable
intervertebral	bodies of vertebrae	variable

Fibrous joint

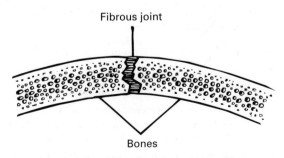

Bones

Fig. 4.16 A fibrous joint. (From Wilson 1990, with permission.)

The junction between the axon of one neurone and the dendrite of another is called a synapse. Chemical neurotransmitters released at the synapse allow the transmission of the impulse from neurone to neurone (see Fig. 4.18). Where a nerve fibre terminates in a muscle cell, at the neuromuscular junction, the transmission process is similar to that at the synapse.

Neurones can be classified according to their function:

1. In motor or efferent neurones, axons transmit impulses from the CNS to muscles or glands.
2. In sensory or afferent neurones, axons transmit impulses from the periphery of the body to the brain or spinal cord.

Nerve impulses

An impulse is the result of either a chemical, electrical or mechanical change to the neurone. This is called the stimulus. The stimulus alters the permeability of the cell membrane which allows the movement of sodium ions into the nerve cell and thus generates an electrical current. The speed of conduction of an impulse depends on the size of the nerve fibre and on whether it is covered by myelin. Myelinated fibres conduct impulses quicker than non-myelinated fibres.

Central nervous system

The central nervous system consists of the brain and spinal cord. The largest part of the brain is the cerebrum which is divided into two hemispheres – one hemisphere is dominant since it appears to take a 'lead' role resulting in the limbs on one side of the body becoming dominant. Each hemisphere has a surface layer of grey matter with white matter below. This is in contrast to the spinal cord where the white matter encloses a core of grey matter.

The brain

The cerebral cortex contains:

- Primary sensory areas – these are receptive areas for incoming impulses
- Primary motor areas – these send out impulses to stimulate action responses, i.e. muscle contraction and glandular secretion

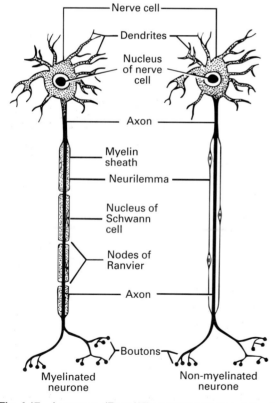

Fig. 4.17 A neurone. (From Wilson 1990, with permission.)

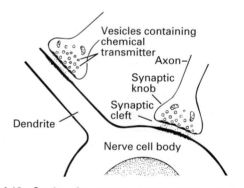

Fig. 4.18 Section of a synapse, greatly enlarged. (From Wilson 1990, with permission.)

- Association areas – these have a generalized function in the smooth working between sensory and motor centres.

The motor area initiates all voluntary movement of the body and is positioned in the frontal lobe anterior to the cerebral fissure. In general, the motor area of one hemisphere controls the movement on the opposite side of the body. The body muscles are represented on the motor strip in the area of the longitudinal fissure (see Fig. 4.19). The amount of brain surface related to a specific part of the body is proportional to the activity rather than the size of the part. Sensory impulses concerned with touch, pressure, pain, temperature and body position are transmitted to the parietal lobe which is posterior to the central fissure. Similar to the motor area, lower body sensations are received at the median portion of the sensory strip. Impulses from the head are received at the lowest part of the strip (see Fig. 4.20).

Other key cerebral functions include the visual areas in the occipital lobe; auditory areas in the temporal lobe; memory, personality, emotional reaction, initiative and responsibility in the frontal lobe.

Basal ganglia are areas of grey matter embedded within the white matter of each cerebral hemisphere, near the thalamus. Basal ganglia play a vital role in the control of voluntary motor activity. They have nerve connections with the motor cortical areas as well as the thalamus, which in turn has connections with the cerebellum. The ganglia give rise to extrapyramidal pathways to skeletal muscle. Basal ganglia appear to exert an inhibitory influence on muscle tone. Damage to them can cause motor disorders which lead to increased muscle activity.

Other parts of the brain include the midbrain, pons varolii, medulla oblongata and the cerebellum or hindbrain.

The brain requires a continuous flow of blood to provide the quantities of glucose and oxygen it needs to function. This need is the same whether the individual is mentally active or asleep. Brain cells are very sensitive to hypoxia; irreversible brain damage occurs if the blood

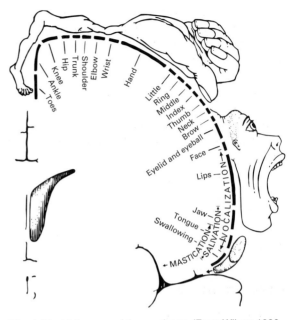

Fig. 4.19 Motor area of the cerebrum. (From Wilson 1990, with permission.)

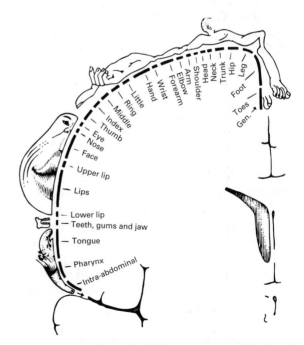

Fig. 4.20 Body representation in sensory area of cerebrum. (From Wilson 1990, with permission.)

supply is interrupted for 2–6 minutes. The brain and spinal cord are surrounded by the meninges which protect and assist in the passage of nutrients to the brain cells.

The spinal cord

The spinal cord is a cylindrical structure composed of grey and white matter enclosed within the vertebral canal. It extends from the medulla oblongata at the base of the skull to the level of the first or second lumbar vertebra. A central canal extends the full length of the cord. It contains cerebrospinal fluid and is continuous with the ventricles of the brain. The functions of the spinal cord are:

- To carry impulses via sensory nerve fibres through ascending tracts to the brain (see Fig. 4.21)
- To carry impulses from the brain via motor nerve fibres down the descending tracts to muscle or glands (see Fig. 4.22)
- To act as a centre for reflex actions.

The cell bodies (grey matter) are found in the interior of the spinal cord in an H shape. The nerve fibres (white matter) are peripheral to the cell bodies. Afferent impulses are received by neurones in the posterior horn of the grey matter. Efferent impulses are discharged by neurones in the anterior horn of the grey matter. Neurones within the grey matter transmit impulses from one half of the cord to the other, and to other levels of the CNS. Nerve impulses from the spinal cord leave via 31 pairs of posterior (sensory afferent fibres) and anterior roots (motor efferent fibres). At the intervertebral foramen the posterior and anterior roots meet to form a spinal nerve. The nerve fibres, on leaving the cord, form enlargements in the cervical and lumbar areas; these enlargements are called plexuses. The cervical plexus is associated with supplying the upper limb (see Fig. 4.23). The lumbar plexus is associated with supplying the lower limb.

Peripheral nervous system

The peripheral nervous system is composed of

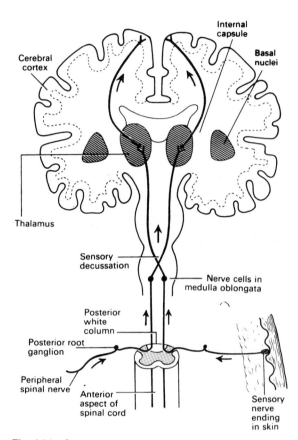

Fig. 4.21 Sensory nerve pathway from the skin to the cerebrum. (From Wilson 1990, with permission.)

nerves and ganglia. There are two main groups of peripheral nerves: cranial and spinal.

Cranial nerves

There are 12 pairs of cranial nerves which emerge from the inferior surface of the brain. Some of these nerves have mainly motor fibres, some have sensory fibres and some are mixed, having both sensory and motor fibres. Cell bodies of the motor fibres form nuclei within the brain stem. Sensory fibres originate from groups of cells outside the CNS and are called ganglia. Exceptions are the olfactory fibres which originate from the nasal mucosa and the optic fibres which originate from the retina of the eyeball.

The origins and functions of cranial nerves are given in Table 4.5.

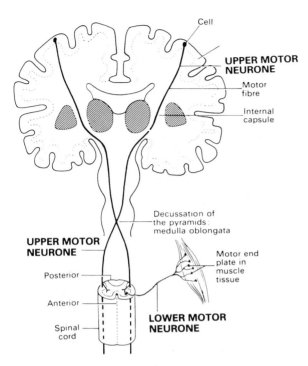

Fig. 4.22 Motor nerve pathways: upper and lower motor neurones. (From Wilson 1990, with permission.)

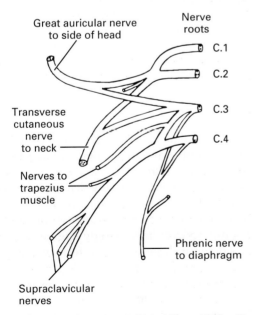

Fig. 4.23 The cervical plexus. (From Wilson 1990, with permission.)

Spinal nerves

There are 31 pairs of nerves which arise from the spinal cord: eight cervical pairs, 12 thoracic pairs, five lumbar pairs, five sacral pairs and one coccygeal pair.

All spinal nerves are mixed nerves and have two origins: the anterior and posterior roots. After leaving the vertebral canal each spinal nerve passes through the intervertebral foramen and divides into two branches called the anterior and posterior rami (see Fig. 4.24). The posterior ramus then divides into smaller branches which supply the muscles and skin of the back portion of the head, neck and trunk. The anterior ramus divides into networks to supply all the structures of the extremities and the front portion of the trunk.

Four main plexuses are formed by the division of the anterior rami:

1. Cervical plexus: this supplies muscles of the neck and shoulder and the phrenic nerve supplies the diaphragm.
2. Brachial plexus: the median, radial and ulnar nerves supply the arms.
3. Lumbar plexus: the femoral, saphenous and obturator nerves supply the lower abdominal wall, external genitalia and part of the thigh and leg.
4. Sacral plexus: this supplies the buttocks, perineum and lower extremities. The largest and longest nerve in the body, the sciatic nerve, arises from the sacral plexus.

The autonomic nervous system

The autonomic nervous system carries efferent fibres and causes involuntary responses to control visceral function within the body. It exerts an influence on arterial blood pressure, sweating and body temperatures, gastric and intestinal mobility and secretion and urinary bladder emptying. It is controlled by groups of nerve cells in the brain stem, hypothalamus and spinal cord. It subdivides into the parasympathetic system and the sympathetic system.

Parasympathetic nervous system

The parasympathetic system has preganglionic

Table 4.5 Origin and function of the cranial nerves (from Wilson 1990, with permission)

Name and number	Central connection	Peripheral connection	Function
I Olfactory (sensory)	smell area in temporal lobe of cerebrum through olfactory bulb	mucous membrane in roof of nose	sense of smell
II Optic (sensory)	sight area in occipital lobe of cerebrum cerebellum	retina of the eyes	sense of sight balance
III Oculomotor (motor)	nerve cells near floor of aqueduct of midbrain	superior, inferior and medial rectus muscles of the eye ciliary muscles of the eye circular muscle fibres of the iris	Moving the eyeball focusing regulating the size of the pupil
IV Trochlear (motor)	nerve cells near floor of aqueduct of midbrain	superior oblique muscles of the eyes	movement of the eyeball
V Trigeminal (mixed)	motor fibres from the pons varolii sensory fibres from the trigeminal ganglion	muscles of mastication sensory to gums, cheek, lower jaw, iris, cornea	chewing sensation from the face
VI Abducent (motor)	floor of fourth ventricle	lateral rectus muscle of the eye	movement of the eye
VII Facial (mixed)	pons varolii	sensory fibres to the tongue motor fibres to the muscles of the face	sense of taste movements of facial expression
VIII Vestibulocochlear (sensory) vestibular cochlear	cerebellum hearing area of cerebrum	semicircular canals in the inner ear organ of Corti in cochlea	maintenance of balance sense of hearing
IX Glossopharyngeal (mixed)	medulla oblongata	parotid glands back of tongue and pharynx	secretion of saliva sense of taste movement of pharynx
X Vagus (mixed)	medulla oblongata	pharynx, larynx; organs, glands, ducts, blood vessels in the thorax and abdomen	movement and secretion
XI Accessory (motor)	medulla oblongata	sternocleidomastoid, trapezius, laryngeal and pharyngeal muscles	movement of the head, shoulders, pharynx and larynx
XII Hypoglossal (motor)	medulla oblongata	tongue	movement of tongue

and postganglionic fibres (see Fig. 4.25). Postganglionic fibres are short and located within organs, for example the gastrointestinal tract. The effects of the parasympathetic system are associated with inactivity, restoring and conserving body energy and elimination of body waste.

Sympathetic nervous system

The sympathetic nervous system originates within the thoracic and lumbar regions of the spinal cord. Sympathetic nerves leave the spinal cord via the anterior roots and form the grey communicating rami of the thoracic and lumbar nerves. Immediately outside the spinal cord there are two interconnected chains of sympathetic ganglia (see Fig. 4.26).

Stimulation of the sympathetic system results in stimulation of the medulla of the adrenal glands which increases the secretion of adrenaline and noradrenaline, thereby augmenting the body's defence response. The effects of the sympathetic system are generalized physiological responses to stress, strong emotion, severe pain, cold or any threat to the body. The purpose of such a response is mobilization of body resources for defensive action.

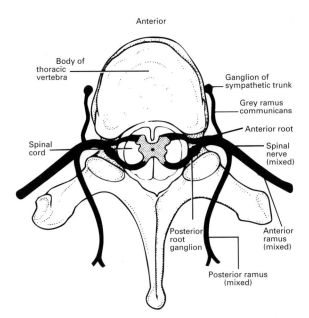

Fig. 4.24 Anterior and posterior rami. (From Wilson 1990, with permission.)

The neurotransmitter that is released by the preganglionic fibres of both sympathetic and parasympathetic systems is acetylcholine. At neuro-effector junctions the neurotransmitter differs in the two systems. In the parasympathetic system the postganglionic fibre releases acetylcholine and in the sympathetic system noradrenaline is released. The sympathetic and parasympathetic systems exert opposing influences upon their target organs.

Reflexes

Reflexes are defence mechanisms, i.e. they are rapid automatic responses to painful and/or potentially harmful situations; for example, the blink reflex to protect the eye from a foreign body. The reflex process functions via the reflex arc, an involuntary fixed motor response to a sensory stimulus (see Fig. 4.27).

The reflex arc consists of:

- A sensory or receptor neurone (afferent nerve) which is sensitive to specific stimuli and integrates centres within the CNS at any level below the cerebral cortex

- A motor neurone (efferent nerve) within the muscular or glandular tissue.

The reflex process

A receptor is stimulated by a change in the environment – for example, stretching a tendon, or a pressure or temperature change – and produces an impulse in the afferent nerve fibre. The impulse travels through the cell body of the sensory neurone and along its axon to the CNS. It may pass through a number of connecting neurones before it excites a motor efferent neurone whose axon transmits impulses out of the CNS to the efferent tissue or organ. Hence, a muscle may contract or a gland produce a secretion.

The knee jerk is an example of a stretch reflex; there are two neurones involved. The cell of the lower motor neurone (a motor nerve cell with its cell body outside the central nervous system) is stimulated by the sensory neurone which responds to tapping of the stretched tendon below the knee. No connector neurone is involved. The lower motor nerve stimulates the muscle of the thigh which contracts and thus kicks the foot forward. The knee jerk is a test used in orthopaedics to assess the integrity of the reflex arc.

AGEING

Ageing is a normal and continual process which occurs throughout life. Although it is generally accepted that there is some decline in function in the organs and tissues of the aged body, ageing is not inevitably accompanied by disease or biological malfunction. Some of the decline is due to progressive loss of body cells. This need not be significant in health terms, since most body systems have considerable spare capacity. For example, we possess two kidneys when the body can adequately function with only one healthy kidney.

In making a nursing assessment of an elderly person, it is essential that the orthopaedic nurse is meticulous in taking the patient's history and that she carries out an accurate physical examination. She must be able to differentiate between the ageing process and pathological change.

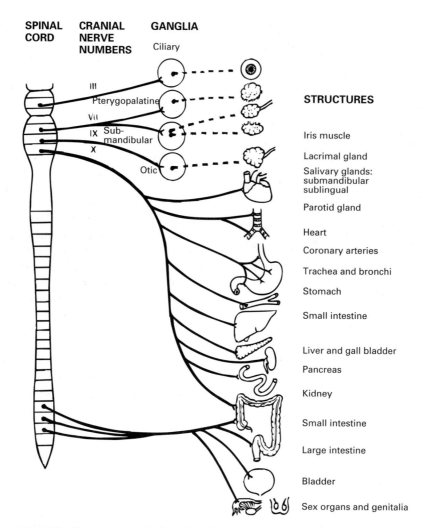

Fig. 4.25 The parasympathetic outflow. (From Wilson 1990, with permission.)

Ageing theories

Numerous theories have been put forward to explain ageing and the varied times of onset of the manifestations of ageing. Sociological, psychological and biological studies have been undertaken which provide different perspectives on the ageing process. Sociological studies on ageing cover changes in lifestyle, family roles and the individual's activities and interests; psychological studies examine the individual's capacity to adapt to environmental demands; and biological studies cover time-related physical changes over which the individual has little control.

Biological theories

From a biological perspective, the health of the individual depends on the efficient functioning of body cells and tissues in all body systems. In health, such functioning is ensured by a process called homeostasis. However, with age there is

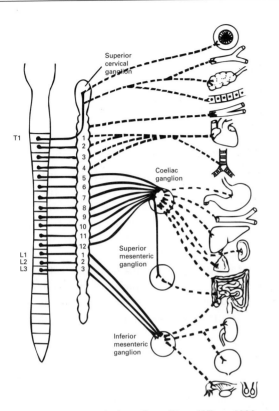

Fig. 4.26 The sympathetic outflow. (From Wilson 1990, with permission.)

a decline in the adaptive ability of the body to cope with change. This means that the elderly person may maintain homeostasis, but with increasing difficulty as the years pass. Systems which normally function effectively may be less efficient under stress conditions and the return to the normal state may be slower.

Irreversible changes occur progressively and do not affect all body systems equally, nor are such changes chronologically related. External appearance can be misleading, masking major internal changes which may be the result of environment stressors or lifestyle.

Cellular change theory Damage to the DNA and faults which occur during cellular divisions produce mutations. It has been postulated that ageing and death may be due to a build-up of such mutated cells so that the individual is no longer able to maintain life.

Scientific evidence has established that chromosomal errors increase with age, but no study has as yet identified them as being responsible for ageing. Some theorists have suggested that man has a biological 'clock' which is programmed so that the individual develops, ages and dies according to a personal timing device.

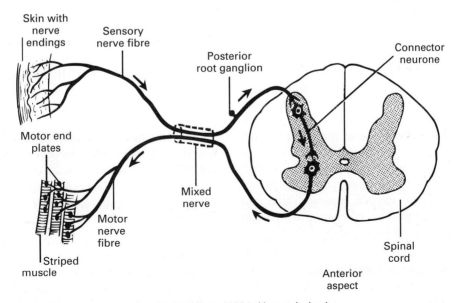

Fig. 4.27 A single reflex arc. (From Wilson 1990, with permission.)

Immune theory Theories associated with the immune system suggest that normal ageing is the result of a decrease in immunological efficiency, which then leads to general impairment of function throughout body tissues. Various studies of the activities of different body cells have been undertaken and evidence suggests that major change occurs in T-cells and in the responsiveness of natural antibodies. There is a decline in both humoral and cell-mediated immunity with age, and a loss of lymphoid tissue from bone marrow, the lymph nodes, the spleen and the thymus. Unfortunately, immune theories offer a perspective on ageing without fully explaining it.

Free radical theory This theory, postulated by Harmon in 1956, states that free radicals are central agents in producing changes at tissue, cellular and subcellular levels. Free radicals are produced normally during certain metabolic processes in the body. They are highly reactive and unstable due to the presence of unpaired electrons. With their production there is a large increase in free energy which leads to the damage of adjacent molecules. The accumulation of this damage leads to a decline in function which is seen in the ageing process.

Organisms have developed enzymes for scavenging free radicals and destroying the potentially harmful products before further damage can occur. When molecules are attacked, fluorescent pigments are produced; hence the development of so-called 'age pigments'.

The free radical theory suggests that ageing is potentially treatable, in that chemical antioxidants should be able to prevent oxidative damage. Vitamins C and E are examples of chemical antioxidants which are capable of interrupting free radical reactions. As yet there is no evidence to suggest that these vitamins have any such benefit.

It is not yet possible to identify any one theory that can adequately explain ageing. What can be described are the signs of change which can be observed in normal individuals as they age.

Ageing and the skeletal system

The normal ageing process need not limit movement. Mobility is, to some extent, affected by personal lifestyle and the degree of activity that the individual has maintained throughout his life, although some limitation of mobility may occur as a result of fear, e.g. the fear of falling. Ageing does, however, lead to changes in balance, cartilage and bone tissue.

Changes in balance

The maintenance of balance relies on integrating responses from the visual system, vestibular system in the inner ear and the proprioceptors in muscles and joints. Older people require greater angular movement in joints for proprioception to be achieved.

Gait disorders are not usually a feature of ageing but are more likely to be an indicator of underlying pathology such as a stroke, peripheral neuropathy or vitamin B_{12} deficiency.

Cartilaginous changes

The normal elastic properties of cartilage may be lost because of an increase in water loss and the deposition of fibres. The increased fibre density in connective tissue and cartilage produces a 'mesh' for the deposition of calcium. This accounts for the increased calcification of cartilage with ageing.

Hyaline cartilage loses fluid and is converted to fibrocartilage. Articular cartilage changes and elasticity is lost. Thinning occurs over weight-bearing areas, affecting function; for example, changes in the menisci of the knee joint inhibit free movement. Many joints of the body become stiffened with age.

Loss of water from cartilage in the intervertebral discs leads to compaction of the vertebrae and shrinkage of the spinal column, which is seen as a loss in height. Height loss is also affected by joint changes and by the flattening of the arch of the foot.

Bone changes

Osteoporosis is an imbalance between bone reabsorption and formation and is a normal ageing process. If severe it may cause fractures, and can also lead to bowing of the long bones and to an increase in spinal curvature due to vertebral collapse.

Ageing and muscle

Most loss of lean body mass occurs in the muscle. Muscle cells display evidence of ageing with an increase in lipid content. Muscle fibres are reduced in number and size, and such changes result in a degree of limitation in the range of movement, which is produced by contraction. The size of individual muscles and the degree of loss of muscle strength vary among the muscle groups. The stiffening of joints and the cartilaginous changes mean that more muscular work is required in many body functions, for example breathing. Periods of immobility, for example bedrest, can lead to disuse atrophy and muscle wasting in the elderly.

Ageing and the nervous system

Brain weight and volume have been shown to decline with age, although this may not be significant. A reduction occurs in cortical areas where the sulci broaden out and the gyri flatten.

Cells are also lost from the cerebral cortex and the cerebellum, although this usually starts later in the cerebellum than in the cerebrum. Major cerebellar change affects the axons, with loss of myelin.

Cerebral blood flow decreases with age, but oxygen extraction from the blood is increased as more oxygen is released from the haemoglobin. The vertebral arteries tend to become tortuous because of changes in the vertebral and intervertebral discs, and they may become kinked with neck movement. This leads to transient ischaemic attacks.

In the peripheral nerves, the number of large fibres reduces, especially in the dorsal roots of the lumbosacral region. As a result, the velocity of conduction of nerve impulses is reduced. Some reflexes, for example the Achilles tendon reflexes, are depressed and reaction time is longer. Part of this deterioration is due to nerve changes and part to a reduction of muscle power and stiffer joints.

Autonomic nervous system dysfunctions are also evident with age, for example, postural hypotension, impaired thermoregulation and gastrointestinal function, urinary incontinence and impaired penile erection.

REFERENCES

Gunn C 1992 Bones and joints, 2nd edn. Churchill Livingstone, Edinburgh
Harman D 1956 Ageing: a theory based on the free radical and radiation chemistry. Journal of Gerentology 11: 298–300
MacKenna B R, Callander R 1990 Illustrated physiology, 5th edn. Churchill Livingstone, Edinburgh, p 270, 284
Powell M 1986 Orthopaedic nursing and rehabilitation. Churchill Livingstone, Edinburgh
Wilson K 1990 Ross & Wilson Anatomy and physiology in health and illness, 7th edn. Churchill Livingstone, London, p 22–23, 241–269, 353–382

FURTHER READING

Atkinson R L, Atkinson R C, Smith E E, Hilgard E R 1987 Introduction to psychology, 9th edn. Harcourt, Brace & Jovanovich, New York
Ebersole P, Hess P 1990 Toward healthy ageing. Human needs and nursing response. C V Mosby, St Louis, MO
Hinchliffe S, Montague S 1988 Physiology for nursing practice. Bailliere Tindall, London
Hubbard J L, Mechan D J 1987 Physiology for health care students. Churchill Livingstone, Edinburgh
Redfern S J 1991 Nursing elderly people. Churchill Livingstone, Edinburgh
Seeley R R, Stephens T D, Tate P 1989 Anatomy and physiology. Times Mirror/Mosby College, Boston
Tortora G J, Anagnostakos N P 1990 Principles of anatomy and physiology, 6th edn. Harper & Row, London
Royle J A, Walsh M 1992 Watson's medical–surgical nursing and related physiology, 4th edn. Bailliere Tindall, London

5

Why move?

Peter S. Davis

This chapter explores the concepts of mobility and nursing diagnosis. These concepts are then applied to specific patient problems related to mobilizing: pressure sore and deep vein thrombosis risk, problems related to the locomotor system, elimination, eating and drinking, personal cleansing, breathing, sleep and rest, problems related to nutrition, and self-image.

People tend to take being able to move for granted. It is not until they temporarily or permanently suffer restrictions to their mobility that they realize what the effects of changes, such as impaired physical mobility, mean to them as individuals. Orthopaedic nurses use the terms mobility, reduced mobility and immobility quite specifically; reduced mobility and immobility are perceived predominantly as physical in origin, but it must be emphasized that they are physical, psychological and social in their effects. The individual with hands and wrists affected by rheumatoid arthritis suffers impaired physical mobility and is often unable to use his hands for long periods without having to stop due to pain (activity intolerance). The physical effects of decreased range of movement, loss of muscle strength and pain are exacerbated by the social effects, such as the inability to take part in leisure activities, and the psychological effects, such as altered self-concept due to disfigurement and depression.

Mental health nurses use the terms reduced mobility and immobility more widely. For example, psychological or psychiatric causes of impaired physical mobility may be severe depression, anxiety or some of the catatonic states. Further, some of the reasons for restricting the mobility of these individuals may be social in origin, as the results of the illness may produce antisocial behaviour requiring the individual to be nursed in a secure unit. Orthopaedic wards often have patients with mental health problems as well as problems of an orthopaedic origin. The experience of nursing patients with combined mental health and mobility problems ensures that the nurse's skills and knowledge are tested to their limits. Why is it, for instance, that demented, confused patients frequently get up immediately after hip arthroplasty without any of the encouragement that is necessary for the patient with no mental health problem? It also appears that they suffer little pain, but this is difficult to assess.

It will, by now, be apparent from earlier chapters that models of nursing are crucial in providing direction in orthopaedic nursing. Riehl and Roy (1980) and Aggleton and Chalmers (1989) identify the key parts of a model of nursing; it is necessary to be aware of these in order to fully understand this chapter. Nursing models, however, are not the only frameworks being used by nurses to develop their delivery of care. Informed implementation of research findings and the development of particular nursing skills and roles, such as the clinical nurse specialist, will also affect the quality of nursing care. Underpinning all these developments is the way in which nurses perceive, develop, respond to and implement changes in health care. The most needed and sensible changes supported by committed individuals often fail due to a lack of understanding of the importance of change by everyone involved.

MOBILITY

A review of the US literature between 1963 and 1983 on mobility and impaired mobility by Creason and colleagues (1985) uncovered only 20 articles on the subject. The situation is similar in the UK: a glance at the literature relating to mobility demonstrates that only scant reference is made to mobility and mobilizing, the bulk being devoted to the more negative subjects of immobility and impaired physical mobility. It is significant that mobility is a term used by nurses, for example when they refer to 'mobility problems'; in fact, they mean impaired physical mobility or activity intolerance. Further confusion occurs when mobility is used in a very restricted sense to mean walking, i.e. ambulation: 'mobilizing well' occurs frequently in nursing and medical patient documentation when what is meant is that the individual is getting up and walking well. Accuracy in the terms that are commonly used is necessary; Figure 5.1 contains suggested meanings for common terminology used in this text.

In England and Wales, approximately 10% of the population are physically disabled; this excludes sensory and mental disorders (Royal College of Physicians 1986). Of these people,

Mobility:	This is when an object is 'free to move, able to move or flow easily' (Concise Oxford Dictionary)
Impairment:	A permanent or transitory psychological, physiological or anatomical loss or abnormality of structure or function (WHO 1980)
Disability:	Any restriction or prevention of the performance of an activity, resulting from an impairment, in the manner or within the range considered normal for a human being (WHO 1980)
Handicap:	. . . . a dynamic relationship between the individual and his environment. The degree to which a disability is handicapping depends on the situations experienced by the individual, the attitudes and the expectations of others and the intervention strategies and environmental modifications which are made (OECD 1986)
Rehabilitation:	The restoration of patients to their fullest physical, mental and social capability (Scottish Health Services Council 1972)

Fig. 5.1 Common terms.

20–30% (that is, 2–3% of the total population) will be severely or very severely disabled. A health district with a population of 250 000 is therefore likely to contain about 25 000 disabled people. About 10% of all disabled persons are aged under 45 years, 30% are between 46 and 64 years and 60% are 65 years or older. More women are disabled than men, but only because of their greater life expectancy.

NURSING DIAGNOSIS

Broadly speaking, physical disability and impaired physical mobility are the same in their effects. However, categories of physical disability have been derived from medical diagnoses and are perceived as disabling conditions – e.g. osteoarthritis, stroke, paraplegia, major congenital malformations (Royal College of Physicians 1986). While a medical diagnosis is useful when caring for people with mobility problems, it is not always essential to nursing care. The nursing process should be directed by a model of nursing (see Table 5.1). A medical diagnosis indicates what disease an individual has in order to plan medical care, while a model of nursing, used to formulate a nursing diagnosis, provides a comprehensive picture of the individual's problems in order to plan nursing care. Miller (1989) makes clear that when a high degree of nursing judgement is required to carry out medical orders, the actions taken fall within the scope of nursing practice, being described as inter-dependent nursing interventions. These are a common occurrence in nursing practice, and

the nurse's identification of patient problems through a nursing diagnosis is crucial for their effective implementation.

Using nursing diagnosis as a stage of the nursing process enables nursing practice to be problem-solving and, more importantly, to be problem-finding (Kirk 1986) (see Fig. 5.2).

A helpful way of showing the differences between nursing diagnosis and medical diagnosis is to make a direct comparison between the two (see Table 5.2). The nursing diagnoses or patient problem categories listed are those derived from the human response patterns to health/illness of 'moving' only. There are nine human response patterns (see Fig. 5.3). If, for example, the response pattern of 'feeling' is also considered, then further nursing diagnosis/patient problems may be identified in relation to mobility, e.g. pain, chronic pain, anxiety.

Woolley (1990) suggests that in order to provide an accurate nursing diagnosis the nurse requires an understanding of three domains: first,

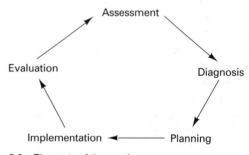

Fig. 5.2   Elements of the nursing process.

Table 5.1   Directors of nursing care

Possible	Preferable
Medical assessment	Nursing assessment
Medical diagnosis	Nursing diagnosis
Planned therapy	Planned care
Implementation, e.g. surgery or prescribing medication	Implementation, e.g. pressure sore prevention, promoting compliance with drug therapy
Evaluation based on progression of disease	Evaluation based on progression of a person as a whole (holism)

Table 5.2   Comparison of nursing and medical diagnoses (from North American Nursing Diagnosis Categories 1988)

Medical diagnosis	Nursing diagnosis
Rheumatoid arthritis	Impaired physical mobility
	Activity intolerance
	Fatigue
	Sleep pattern disturbance
	Diversional activity deficit
	Altered health maintenance
	Feeding self-care deficit
	Bathing/hygiene self-care deficit
	Dressing/grooming self-care deficit
	Toileting self-care deficit
	Impaired home maintenance management

Exchanging	Giving and receiving mutually
Communicating	Sending messages
Relating	Establishing bonds
Valuing	Assigning relative worth
Choosing	Selecting alternatives
Moving	Changing position actively
Perceiving	Receiving of information
Knowing	Understanding the meaning of information
Feeling	Being subjectively aware of information

Fig. 5.3 Nine human response patterns.

the central concepts of the nursing discipline, as reflected in a model of nursing; second, the processes of problem-solving or the nursing process; and third, the foundation of theoretical knowledge on which to base practice. The first two domains have been discussed in this and previous chapters of the text; therefore, a consideration of the theoretical knowledge on which practice is founded will now be considered within a nursing diagnosis framework.

There can be little doubt that moving, mobility, mobilizing, activity, or whatever terms are used, are important to orthopaedic nursing. Kim and co-workers (1984) in their study showed that in the list of the 10 most frequently identified nursing diagnoses, two were decreased activity tolerance (ranked fourth) and impaired physical mobility (ranked tenth). Consideration of the causes or aetiologies of a nursing diagnosis such as impaired physical mobility demonstrates the importance of applying nursing diagnosis to orthopaedic nursing (see Table 5.3). Using the same terminology and, more importantly, agreeing on the definitions of these nursing diagnoses will ensure that as a profession we can communicate more accurately and succinctly between ourselves and our patients.

Mobility as a concept may be considered a blend of activity and rest. Carrying out, or the potential to carry out, both of these elements of mobility is essential to a person's health. The

Table 5.3 Aetiology or causes of impaired physical mobility (For a fuller description of these terms see Creason et al 1985)

Intolerance to activity, decreased strength and endurance
Pain, discomfort
Perceptual/cognitive impairment
Musculoskeletal impairment
Neuromuscular impairment
Psychological impairment
Lack of knowledge

importance of exercise, rest, relaxation and sleep in appropriate quantity and quality should be understood by all nurses as health promoters. The maintenance or promotion of health is a vast topic and cannot be covered in this text but must be considered as a fundamental component of the orthopaedic nurse's role. (For an introduction to health promotion as related to exercise, rest, relaxation and sleep see: Open University 1984 (all areas), Seedhouse 1986 and Gott & O'Brien 1990 (health promotion), and Oswald & Adam 1983 (sleep).)

SELF-EMPOWERMENT

By promoting health and providing quality nursing care, the orthopaedic nurse should aim to empower the patient, but this may be difficult to achieve in environments as varied as the hospital and community or in individuals who are temporarily physically impaired or permanently physically disabled. To be able to empower others, one must be capable of self-empowerment. Using self-empowerment will benefit the person with mobility problems, the nurse as a professional, the nursing profession and society in general, as many of the problems people encounter are due to actual or perceived powerlessness.

Self-empowerment is a process whereby the individual increasingly controls himself and his life, and thus becomes more independent (Fenton 1989); that is, he is able to choose to live within his inherent capacities and means and to follow his own personal values and preferences. To facilitate self-empowerment, nurses need to develop appropriate beliefs and attitudes (see Fig. 5.4). Table 5.4 lists characteristics of the more or less self-empowered individual and

- Each individual is unique, valuable and worthy of respect

- Education, therapy and self-empowerment are value-based

- The more self-empowered a person becomes, the more he will be able to help others to be the same

- Once individuals have learned to respect, love and value themselves, they will be able to respect, love and value others

- It is helpful to differentiate the behaviours which encourage the developing parts of a person from those which serve to anchor them in states of depression, hostility, fear and/or insecurity

- Taking risks and learning from mistakes is effective and valuable

- Everyone has something to teach and something to learn

Fig. 5.4   Beliefs which lead to self-empowerment. (Adapted from Fenton 1989.)

Table 5.4   Comparisons of more or less self-empowered individuals

More self-empowered	Less self-empowered
Proactive	Reactive
Open to change	Closed to change
Considers others in situations of change	Considers only self in situations of change
Assertive	Non-assertive or aggressive
Self-accountable	Blames others
Self-directed	Led by others
Uses feelings	Overwhelmed by or fails to recognize feelings
Learns from mistakes	Debilitated by mistakes
Confronts	Avoids
Realistic	Unrealistic
Seeks alternatives	Tunnel vision
Likes self	Dislikes self
Values others	Negates others
Considers others' needs	Selfish
Interested in the world	Self-centred
Enhances other people's lives	Restricts the lives of others
Can say no	Difficulty in saying no

provides goals and directions for those seeking to promote self-empowerment.

NURSING MODELS

When identifying how three common models of nursing deal with mobility, it becomes evident that the physical and physiological elements of mobility dominate over the sociological and psychological elements:

1. Orem's self care model: universal care requisite of the maintenance of a balance between activity and rest
2. Roper's activities of living model: the activity of mobilizing
3. Roy's adaptation model: the person's need for exercise and rest within the physiological mode.

Orem's model concentrates on the nurse–patient relationship and Roy's on the individual and his response to himself and his environment. Their frameworks, however, consider mobility in such a way that it is difficult to relate mobility meaningfully to other aspects of the model.

Roper, Logan and Tierney's activities of living model allows for the relationships between the other elements of the model and mobilizing to be taken into account; for example, mobilizing may be considered with respect to:

- The factors influencing it – i.e. physical, psychological, sociocultural, environmental and politico-economic
- The life span: conception to death
- Dependence–independence
- The other activities of living
- A systematic approach to individualizing nursing.

Unfortunately, Roper's model tells us little about how the nurse should perceive the individual (see Fig. 5.5). However, by blending an activities of living model with an ethos of self-empowerment, it is possible to glean the essence of the goal of self-care from Orem's model and the essence of promoting the best possible adaptation choices by individuals in Roy's model. The further addition of problem identification/ nursing diagnosis to Roper's systematic approach to individualizing nursing, which has an inherent problem-solving approach, would also be of benefit (see Fig. 5.6).

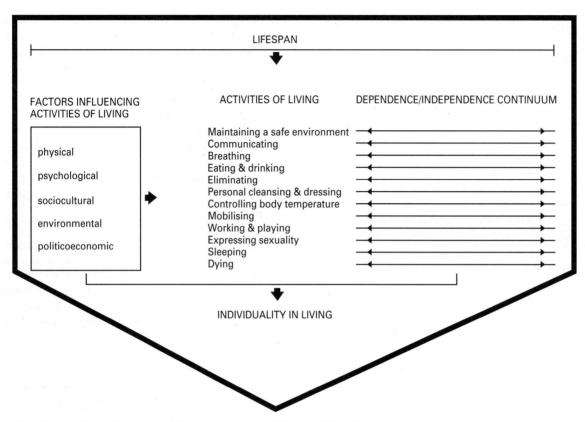

Fig. 5.5 Activities of living model. (From Roper, Logan & Tierney 1990, with permission.)

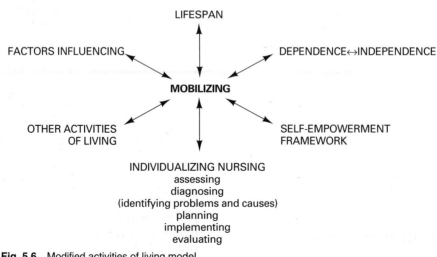

Fig. 5.6 Modified activities of living model.

PATIENT PROBLEMS RELATED TO MOBILIZING

The modified activities of living model of nursing may be used to provide an overview of the theoretical knowledge and practical skills that are fundamental and essential to caring for patients with problems concerned with mobilizing. Other chapters relate this knowledge and nursing skills to more specific patient problems. The remainder of this chapter now addresses some of the more fundamental and essential nursing care related to patient problems.

Pressure sores

The problem of impaired skin integrity is the potential or actual disruption or destruction of skin layers, usually due to reduced or absent mobility. The end result is a pressure sore, which is a localized area of dead tissue resulting from disruption and/or occlusion of the blood supply by pressure or other mechanical forces.

Pressure sores are an ancient, extensive, significant and perennial problem. Barton and Barton (1981) refer to a prevalence figure of 30 000 hospital patients with pressure sores at any one time in the UK, and a similar prevalence is thought to exist in the community (Hibbert 1980). Versluysen (1986) found, in her one hospital study, that 32% of patients in the three orthopaedic wards developed pressure sores, although this figure has been questioned.

Pressure sores are due to the interaction of many factors. These factors may be divided into those characteristics that are specific to the individual patient, and those which are derived from the patient's environment.

Patient characteristics

Crow (1988) proposes that two of the most important patient characteristics that predispose a patient to pressure sores are age and reduced physical activity. Other characteristics appear to be derived from these two; for example, vascular factors, such as arteriosclerosis, are predominantly age-related.

Methods of calculating pressure sore risk are based on identifying the specific factors of the individual patient which predispose him to pressure sore development. Examples of these factors are given in Table 5.5. Medical diagnoses are absent from this table, as they do not specifically identify the nature of the patient problem. They are useful, however, as indicators of what the problems are likely to be; for example, the medical diagnosis of diabetes indicates that altered nutrition, peripheral tissue perfusion and sensibility together with pain may be potential or actual patient problems.

External loads

The most important external factor predisposing to pressure sores is external loads. These loads have been shown to close the microcirculation and lymphatic system. Crow (1988) suggests that

Table 5.5 Factors predisposing to pressure sore development; ROM = range of movement

Related to:	Problem/nursing diagnosis
Individual patient-specific factors	
Mobilizing	activity intolerance, pain, sensory alterations, decreased muscle strength, fatigue, lack of motivation, fear, limited ROM, imposed restriction of movement (e.g. splints, traction, prescribed bedrest etc.), powerlessness, knowledge deficit
Eating and drinking	feeding self-care deficit, altered nutrition (more or less than body requirements), fluid volume deficit
Eliminating	altered patterns of urinary or faecal elimination; particularly incontinence
Sleeping	Fatigue and sleep pattern disturbance e.g. leading to reduced movement caused by taking anxiolytics and narcotics
Cleansing and dressing	bathing and hygiene self-care deficit
Breathing	altered tissue perfusion (peripheral), e.g. due to smoking
Controlling body temperature	hypothermia, hyperthermia
Environmental factors	
Compressive pressure	
Shearing pressure	

pressures of 60 mmHg can be withstood by patients, whereas Judd (1989) states that pressures greater than 32 mmHg on the skin for 1.5–2 hours in immobile patients can lead to damage. However, capillary pressure varies with posture as well as with blood pressure fluctuations, so that it is misleading to give a set figure for soft tissue ischaemic pressure; this probably accounts for the contradiction in the above figures.

There are thought to be three principal forms of mechanical force acting on body tissues: compression, shear and tension. Compression is the force exerted perpendicularly over a given area, divided by that area; the greater the pressure on the skin, the more the tissues are distorted. The duration of the pressure is as important as its intensity, and short periods of very high pressure – for example, sitting on a hard bed pan – can be as damaging as prolonged periods at lower pressures. The areas of the body where the skeletal bony prominences are subjected to concentrated loading are those most likely to be the sites of pressure sores (see Fig. 5.7).

Shear is the force exerted parallel or at an angle to the skin surface, causing the skin layers and tissues to move laterally and producing severe distortion. This occurs particularly where there is friction between the skin and, for example, the bed sheets. The frictional forces hold the upper layers of the skin stationary whilst the skeleton and the subcutis move. These forces stretch and squeeze the microvessels, leading to capillary and venule disruption as well as to tis-

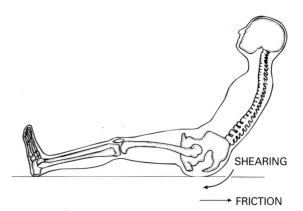

Fig. 5.8 Semirecumbent position and subjection to shearing forces.

sue ischaemia. The lymphatics are also damaged, thus accelerating tissue necrosis (see Fig. 5.8).

Skin tension has a similar effect to shear. It is seen when very tacky adhesive tape is used causing blisters due to tension on the skin.

The incidence of pressure sores for each at-risk body location is given in Table 5.6, based on the work of Locket (1983). It is interesting to note that 93% of pressure sores occur in the pelvic region or below and that Locket does not include the head. The omission of the head is an important error, as the occipital area in particular is prone to pressure sore development.

Grading of pressure sores

A number of different grading systems can be used to assess pressure sores according to their location, size and severity. The purpose of these classifications is to evaluate accurately and to document the progress of the sore. Lowthian (1987) probably provides the clearest, most usable classification (see Fig. 5.9).

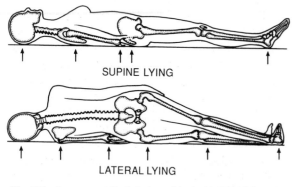

Fig. 5.7 Areas most likely to be subjected to harmful pressure.

Table 5.6 Incidence of pressure sores

Location	Incidence (%)
Sacrum	31
Buttocks	27
Heels	20
Trochanters	10
Lower limbs	5
Trunk	4
Upper limbs	3

Grade 0 = Potential sores	Inflammation with local heat, erythema, oedema and possible induration – more than 15 mm in diameter
Grade 1 = Incipient sores	Blood under the skin or in a blister, or black (necrotic) discoloration under the skin – more than 5 mm diameter; or clear blister/bulla more than 15 mm diameter
Grade 2 = Superficial sores (open)	A break in the skin (epidermis) which may include some damage to the dermis but without black discoloration – more than 5 mm diameter
Grade 3 = Medium sores (open)	Destruction of the skin (epidermis and dermis) without an obvious cavity, but possibly with black discoloration (possibly a slough) – more than 5 mm diameter
Grade 4 = Deep sores (open)	Penetration of the skin (epidermis and dermis) with a clearly visible cavity (with or without necrotic tissue) – more than 5 mm diameter at the surface
Grade 5 = Sinus/bursal sores	Necrotic, possibly infected possibly suppurating sore – more than 40 mm diameter overall, but with either no skin opening or less than 15 mm diameter

Fig. 5.9 Lowthian's (1985) classification of pressure sores.

Pressure sore risk assessment

A literature search reveals that as many as 15 risk scales have been developed between 1962 and 1987. Of these, only two have been developed specifically for the orthopaedic patient, the pressure sore prediction score (PSPS) (Lowthian 1976) being the most popular, and only Norton's and Lowthian's scales have been fully researched and validated by prospective studies. (For details of the Lowthian PSPS see Figs 5.10 and 5.11.) Barratt (1987) has investigated the claims of the developers of several risk calculators, and questions their accuracy.

Interestingly, the PSPS and the pressure sore grading system of Lowthian can be used at hospital and unit level to provide an overall picture of patient risk and progress. These data can be further analysed to assess nursing workload levels in order to determine unit staffing needs and skill mix for spans of duty. Further, the data can be used to predict the number and types of supports, such as special beds, that the patients require (see Lowthian 1989).

The frequency with which pressure sore risk assessments are made depends on the patient's general condition and whether there are any sudden changes involving himself and his environment, such as a general anaesthetic and surgery. These assessments can be made using risk calculators in any environment, i.e. hospital, community and long-stay units, and whenever possible patients should be taught to identify their own risks and take appropriate action.

Methods of relieving pressure

Boore and colleagues (1987) identify two mechanisms for relieving pressure:

1. That which aids natural behaviour
2. That which uses devices which redistribute pressure.

Devices which mechanically alter the patient's position should be added to Boore's categories.

Aiding natural behaviour The nurse may aid natural behaviour by moving the patient or by teaching and assisting the patient to move. It is essential that the nurse assesses the patient's ability to move himself and enables him to do this whenever possible, rather than automatically moving or transferring him and putting both herself and the patient at risk of injury.

The effect of movement is to relieve pressure from one area and to transfer it to another, and this must be continued day and night. Lowthian (1979) has developed a 24-hour turning clock

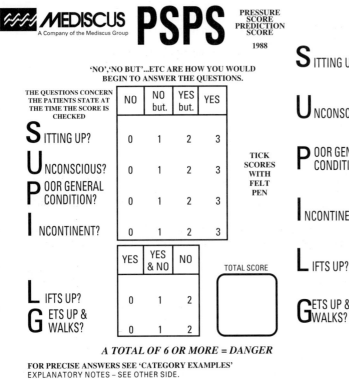

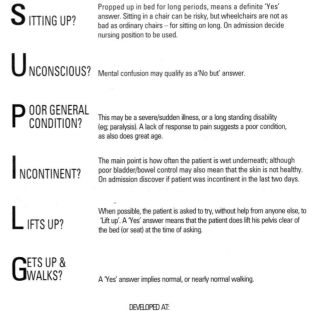

Fig. 5.10 The pressure sore prediction score.

for bed-bound and chair-fast patients. The previous position of the patient must be recorded to ensure that each area of the body is subjected to the minimum period of pressure possible. The use of these schedules is strongly recommended for high-risk patients, as although they may be difficult to maintain, Barton and Barton (1981) have shown that once a pressure sore has developed, effective treatment requires a 50% increase in nursing time.

Nursing interventions to promote patient self-help may be as straightforward as providing an overhead trapeze device or encouraging wheelchair patients to adjust their position frequently by doing push-ups.

Devices to redistribute pressure or mechanically alter a position These devices fall into three categories (Torrance 1981):

1. The surface area utilized to support the body is increased or the area being compressed is varied.

2. Aid is provided when the patient is turned.
3. Specific areas are supported.

Increasingly, researchers and authors are producing comparative lists of these devices to help the nurse and patient make an appropriate choice (Torrance 1981, David 1986, Boore 1987, Pritchard & David 1988). These are a very useful resource but are often incomplete and biased by personal preference or manufacturers' involvement. An example of these lists is given in Table 5.7.

Devices that increase the surface area utilized to support the body may be in the form of foam mattresses such as the combination foam mattress (Vaperm), which has different densities of foam, or mattresses made from slashed foam or rigid egg-box type foam. Scales and co-workers (1982) have shown that these Vaperm mattresses reduce the pressure around a load by 50% compared to the standard DHSS mattress.

Mattresses and cushions filled with various

Sitting up?
Yes: propped up in bed most of the day; sits up both day and night
Yes but: for short periods only, although spends long periods in fixed chair; lies down for long periods
No but: occasionally sits in a chair; sits in a self-propelled chair (long periods) but flat when in bed
No: bedfast and nursed flat; only sits up when in a chair – short periods

Unconscious?
Yes: deeply unconscious; does not respond to pain
Yes but: rousable – responds to commands or pain
No but: confused; withdrawn; excessive sleeping; semiconscious at times
No: fully conscious and orientated; fully conscious and slightly confused

Poor general condition?
Yes: seriously or critically ill; terminal (acute) illness; recent paraplegic; recent hemiplegic; quadraplegic; emaciated and cachectic; severe general infection; severe multiple sclerosis; iliac thrombosis; severe uraemia; severe injuries including legs or pelvis; on narcotics; Hansen's disease; extensive loss of pain or sensibility; limited mobility plus great age
Yes but: general condition could be worse; fair condition but some injuries to lower half of body; severe injuries but free movement of lower half of body; young paraplegic; active hemiplegic; well-established disease or disability
No but: elderly and thin or obese; restricted movement of lower extremities; recent operation under general anaesthetic; on steroids; on chemotherapy; pyrexial; anorexic; arthritic; diabetic; some neuropathy; some arterial disease
No: fairly good general condition – awaiting minor operation; fairly fit – awaiting discharge; minor local or mental disease; disease confined to upper extremities

Incontinent?
Yes: continual dribble or leak; frequent urine or faecal incontinence or both
Yes but: small amounts at infrequent intervals; urine only and infrequent; faecal (infrequent) but some leaks from catheter or urinal
No but: sometimes wets bed or spills urinal; occasional 'accidents' with attached urinal; occasional leaks from indwelling catheter; occasional faecal accidents
No: no incontinence or 'accidents' recently; indwelling catheter or stoma, but no leaks or 'accidents'

Lifts up?
No: unable to lift pelvis; can neither help with lift nor shuffle
Yes and no: can only lift pelvis with some effort, and soon tires; seldom lifts self; can lift with help; lifts slightly – shuffles into new position
Yes: lifts all of body clear of support; easily lifts pelvis clear

Gets up and walks?
No: bedfast or chairfast; stands and shuffles – with help and encouragement
Yes and no: has difficulty walking with aid; walks with help and encouragement; soon tires; can only walk to toilet
Yes: fully ambulant; slight impediment; uses walking aids with no difficulty

Fig. 5.11 Pressure sore prediction score category examples. (Reproduced with the permission of Peter Lowthian, Royal National Orthopaedic Hospital NHS Trust, Stanmore.)

other materials may also be used – i.e. air, polystyrene beads, fibres, gels and water. For example, low air-loss beds support the patient on sacks of a flexible vapour-permeable material with air pumped into the sacks. Fluidized air beds, such as Clinitron, also require pumped air to function.

Devices that vary the area being compressed include alternating-pressure beds such as the ripple mattress and air wave system. Large air-cell double layer mattresses have been shown to be more effective than small-cell ones (Crawl 1988).

Various pads and devices have been devel-

Table 5.7 Examples of devices to redistribute pressure (adapted from Boore et al 1987)

Mode of action	Equipment
Beds, mattresses and cushions	
Can equalize pressure over most of the support surface	water flotation bed low air loss bed fluidized air bed (Clinitron) individually shaped foam or matrix support
Can spread the load over a large area	low pressure air bed net suspension bed water mattress, bed and cushion slit foam mattress Roho mattress and cushion polystyrene beads silicone gel cushion
Alter the area subject to pressure	alternating pressure beds: ripple, pulsair, airwave
Other	
Prevent contamination with urine	special incontinence sheets
Absorb moisture	bead pads sheepskin, absorbs water vapour only
Protect bony prominences	heel and elbow pads: sheepskin, synthetic sheepskin and foam foam pads gel pads

oped from materials such as sheep skin and foam to protect specific areas of the body like the heels and elbows.

Beds to aid turning can be motorized or manual, and can turn the patient through the vertical or horizontal axis. Examples are the circoelectric bed, the wedge turning frame, and turning and tilting beds.

Unfortunately, knowing about methods and devices to systematically prevent pressure sore development does not guarantee their use. Ritualized care such as massaging with soap, causing damage to the skin (Torrance 1981) and ill-informed use of harmful devices such as ring cushions to sit on (Crew 1987), should cease.

Treating and dressing pressure sores

Under appropriate conditions pressure sores will heal, but all the preventative measures described in the previous section must be considered and implemented as necessary throughout the healing process to prevent a recurrence or the development of further sores.

An understanding of wound healing, as described in Chapter 8, is necessary. Before wound healing can occur, any necrotic tissue should be removed to produce a healthy granulation bed. This wound debridement can be achieved surgically, enzymatically or chemically. Pritchard and David (1988) and Torrance (1981) summarize a selection of dressings used in the treatment of pressure sores, giving their use, advantages and disadvantages. Other therapeutic measures include ultrasound, infrared, ultraviolet and laser treatment.

For a successful outcome, it is essential that the prevention and treatment of pressure sores are carried out within a holistic framework. The skin and underlying tissues are unlikely to remain healthy or to heal readily if the patient's nutritional status is poor or if he is suffering from sleep disturbance. (Sleep is important in the restorative and repair processes of the body (Oswald & Adam 1983).)

Deep vein thrombosis

Impaired physical mobility may give rise to circulatory stasis in the patient. If he has also experienced injury or trauma to the circulatory system and an alteration in blood chemistry, he is in danger of developing deep vein thrombosis (DVT). If the thrombus or part of it becomes dislodged and begins to float in the venous system, potentially fatal pulmonary embolism may occur when the clot blocks one of the pulmonary vessels. In 10–15% of hospital deaths, autopsies confirm pulmonary embolism as the major cause, making it one of the most common causes of hospital mortality (Kendall et al 1986). Not every patient who suffers from DVT will develop pulmonary embolism. However, a review by Kendall and associates showed that the incidence of DVT is suprisingly high: 50% of patients undergoing major orthopaedic surgery or suffering trauma to the pelvis, hip or knee develop calf vein thrombosis, while 20% develop proximal vein thrombosis. (It must be remembered that clot formation above the knee is more often fatal.)

As long ago as 1856, Virchow identified three main causal factors in the formation of blood clots (see Love 1990). However, it is the combination of these factors that influences clot formation; each factor on its own has little effect (see Fig. 5.12). Further, many thrombi go undetected and are relatively harmless.

Trauma may be caused by accidents, surgery or inflammation of the veins; the subsequent damage to the vein and valve cusp encourages coagulation at the site.

Blood chemistry may be affected by drugs (for example, the oral contraceptive pill), the presence of malignancy or any tissue damage. Tissue damage elicits a protective response termed the 'acute phase reaction' (see Love 1990). As a result of this the blood becomes hypercoagulable as a protection against further blood loss; the effect lasts from 3 to 11 days.

Stasis is associated most commonly with imposed restriction of movement – for example, after surgery or due to external devices such as splints or casts, when the calf muscles are unable to pump blood through the veins as they do in normal activity and the rate of venous return slows significantly. Blood pools in the valve cusps, leading to coagulation.

In common with pressure sores, deep vein thrombosis may also be due to many other factors

which are either specific to the individual patient or general and related to the environment.

Patient characteristics

Age and reduced physical activity are, again, both important characteristics that increase the risk of DVT developing. Calculation of the patient risk is based on assessing many of the patient's individual characteristics. Examples of these predisposing factors are given in Table 5.8.

Environmental factors

Environmental factors include:

- compressive pressure, particularly in specific regions of the body (for example long socks with garter supports)
- surgery of more than 1 hour's length and in certain regions of the body
- the surgical technique used.

Stamatakis and co-workers (1977) showed that during total hip replacement surgery the femoral vein becomes distorted. This led to 51% of the

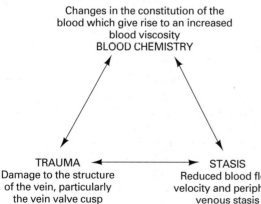

Fig. 5.12 Virchow's triad.

Table 5.8 Factors predisposing to deep vein thrombosis (DVT)

Related to:	Problem/nursing diagnosis
Individual patient-specific factors	
Mobilizing	Activity intolerance, pain, decreased muscle strength, fatigue, lack of motivation, fear, limited ROM, imposed restriction of movement (e.g. splints, traction, prescribed bedrest etc.), powerlessness, knowledge deficit
Eating and drinking	Altered nutrition (more than body requirements, causing obesity), fluid volume deficit
Breathing	Ineffective breathing pattern
Controlling body temperature	Hypothermia
Expressing sexuality	Altered hormonal status, e.g. due to contraceptive pill, pregnancy
Other	Presence of malignancy, previous history of DVT
Environmental factors	
Compressive pressure	
Surgery; length and nature	

160 patients studied developing DVT in the femoral vein.

Risk assessment and detection

Recognition of predisposing factors is important in identifying the at-risk patient. Unfortunately, as yet there are no validated quantitative risk calculators for nurses to use, as there are for pressure sores. As an undetected DVT may lead to pulmonary embolism, early detection of its occurrence is essential. Love (1990) identifies four methods for the detection of DVT which are substantially a part of nursing care (see Table 5.9). Iodine labelling and scanning, phlebography and Doppler ultrasound investigations help to confirm and gauge the extent of the thrombosis. Unfortunately, in up to 80% of affected patients the pulmonary embolism is not detected.

Table 5.9 Methods for the detection of deep vein thrombosis (DVT) (adapted with permission from Love 1990)

Test	Purpose and method	Advantages	Disadvantages
Visual examination of the limb	Perform a daily visual assessment for discoloration of the skin and signs of redness in the distribution of the tibial, popliteal and femoral veins. A mirror can be used if visual access is made difficult by restricted positioning	Non-invasive procedure which can be carried out by nurses	Cannot be done if the lower limb is bandaged or encased in a cast
Assessment of pain and/or discomfort	Regularly assess the patient's level of comfort. Ask the patient to specify the exact location of pain or discomfort. Identify sources of discomfort or pain in the distribution of the tibial, popliteal, femoral and iliac veins. Locate pain source to calf muscle, behind the knee, at the back of the leg or in the groin region	Non-invasive procedure which can be carried out by nurses	The patient's complaint may not be fully appreciated. Delay in identifying the cause may occur if the first recourse is to administer analgesic agents. The patient may have other sources of pain which are confusing the situation
Four-hourly temperature	Be suspicious of all unexplained low-grade pyrexia	Non-invasive procedure which can be carried out by nurses	There are many causes of low-grade pyrexia other than DVT
Homans' sign	Examine for sharp pain or discomfort in the calf when the patient's foot is dorsiflexed. Eliminate the possibility of pain or discomfort arising from other sources such as a Baker's cyst	Non-invasive procedure which can be carried out by nurses	DVT needs to be in an advanced stage before the test is positive. Can only be used to detect calf vein thrombosis. Does not detect the potentially fatal femoral and iliac vein thrombosis. Cannot be done if the lower limb is bandaged or encased in a cast. There are other causes of calf pain, such as a Baker's cyst
Calf measurement	Take and record measurements of the calf in cm. A baseline measurement needs to be established preoperatively. The same position needs to be used on each occasion. Take measurements daily throughout the risk period. Eliminate the possibility of swelling arising from other sources	Non-invasive procedure which can be carried out by nurses	Cannot be done if lower limb is bandaged or encased in a cast, or there are other causes of calf swelling. Distortions occur unless the same position on the calf is used each time. A baseline measurement needs to be known

Methods of prevention

All patients at risk of developing DVT should be identified and prophylaxis implemented. However, there is much debate about which of the wide variety of prophylactic measures have optimum results with minimum risk. Broadly, preventative measures fall into two groups:

1. Those that alter the blood chemistry through antithrombotic agents
2. Those aimed at promoting blood flow.

Love (1990) identifies the same methods of prevention: operating through pharmacological means or producing the desired effects mechanically (Table 5.10).

Pharmacological measures, such as subcutaneous low-dose heparin, are an effective and popular method of prophylaxis. However, local allergies and haematomas may occur and excessive bleeding may be a complication. Several other drugs such as aspirin, which reduce platelet stickiness, have also been used to reduce the incidence of DVT.

Active methods of promoting blood flow are initiated by the patient. These include early ambulation with weight-bearing, methods which simulate weight-bearing, and deep breathing. They require the patient to be well-informed and motivated.

Passive methods of promoting blood flow include compression stockings, lower limb elevation and pneumatic compression. Compression stockings must be used correctly; otherwise, they may become a cause rather than a preventer of DVT. It is therefore important to understand the principles of the stockings' effect and to follow the manufacturer's instructions on their use and fitting.

Utilizing the calf muscle pump, as when the foot is alternately dorsi- and plantarflexed, improves the venous return. However, Gardner and Fox (1983) discovered that a venous pump also exists in the sole of the foot, and showed that a significant pumping action is produced by applying the normal load of the body weight to the foot. This action occurs even in the paraplegic patient whose calf muscles are paralysed.

This is significant, as encouraging patients to dorsi- and plantarflex the ankle to utilize the calf muscle pump will not be effective unless pressure is applied to the sole of the foot to open up the deep plantar veins which empty up into the calf. This may be achieved artificially if patients are unable to weight-bear, by using pneumatic venous foot pumps or a foot board. Gardner and colleagues (1990) have subsequently shown that machines used to produce impulse pumping have such a marked effect on the microcirculation that they produce other benefits such as a reduction in swelling, prevention of compartment syndrome and relief of pain as well as prevention of deep venous thrombosis.

Treating deep vein thrombosis

Once detected, the patient with a DVT or pulmonary embolus will require anticoagulation therapy and possibly surgical or other interventions to disperse or remove the thrombus. Anticoagulation is a prophylactic measure to ensure that no further episodes of DVT occur, but it also creates potential or actual problems for the patient who must be well-informed about possible side-effects and about recommendations and contraindications while on this long-term therapy. Figure 5.13, adapted from Ford (1987), is an example of the information the patient will require. Nursing care must incorporate the same information in its care plans to ensure that the nurse is able to detect complications at an early stage, promote desirable patient behaviour and ensure compliance by empowering the patient.

Problems related to the locomotor system

Creason and co-workers (1985), in their research on the nursing diagnosis of impaired physical mobility, identified what may be termed its causes or effects. Using Creason's framework, four main patient problems may be identified and their cause or effect determined so that nursing interventions may be planned (see Table 5.11).

Table 5.10 Methods of preventing deep vein thrombosis (from Love 1990)

Method	Nursing intervention	Rationale	Cautions
Pharmacological Subcutaneous sodium heparin 5000 IU, 8–12-hourly	A therapeutic dose which achieves peak blood plasma levels at 2 h in the range 0.5–0.2 IU/ml is recommended. A test dose is advised. Observe for evidence of haematuria, spontaneous bruising, haematoma as indicators of heparin overdose. Best protection is achieved when commenced preoperatively	Heparin neutralizes factor X as its prime target. Exerts a direct inhibitory effect on thrombus formation. Efficient and reliable	Heparin is a non-standard preparation so each batch can differ in strength. Not really suitable for injured patients at risk
Mechanical (active) Simulated or actual plantigrade walking, weight-bearing	Inquire if patient can dorsiflex (heel down) and plantarflex (toe down). Use foot board if patient is confined to bed	Prevents peripheral venous stasis. Promotes an increased blood flow velocity. Encourages complete emptying of the vein valve cusps	Condition of stasis return once activity ceases. Patient's physical capabilities may preclude use, especially in the acute phase of care when patient most needs protection
Early ambulation	Inquire if patient is independent with walking and able to initiate own walking activity. Early 'angulation' is not a substitute for ambulation. Full benefits achieved only when done vigorously on a continuous basis. Repeat sequences 5 times half-hourly	Counteracts the detrimental effects of defective venous blood flow patterns characterized by turbulence and eddying	Application often erratic, may be delayed and not feasible on a continuous basis. No exercise, no protection
Deep breathing	Use an incentive spirometer. Use sequence of 5 deep breaths followed by 10 ordinary breaths to avoid hyperventilation. Repeat 5 times half-hourly	Uses 'respiratory' pump. Negative barometric pressures within the pleural cavity exert a sucking force. Normal: −2 to −8 mmHg Deep: −2 to −32 mmHg	Deep breathing usually occurs in response to an oxygen deficit so is unnatural when patient is at rest. As with other active mechanical methods, patient's condition may preclude application, and patient compliance is essential
Mechanical (passive) Graded compression thromboembolic deterrent stockings	Must be measured to provide a graded compressive force of 18 mmHg at the ankle reducing to 8 mmHg at the thigh. Can be used beneath foam back skin extensions. Ensure that circulation and sensation are known to be adequate and that skin is intact. Can be left in place for period of use or changed daily as preferred or indicated. Fabric quality deteriorates with use and washing: use new hosiery for each patient. Fabric care: see instructions	Static compressive force effects an increase in venous blood flow velocity up to 38%. Limits venous distention and encourages complete emptying of the vein valve cusps and segments. Helpful for patients who have varicosed veins or previous injury or surgery to pelvis or lower limb. Provides a continuous resource to counteract the effects of peripheral venous stasis complementary to active treatments	Cannot be used for patients who have been injured or had surgery to lower limb. Hosiery must fit accurately. Application can be difficult. Can embarrass circulation and damage skin if too tight or if hosiery becomes wrinkled
Bed elevation	10° of elevation effects a 30% increase in blood flow velocity	Simple to use	Patient's condition may preclude use
Powered mechanical artefacts	Complement active and non-powered passive forms. Include 'air boots' and, in principle, the continuous passive motion machine	As for active and passive treatment	Availability. Patient's condition may preclude use. May require special expertise

Because the medication you are taking reduces your blood's ability to clot you must take special precautions:

Wear a Medic Alert bracelet or carry a card with information that you are taking anticoagulants
Take your medication at the same time each day, as prescribed
Keep all appointments for blood tests
Increase or decrease your medication only as directed by your doctor
If you do cut yourself, immediately apply pressure directly to the wound with a clean dressing or cloth for 5 to
     10 minutes. If possible elevate the part cut. If the bleeding does not stop go to your nearest hospital accident
     and emergency department immediately.
Tell your dentist you are on anticoagulants on each visit
Always check with your doctor before taking any new medication
Never take aspirin or other medication that contains aspirin. Read all labels carefully
Avoid alchoholic beverages – they may alter your blood clotting time. Ask your doctor for specific advice
Immediately report any of the following to your doctor:
     nosebleeds
     coughing up red to black mucus
     bruises that persist longer than usual or that increase in size
     bleeding gums
     blood in your urine or stools (which may be bright red or tarry)
     weariness
     dizziness, faintness
     anxiety and apprehension
     irritability
     confusion

Fig. 5.13   Information for patients on anticoagulant therapy.

Table 5.11   Problems related to the locomotor system and reduced mobility

Patient problem	Definition	Cause or effect
Reluctance to attempt movement	Perceived inability or reluctance to perform a desired activity	Pain, fear, lack of motivation, fatigue, lack of knowledge
Limited range of movement (ROM)	Limitation of joint function not due to denervation or assistive devices	Contractures, dislocation, infection, stiffness
Decreased muscle strength, control and/or mass	Decreased muscle strength, decreased control related to peripheral degeneration and decreased mass related to atrophy of single muscle or groups	Generalized, localized, spastic, flaccid, atrophy (disuse), positional, weakness
Impaired coordination	Lack of ability to coordinate movement by loss of all or part of the brain's control	Tremor, spasticity, proprioception, gait

Reluctance to attempt movement

There may be many reasons why a patient feels reluctant to move. The patient may be in pain, and this should be addressed as quickly as possible and reduced to a level acceptable to the patient (see Ch. 7). Frequently the patient is afraid that moving will cause pain or will cause him damage or harm. A knowledgeable, confident and reassuring approach is required by the nurse to encourage and support a patient at these times. Persuasion and support rather than coercion are needed. If the patient feels in control of the situation through understanding the reasons for the movements and their therapeutic effects, then progress will be accelerated and complications reduced.

As Crowe (1988) makes clear, the patient must have the desire to move; the motivation has to come from him, but may be promoted or extinguished by the nurse. Maslow (1954) developed a theory of man's drive to meet physical, social and psychological needs based on the individual's motivation to achieve his potential. It is relatively straightforward for a nurse and patient to identify and satisfy basic physiological needs, such as eating and drinking or breathing, but more difficult to satisfy psychological needs such as a high self-esteem. Nurses can help the patient satisfy both his basic and more complex psychological needs by empowering him with the drive and desire to meet these needs and then allowing him to achieve his potential. The arthritic individual may well allow the nurse to do everything for him as this is easier and quicker for both patient and nurse. However, in this situation the individual will tend to become demotivated and dependent.

Limited range of movement

Joints which are not put through a range of movement at regular intervals will become stiff and eventually a contracture will occur. This is due to the ligaments and tendons, in particular, not being stretched and thus becoming denser, contracted and less elastic. For example, wearing shoes with high heels for a period of time reduces the range of dorsiflexion of the ankle; the Achilles tendon shortens and contracts, causing ankle stiffness. When flat shoes are worn again the stretching of the Achilles tendon can often be felt. If the contraction is significant or the individual elderly, the tendon may become painful, damaged or even torn when full dorsiflexion is imposed by the flat shoes which again allow full range of movement.

Generally, the patient's joints should be rested in a neutral, functional position as far as possible. This prevents damage due to prolonged hyperextension or flexion. The wrist, for example, has a neutral position of 30° of extension, and thus splints used for immobilizing the wrist in neutral should produce this degree of extension with slight ulnar deviation, and allow the metacarpophalangeal joints to rest in a position of 90° of flexion, as though the patient was gripping a tumbler. These neutral positions are therefore not only optimum for the prevention of

joint contractures but are also functional for the individual who will still be able to feed himself and take a drink.

Decreased muscle strength, control and/or mass

Many of the patient problems so far discussed require a close working relationship between the nurse, physiotherapist, occupational therapist and patient. The skill of the health care professional is in getting the balance between activity and rest right, at any point in time, so that the patient can achieve an optimum rate of recovery and degree of comfort, with minimal complications.

Active exercises Powell (1986) proposes that exercises have four main purposes:

1. To retain movements to prevent stiffness in joints and maintain normal tone in the muscles controlling them
2. To restore movements which have been lost owing to disuse, injury or disease
3. To redevelop muscles and to restore muscle balance which has been lost through disuse, injury or disease
4. To retain the memory of movement patterns and to regain functional control in general.

These exercises all require patient cooperation and participation and may be classified according to the degree of participation and the degree (or lack) of movement required:

- Free active exercises are carried out by the patient on his own. Their aim is to gain or retain joint movement and strengthen muscles. As previously discussed, they also stimulate and assist the circulatory system to prevent circulatory stasis.
- Isometric exercises (static contractions) are performed by the patient on his own. They produce muscular contractions without movement of the joint(s). They may be performed, for example, by the patient with a leg immobilized in a plaster of Paris cylinder, to maintain the tone and strength of the quadricep muscles so that recovery is speeded up and circulatory stasis reduced.

- Assisted active exercises are active movements performed by the patient but with the assistance of a health care professional such as a physiotherapist or nurse, or a mechanical device or the patient's sound limb.
- Resisted active exercises are carried out by the patient against a resistance such as a footboard or weight attached to a limb or against the physiotherapist or nurse herself.

Individuals should be provided with written instructions of exercise programmes to prevent joint and muscle deterioration due to disuse and to enable them to continue progressive rehabilitation once discharged from hospital. Many day centres now provide exercise classes for the elderly to enable them to maintain muscle strength and range of joint movement, and so help them avoid the potential problems of reduced physical mobility and improve their quality of life. For instance, to strengthen an individual's shoulder, he may be given a programme of exercises which he is expected to perform twice daily (see Fig. 5.14).

Passive movement Passive movements are not performed by the patient. The physiotherapist or nurse, or a mechanical device such as a continuous passive mobilizer, puts the patient's joint(s) through a range of movement and stretches his muscles.

These movements are necessary for patients with impaired physical mobility due to conditions such as polyneuritis, multiple sclerosis or motor neuron disease. They aim to prevent tightness and contractures of joints and muscles. The nurse is usually instructed and assisted by the physiotherapist when performing them for the patient. Downie and Kennedy (1980) have produced an excellent text on these movements, emphasizing that care must be taken when carrying them out. This is because joints and tissues may be easily damaged by excessive vigour or overextending the range of movement of the relatively unprotected joints and muscles, as all the soft tissues of the joints and the muscles are weakened due to disuse.

Problems with elimination

Impaired physical mobility may cause a toileting self-care deficit, such as inability to maintain or achieve continence, and may also lead to constipation, renal calculi and urinary tract infection. These problems may be further exacerbated by therapies or nursing interventions such as the drugs given for pain management, premedications, or restricted fluid intake before and after surgery. The lack of privacy and the discomfort of using bed-pans, commodes and urinals while confined to bed only add to the patient's difficulties.

Environment and positioning

Whether the patient is at home or in hospital, his inability to eliminate without assistance leads to an inevitable loss of privacy and dignity and causes discomfort. Anderson (1978) paints a vivid picture of these problems. 'There you sit, enveloped in the array of white screening that surrounds your bed, but offers no privacy whatsoever. Perched in an uncomfortable and impossible position, the great trial of concentration and effort begins'.

Western culture and basic human anatomy and physiology ensure that patients are unprepared for eliminating while in bed, in the presence of others and into strange receptacles.

---

1. Standing upright, with your arms straight by your sides, raise your right arm forward and upward above your head, as far as possible. Return to resting position and repeat with your left arm

2. Standing upright, with your arms straight by your sides, raise your right arm sideways and upward above your head, as far as possible. Return to resting position and repeat with your left arm

3. Standing upright, with your arms straight by your sides, raise your right arm sideways to shoulder level. Then bring your arm across your body, bending your elbow at the same time, to touch your left shoulder if possible. Return to resting position and repeat with your left arm

Fig. 5.14 Exercises to strengthen the shoulder.

Postures such as lying, and restriction of movement and position due to casts or traction, add to the problem. This makes it difficult for the individual to relax sufficiently to be able to urinate. As defaecation occurs best in a squatting position, this function is also inhibited by environmental and positioning restrictions and therefore may lead to constipation.

Psychological stimuli such as running taps may help a patient to urinate but other interventions should also be carried out to help alleviate inhibiting factors. For example, the nurse should:

- Ensure maximum privacy for the patient when he is using a bed pan
- Allow the patient to communicate that he has finished or needs assistance – for example by giving him a call bell – rather than keep checking
- Ensure that the patient is comfortable and feels safe
- Provide toilet paper and leave it within reach
- Whenever possible allow the patient to use the toilet or commode rather than bed-pan or urinal
- Provide hand-washing facilities.

Constipation

Constipation is the reduction in the frequency of defaecation from what is normal for an individual, with an associated difficulty in passing faeces (Boore et al 1987). There can be little doubt that constipation is a significant problem both for the patient with reduced mobility and for the orthopaedic nurse. For the former it is uncomfortable and distressing; for the latter it consumes both time and resources.

In patients with orthopaedic conditions, reduced mobility or the therapeutic interventions involved in treatment often lead to reduced food or fluid intake; for instance, a patient may have difficulty in eating and drinking owing to pain on movement or limited range or movement. Medication such as antibiotics may also lead to anorexia, nausea and even vomiting. The resulting insufficient food intake fails to stimulate peristalsis, and dehydration produces small,

hard, dry stools which irritate the colon, causing spasm and a failure to stimulate normal colonic motility.

A nursing assessment is made by recording bowel motions and habits to establish a deviation from the individual's norm. A nursing diagnosis identifies the probable cause of the problem, and a care plan in the form of dietary modifications, such as increasing fibre or daily fluid intake to approximately 2 litres for adults, may be all that is necessary. Alleviation of the problem may be achieved directly by assisting the patient with eating and drinking, or through the provision of aids or patient education. In some cases it may be necessary to alleviate constipation with laxatives or enemas; however, their regular use is not recommended.

Diarrhoea

Diarrhoea is often due to a change in diet or to antibiotic therapy. Simply altering the diet, or reducing the patient's anxiety by informing him that antibiotics are causing the problem, may be all that is required. However, if diarrhoea is profuse and lasts for more than a day or two, urgent action must be taken as the resultant dehydration may be life-threatening.

Diarrhoea as a result of conditions such as pseudomembranous colitis, which is induced by antibiotic therapy, must be suspected by nurses if the condition is of sudden onset and is severe. Seal and Borriello (1983) explain that the discovery of *Clostridium difficile* as the infective organism in pseudomembranous colitis, which is due to the patient's disrupted gastrointestinal flora resulting from antibiotic therapy, indicates that the condition has infective properties. As the majority of orthopaedic patients undergoing surgery have prophylactic antibiotic cover, the problem can spread quickly through a ward of susceptible patients.

Retention and difficulties in micturition

Difficulties in defaecating generally develop over days and do not require urgent nursing interventions. On the other hand, micturition problems and urinary retention often develop over minutes or hours and require more immediate attention.

Urinary tract infection due to urinary stasis, and urinary retention as a result of surgery or a general anaesthetic are common in patients with orthopaedic conditions. The effects of urinary stasis may be minimized by ensuring that the adult patient drinks at least 2 litres of fluid per day, providing that no other medical or nursing diagnosis contraindicates this. If, however, the patient is unable to urinate, then urethral catheterization may be necessary. Because there is a high risk of infection from both the catheterization procedure itself and from leaving an indwelling catheter in situ, the nurse must ensure that all other reasonable nursing interventions have been attempted before this is carried out. (See Ch. 8 for risks of urethral catheterization and prevention of infection.)

Urinary incontinence as a consequence of impaired physical mobility due to an orthopaedic condition, together with the potential ill-health of elderly patients, is not an uncommon combination. In this respect, it is essential that orthopaedic nurses develop the skills necessary for caring for the elderly with continence problems, and they should form close links with nurses directly involved in the health care of the elderly.

Problems eating and drinking

Good nutrition is fundamental to physical well-being and is important for many activities of living, including elimination as already discussed. However, poor nutrition must not be confused with self-care deficits in feeding which are more specific in nature and related to problems of mobility.

Self-care deficits in feeding may be due to the following:

1. The individual's physical disability
2. Motivational factors, such as the individual's appetite and his compliance with cultural and religious customs, e.g. eating and fasting at set times, and the presentation and prohibition of certain types of food and drink

3. The individual's position for eating and drinking
4. The availability of assistance when eating and drinking.

Physical disability

To overcome an individual's self-care deficit in feeding, the orthopaedic nurse must have empathy, patience, resilience and common sense. Arthritic patients, for example, suffer from deformity and pain. If these are severe and involve the joints of the hand, then holding cutlery may be difficult for them. Painful joints with limited ranges of movement affect the shoulder and elbow and this reduces grip strength. Items of food that are easiest to eat are those that can be picked up in the fingers (Wainwright 1978). Arthritic patients tend to use both hands to support cups while drinking, and built up handles on cutlery can help a weak grip. (See Michael Mandelstam (1990) *How to Get Equipment for Disability* for information on how to assess the disabled individual and decide on and obtain appropriate aids to help him eat and drink in hospital and the community; there are also details on the rights of disabled individuals.) The provision of sandwiches for some meals may be a simple but effective solution to many feeding problems.

Motivational factors

Henley (1987) warns that we should not underestimate the psychological importance of giving the patient familiar food or food which he considers healthy. Many people adhere strictly to religious restrictions on the consumption of some types of food. For example, a devout Muslim would not feel able to eat a salad from which a slice of ham had merely been removed.

It is essential that the orthopaedic nurse obtain as much information as possible from the individual, and that she is prepared to be flexible and innovative. An individual's appetite may have been good or bad throughout his life and may remain unchanged with age. He may have his own food and drink likes and dislikes which must be taken into account. Illness may produce anorexia or nausea.

Positioning for eating and drinking

As eating and drinking are social events, efforts must be made to enable the patient and his family to eat together if he is at home or for patients to eat together in a hospital environment. However, coercion must not be used on those individuals who do not wish to eat with others as this can be stressful and embarrassing for them.

The patient's position is important, as poor positioning – for example, eating from a plate that is balanced on a lap or not sitting upright in bed – may give rise to feeding difficulties. Special chairs and beds are available to ease these problems, but common sense suffices in many instances: a few carefully positioned pillows are often all that is required.

Availability of assistance

Some individuals will require assistance in feeding from carers such as nurses or relatives. This may vary from arranging and cutting up food to inserting food into the patient's mouth. Whenever possible, the individual's ability to feed himself must be maintained, and it is in achieving this that the knowledge and skills of the orthopaedic nurse may be fully utilized. An individual who has undergone spinal surgery and is confined to a supine position is still able to use his arms. With mirrors, careful selection and preparation of food and drink, and the use of suitable utensils and aids, these patients are able to feed themselves. This gives them more control over their situation and is psychologically beneficial.

Problems of personal cleansing and dressing

Bathing, grooming and dressing are all personal and private aspects of everyday life. One of the stabilizing and often pleasurable aspects of daily living is removed if the individual is unable to carry out these activities. Dressing, in particular,

is one way for people to demonstrate individuality and show that they have control of their lives and possess decision-making capabilities. All these activities also reflect, to some extent, people's social and economic position and niche in life.

The inability of people with orthopaedic conditions to perform personal cleansing and dressing activities is predominantly due to impaired physical mobility as a result of:

- pain on movement
- prescribed restrictions, such as plaster of Paris casts or bedrest
- limited range of movement
- reduced muscle strength
- the lack of a desire to move.

Personal cleansing

Whenever possible, the individual must be enabled to perform personal cleansing activities independently. With the help of equipment and aids this is often possible (see Mandelstam 1990). For example, a wide-handled tooth brush or glove flannel can give individuals with arthritic hands greater independence; long-handled combs and brushes can also help.

An individual with impaired physical mobility may not be able to take a bath independently. Roper (1988) describes a variety of aids and equipment that are available to assist individuals and nurses in the performance of this activity. These may range from bath seats and hand rails to hoists and even special baths and shower units. However, some orthopaedic patients are unable to move or be moved from their beds. In hospital and the community this problem demands imagination, tact and time from the orthopaedic nurse. Each patient will have individual needs, idiosyncracies and levels of dependence. It may be that a towel bath, as described by Wright (1990), is more appropriate and comforting to the patient than the usual bed bath. Special basins are available for washing patients' hair while they are in bed.

Sexuality is often expressed through the way people groom, dress and maintain their hygiene.

The male patient who wishes to, but cannot, shave daily must be given assistance or be shaved by the nurse. Mirrors should be available to enable women and men to groom and make up or shave themselves if possible, or to see the results of the nurse's attention.

Menstruation may create problems for women with impaired physical mobility or with pre-scribed restrictions to movement such as traction with a Thomas splint or hip spica casts. Sensitive assistance with the positioning of sanitary pads is required.

Dressing

The majority of able-bodied people dress daily without giving a thought to the strength, supple-ness, stamina and agility that it requires. Cloth-ing and footwear for the orthopaedic patient may need to be adapted from readily available items, or to be specially manufactured. The indi-vidual's need may be temporary as, for example, when an arm is in a sling or following foot surgery, or permanent, for example when an artificial limb is fitted or the individual has rheumatoid arthritis.

The Disabled Living Foundation, RADAR (Royal Association for Disability and Rehabilita-tion) and other similar bodies provide a wealth of information on availability, designs and costs of clothing and footwear. In addition, there are aids to assist dressing such as shoe horns and stocking aids. Mandelstam (1990) provides an extensive list of manufacturers of clothing, foot-wear and aids.

Patients in hospital or at home should, when possible and appropriate, be able to wear their own clothing and maintain their own routines of dressing and undressing. General principles to consider when assisting the patient to decide on appropriate clothing and footwear are:

- ease of putting on and removing
- cost
- aesthetic quality and style
- comfort
- ease of washing and cleaning
- safety

- non-restrictiveness, for general mobility and therapeutic exercises
- warmth (but not excessive)
- versatility, adaptability and repairability.

Developments such as Velcro fastening, elastic laces and the style of many of today's clothes and shoes help to ensure, with careful selection and adaptation, that dressing and undressing are potentially easier and less painful and frustrat-ing for those with impaired physical mobility.

The mass production of sports and leisure wear has meant that stylish, comfortable, wash-able and relatively cheap clothing and footwear are now available for all ages. The latest develop-ments in materials, particularly for shoes, enable orthotists now to produce items that are comfort-able and acceptable to wear.

Problems of breathing

The absence of breathing is obviously serious, as in respiratory arrest or apnoea. Other problems may occur in breathing and the gaseous ex-change in the lungs owing to:

- the quality of breathing
- the quality of the breathed air
- the condition of the individual's lungs and cardiopulmonary system.

The activity of breathing

Ideally the lungs should be able to expand easily on inspiration and the lung bases should be aerated regularly by taking deep breaths. There are several reasons why this may not occur in orthopaedic patients:

1. Impaired physical mobility, which may be:
   a. local, such as when wearing a tight plaster jacket
   b. general, for example owing to conditions such as rheumatoid arthritis or to prescribed therapy such as bedrest
2. Posture: lung expansion is easiest in the upright position
3. Pain and its management
4. Physical deformity
5. Surgery.

Pain prevents deep breathing and coughing. Also some analgesics, such as morphine, depress the respiratory centre and reduce the depth and rate of breathing. Physical deformities such as scoliosis and the effects of ankylosing spondilitis reduce lung expansion. General anaesthetic agents reduce respiratory function by depressing breathing and paralysing the cilia of the respiratory tract that keep the lungs clear of mucus and debris.

Deep breathing By encouraging regular deep breathing, more oxygen enters the bloodstream to respond to increased metabolic demands, perhaps following injury or surgery. Additionally, the lung bases are aerated which prevents the mucous secretions stagnating in them as dilatation of the bronchioles and alveolae also occurs. If this does not occur, the stagnant secretions can solidify and act as a mucous plug in the bronchioles. This plug is difficult to expectorate; the air distal to the plug is absorbed but fluid still exudes from the walls of the alveolae, providing an ideal medium for bacterial growth. The resultant chest infection may further reduce gaseous exchange.

The orthopaedic nurse needs to work closely with, and often under the guidance of, the physiotherapist in teaching the patient deep breathing exercises and helping him maintain them.

Powell (1986) advises that the nurse should place her hands on either side of the patient's thorax and instruct the patient to breathe in so as to push the hands away, and then breathe out and relax. After each deep breath, taken slowly, there should be complete relaxation and the procedure should be repeated 5 or 6 times. The patient can place his own hand below the sternum and if the exercises are performed correctly, he should feel a significant movement of the hand as compared to shallow breathing. Once taught, these exercises can be performed hourly by the patient at home or in hospital, with monitoring by the nurse. More specialized breathing exercises may need to be taught by the physiotherapist; or the patient may need to be assisted by equipment such as patient-activated positive pressure ventilation or spirometers that gauge lung ventilation improvements and allow the

patient to see his progress, adding a competitive and fun component to the exercises.

Posture The upright position allows greater diaphragmatic freedom and thus encourages increased ventilation of the lungs with less effort from the patient, as the abdominal contents drop with the assistance of gravity on inspiration. As Boylan and Brown (1985) describe clearly, inspiration is an active process whereas expiration is passive. Therefore, inspiration requires greater energy and motivation from the patient and is more tiring. Often the orthopaedic nurse needs to be innovative and flexible, as the patient's condition or therapy may prevent or make difficult the achievement of this posture. The patient must be encouraged to be up and walking as soon as possible. Sitting upright, well supported, in a chair is also beneficial. However, if the patient is confined to bed, then the upright sitting position, well supported by pillows, may be the only possible solution. The patient must be upright, as the slumped position is even more detrimental to diaphragmatic freedom than lying flat. To help minimize the risk of the patient sliding down the bed, the foot of the bed should be elevated by 5–10°. This not only maintains the patient in a more upright position, but reduces the risk of sacral pressure sore development, as shear forces are markedly reduced.

Heavy bedclothes tucked in tightly around the chest also impede good lung ventilation. Therefore, bedclothes should be loose, light and should allow freedom of movement.

Quality of the breathed air An environment which is airy, well-ventilated and with a constant warm temperature is pleasant and psychologically beneficial to the individual. The opposite can be harmful to physical, social and psychological health. For example, a hot, stuffy, smoky atmosphere for even a short period of time can produce coughing, sore throat, headache, tiredness and lethargy.

Impaired physical mobility may reduce the individual's ability to control his environment and thus makes him dependent on the nurse. However, whenever possible, he should be encouraged to be outside in the fresh air as this will have psychological benefits as well.

Good ventilation keeps unpleasant odours to a minimum but also reduces the prevalence of airborne bacteria and viruses that may cause illness. Pleasant-smelling aromas from oils will encourage deep breathing but have also been shown to have therapeutic benefits. Lavendar, for example, helps relaxation and promotes sleep. Aromatherapy, which is the use of essential oils in this way, is not new and dates back to the Ancient Egyptians who used them for religious as well as medical reasons.

The individual   So far, general principles and the environment have been considered with respect to breathing and its relationship to impaired physical mobility. The individual with an orthopaedic condition may have an unrelated breathing problem which is exacerbated by the condition or its therapy. As many individuals with orthopaedic problems are elderly they:

- are more likely to suffer from conditions such as chronic bronchitis
- have poorer lung ventilation due to the normal ageing process; in the elderly there is:
  — a reduction of vital capacity by 25%
  — a reduction of maximum breathing capacity by 50% (between 20 and 80 years of age)
  — increased rigidity of the chest wall
  — reduction of the thoracic volume due to a tendency to stoop, and perhaps kyphosis and/or scoliosis.

An orthopaedic patient may be a smoker and would possibly wish to be given information, encouragement and support to stop or reduce his smoking. This must be his own choice with help from the nurse. The patient's health would benefit generally, but it would also ensure quicker, more efficient therapy and a better quality of life if recovery or cure were not possible. The patient should not be coerced or blamed, as these strategies have been shown to be of no benefit in health promotion.

Adult respiratory distress syndrome (ARDS) is a result of interference with gaseous exchange in the lungs leading to interstitial fibrosis and hyaline membrane formation. In the orthopaedic patient this may be associated with severe soft tissue injury and fat emboli due to fractures. Treatments such as massive blood transfusions, excessive fluid administration and prolonged artificial ventilation may also cause ARDS.

Problems of sleep and rest

Undoubtedly, sleep pattern disturbance causes discomfort and interferes with the desired lifestyle; it may also lead to ill-health or be the result of ill-health. Recovery from orthopaedic conditions and their treatment can be hindered or prevented by a lack of adequate sleep and rest. Oswald and Adam (1984) have shown that sleep is essential to the healing process.

Since nurses tend to spend more time in close contact with orthopaedic patients than do other health care professionals, the responsibility for dealing with sleep pattern disturbance rests largely with them. Because of their limited understanding of the nature of sleep and rest, reinforced by general attitudes which belittle their importance, nursing and medical staff care relatively poorly for individuals with problems of sleep pattern disturbance. How many times a night is an arthritic patient awakened by the pain of diseased joints as he attempts to make a positional change or is unable to relax and rest as he finds it impossible to achieve a comfortable position? The anxieties of having arthritis and not knowing what the future holds further affect his sleep and rest.

Functions of sleep

Sleep and rest as periods of relative immobility are essential to our functioning in preparation for our periods of mobility. Although there is still much debate about the exact nature and function of sleep, there are areas of general agreement. Sleep is considered to be restorative, being important in tissue renewal and in the growth of body cells in children (see Webster & Thompson 1986, Closs 1988). Horne (1983) suggests that sleep is necessary only for brain cell restitution and that physical rest will suffice to allow the restoration of other body cells. In either

Table 5.12 Effects of sleep pattern disturbance

Difficulty falling asleep
Awakening earlier or later than desired
Interrupted sleep
Not feeling well-rested
Malaise
Tiredness
Lethargy
Restlessness
Irritability
Sensitivity to pain and discomfort
Listlessnes
Apathy
Slow reaction

case, sleep and rest are fundamental activities of living.

Individuals vary in the length and quality of the sleep and rest that they require. However, sleep pattern disturbance in all individuals leads to specific adverse effects (see Table 5.12). All these effects may be of importance to the orthopaedic patient and should be prevented or identified and overcome by the health care team and particularly by the orthopaedic nurse working with the patient. Sleep pattern disturbance often forms part of an interrelated complex cycle of cause and effect. For example, many patients state that they would be able to cope with the pain and discomfort of their condition, such as rheumatoid or osteoarthritis, if only they could get a good night's sleep. Somehow this cycle of pain and lack of sleep and rest (see Fig. 5.15) must be overcome.

Promoting sleep and rest

Pain is probably the most significant cause of sleep pattern disturbance in individuals with orthopaedic problems. Medications, such as hypnotics, are not a suitable solution to the long-term chronic pain and sleep disturbance of many orthopaedic patients, owing to the effects of increased tolerance, dependence and side-effects. However, immediately prior to surgery or for a few days post-trauma, they may help in promoting sleep and rest. Nursing interventions in the form of relaxation techniques, such as aromatherapy, massage and instructions on self-relaxation, are preferable and can be used with pain-reducing medication. Increased relaxation will often reduce the necessity for pain-reducing medication. If further sleep-promoting interventions are encouraged (see Fig. 5.16), the quality of sleep may improve dramatically, obviating the need for medication.

Closs (1988), in her review of the research on sleep disturbances in hospital, showed that 78% of patients were awakened at least once during the night. The commonest cause of this was noise. Routines such as drug rounds and lights out at late times were also significant sleep disturbers.

If sleep is accepted as important to the patient's health, recovery and well-being, then orthopaedic nurses must be more knowledgeable and systematic in their nursing care. Individuals vary significantly in their sleep needs and the factors that promote or hinder them. Indeed the same individual's sleep pattern will change through the various stages of his life and from day to day depending on his situation and life events.

Short-term sleep disturbances of a few days, such as those due to the discomfort caused by orthopaedic surgery, are not a significant problem

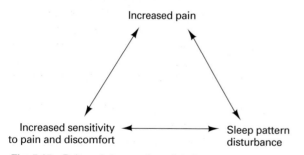

Fig. 5.15 Pain and sleep pattern disturbance.

Reduce or eliminate pain
Reduce or eliminate anxiety and depression
Assist patient to achieve comfortable position
Ensure warmth and dark
Minimize noise
Ensure satisfaction of basic needs such as hunger
  or desire to eliminate
Encourage regular circadian clock, i.e. awaken at
  same time each day.

Fig. 5.16 Sleep-promoting interventions.

for the individual so long as he is reassured that the diminished sleep will have no long-term effects. More important are the chronic sleep problems of many orthopaedic patients. The cause of the sleep pattern disturbance should be identified and then the intervention planned and implemented to reduce or eradicate the problem. The orthopaedic nurse will find it difficult to gauge the extent of the problem or whether interventions were successful unless information is obtained from and about the individual.

Assessing sleep pattern disturbance and evaluating nursing interventions may be achieved relatively easily. Subjective methods used are similar to those for pain management:

- Visual analogue scales
- Questionnaires
- Interviews
- Daily sleep charting.

Self-assessment of sleep by the maintenance of a daily sleep chart can produce useful information about changes in sleep, and gives the individual more control over his care. Recording this information requires little time and effort and is easy to carry out (see Fig. 5.17). It is also important to accept that a patient is satisfied or dissatisfied with his sleep when he says he is, no matter what others may think or feel. In many cases the nurse, with the individual, must make the best of adverse situations. Positioning of patients wearing casts and splints or in traction may be restricted; however, imaginative use of pillows

What time did you go to bed?

before 21.59
22.00 – 22.59
23.00 – 23.59
24.00 – 00.59
01.00 – +

What time did you get up?

before 04.59
05.00 – 05.59
06.00 – 06.59
07.00 – 07.59
08.00 – +

How well did you sleep?

worst ever |_|_|_|_|_|_|_|_|_|_| best ever
　　　　　0　1　2　3　4　5　6　7　8　9　10

Fig. 5.17 Examples of sleep assessments.

and supports together with pain and anxiety-reducing interventions and a quiet, warm, well-ventilated environment will all help to promote and ensure better quality sleep.

Problems of nutrition

Orthopaedic nurses need to have an understanding of normal nutrition, the function of food in life and health, its social and psychological implications, food choices and habits, and current theories and information, so that they can provide a good standard of care.

A normal diet is one supplying all the necessary nutrients for normal body function (Boore et al 1987); that is, it should provide protein for growth, maintenance and repair of the body, fats and carbohydrates for energy, vitamins and minerals to regulate body processes and, most importantly, water. Nutrition should not be confused with eating and drinking, which has been discussed earlier in the chapter. An individual may be capable of eating and drinking but still have problems related to his nutrition.

Boore et al (1987) described in some depth the composition and quantity of a balanced or normal diet. In addition to this, the orthopaedic nurse requires an understanding of several areas of nutrition related more specifically to the orthopaedic patient and how ill health of an orthopaedic nature may be prevented or minimized.

Osteoporosis and diet

Primary osteoporosis has several identifiable risk factors associated with it. One of these is diet, and the most obvious deficiency in the bones of an osteoporotic patient is calcium. With advancing age, less calcium is absorbed from the diet and a decline in the level of oestrogen in women at menopause also decreases the efficiency of calcium absorption (Office of Health Economics 1990).

Studies suggest that increased dietary calcium slows the osteoporotic process, and if a high calcium diet is taken throughout life, the increased peak bone mass provides protection against possible fractures. The peak bone mass is further increased through exercise, which also slows the bone loss process.

The current Department of Health recommended daily allowance of calcium is 500 mg for all adults, but the National Osteoporosis Society suggest 1500 mg for the postmenopausal woman who is not on hormone replacement therapy (National Dairy Council 1990) (see Table 5.13). Nordin and Heaney (1990) suggest that the present evidence shows that a significant component of the osteoporosis affecting postmenopausal women is attributable to a relative or absolute inadequacy of calcium and therefore is potentially and easily preventable. Milk, dairy products and bread are among the richest sources of calcium, providing it in an easily absorbed form. Typical calcium content of foods is given in Figure 5.18.

Vitamin D is important for the absorption of calcium and is obtained from dietary sources or the action of sunlight on the skin. Its deficiency will therefore lead to calcium–deficient, weakened bones. With age, the ability to convert dietary vitamin D to its active form of calcitriol declines, putting the elderly at risk. Others at risk are those who, for whatever reason, are not exposed to enough sunlight, such as the housebound, dark-skinned people (as dark skin filters

2 large (60 g) slices bread, white or fortified wholemeal	660 mg
2 large (60 g) slices non-fortified wholemeal bread	14 mg
⅓ pint (190 ml) silver top milk	225 mg
⅓ pint (190 ml) semi-skimmed milk	231 mg
⅓ pint (190 ml) skimmed milk	236 mg
1 oz (28 g) Cheddar or other hard cheese	207 mg
5 oz (140 g) pot of yogurt	240 mg
3 oz (84 g) cottage cheese	60 mg
4 oz (112 g) ice cream	134 mg
2 oz (56 g) sardines, including bones	220 mg
4 oz (112 g) spring cabbage	34 mg
4 oz (112 g) baked beans	50 mg
1 large orange	58 mg
3 oz (84 g) shelled prawns	126 mg

Fig. 5.18   Typical calcium content of food.

out some of the ultraviolet light essential for vitamin D production), or those who keep themselves covered for cultural or personal reasons. Good sources of vitamin D are oily fish, margarine, eggs and fortified breakfast cereals.

Osteomalacia and childhood rickets are also caused by vitamin D deficiency, which may lead to softening and deformity of the bones.

Obesity

Obesity can give rise to biopsychosocial problems. The extent of these is related to the degree of obesity and the individual's response to it. Nutritional intake is normally regulated in proportion to body stores and is usually reduced to prevent overstorage; in obesity this mechanism in some way does not function correctly. A person may be considered obese when the excess adipose tissue is harmful to health. In adults the height to weight charts used to determine obesity and its degree are derived from life insurance statistics as there is a correlation between obesity and life expectancy. Krause and Mahan (1984) recommend that a person who is 10% in excess of the norm be described as overweight and 20% in excess as obese. Table 5.14 gives acceptable weight ranges for men and women derived from the Royal College of Physicians report on obesity (1983).

In the orthopaedic patient, excess body weight

Table 5.13   Recommended daily calcium (mg/day); HRT = hormone replacement therapy

Population	Department of Health	Osteoporosis Society
Pregnant women (third trimester)	1200	1200
Breast-feeding women	1200	1200
Infants 0–1 years	600	800
Children 1–8 years	600	800
Adolescents 9–14 years	700	1200
Young adults 15–17 years	600	1200
All adults over 18 years	500	—
men and premenopausal women	—	1000
postmenopausal women (on HRT)	—	1000
postmenopausal women (no HRT)	—	1500
men and women over 60 years	—	1200

Table 5.14 Acceptable weights

Height			Weight	
ft	in	cm	lb	kg
Men				
5	5	165	121–152	55–69
5	6	168	124–156	56–71
5	7	170	128–161	58–73
5	8	173	132–166	60–75
5	9	175	136–170	62–77
5	10	178	140–174	64–79
5	11	180	144–179	65–80
6	0	183	148–184	67–83
6	1	185	152–189	69–86
6	2	188	156–194	71–88
6	3	191	160–199	73–90
Women				
4	11	150	94–122	43–55
5	0	152	96–125	44–57
5	1	155	99–128	45–58
5	2	157	102–131	46–59
5	3	160	105–134	48–61
5	4	163	108–138	49–62
5	5	165	111–142	51–65
5	6	168	114–146	52–66
5	7	170	118–150	53–67
5	8	173	122–154	55–69
5	9	175	126–158	58–72
5	10	178	130–163	59–74

may aggravate an existing disease such as osteoarthritis, and by producing conditions such as hypertension may further exacerbate the disease and its treatment. Undoubtedly, excess weight will produce impaired physical mobility. In many cases the individual is locked into a vicious cycle of increasing weight (see Fig. 5.19) which needs to be broken by the concerted effort of the individual and the support and empathy of the health care team, especially the dietitian, doctor and nurse. This effort and support should be provided in hospital and community settings. The orthopaedic nurse needs skills and an understanding of health promotion and its strategies to provide effective dietary therapy which requires the patient to make a commitment to lose weight. Empowering the patient through increasing his knowledge and understanding will increase his control of the situation and improve self-esteem. However, it must be remembered that the patient has a choice and may decide not to lose weight, and must not be blamed or reprimanded for such decisions.

Malnourishment

Silk (1983) identifies two major factors that contribute to malnutrition in hospital patients:

1. Inadequate nutrition prior to admission, i.e. starvation
2. The injury sustained, i.e. trauma, surgery, sepsis and burns.

Each may be an isolated factor, but the two often occur together. The rheumatoid arthritis patient with feeding self-care deficits, depression and anorexia may not be taking adequate nourishment; if he then needs to enter hospital for joint replacement surgery this may lead to further malnutrition during the period prior to and after surgery.

The metabolic changes that occur in response to starvation combine to keep the loss of body constituents to a minimum (see Table 5.15) (Silk 1983). Muscle protein is initially broken down very rapidly, a process known as gluconeogenesis; this will compound the individual's impaired physical mobility problems by reducing his strength. Later, the reduced metabolic rate will lead to lethargy and feelings of tiredness and loss of energy, thus inhibiting the success of any rehabilitation programme.

There are three phases of the metabolic response to injury (see Table 5.16). Nutritional support is most important in the flow phase, and so care is directed toward preventing as much tissue breakdown as possible by providing a balanced input of energy (such as carbohydrates), nitrogen, trace elements and vitamins. In reality, nutritional support during the flow phase can compensate only partially for the breakdown of body tissue during gluconeogenesis. A major aspect of the metabolic changes during the flow phase (see Table 5.17) is that basal energy requirements increase the metabolic rate, for example after multiple fracture, by as much as 25%.

Preventing and minimizing malnourishment

The nurse's role is initially to assess the extent of malnourishment and then to assist and support

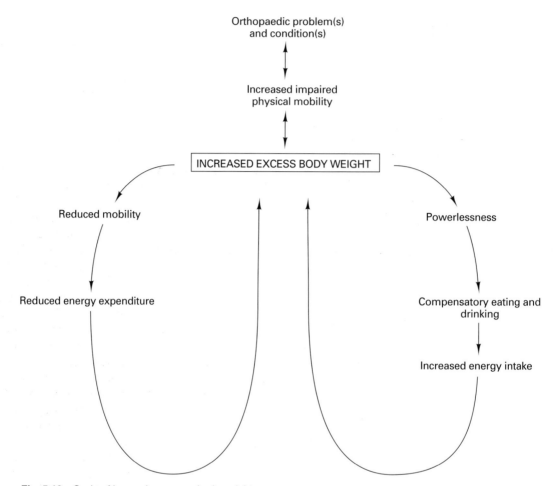

Fig. 5.19 Cycle of increasing excess body weight.

the patient in complying with whatever actions and regimens are suggested or prescribed, and to monitor their effect. Monitoring may be through blood testing or more complex techniques, or by simply weighing the patient regularly. A balanced, nutritional formulation should be compiled, with great care being taken to replace depleted vitamin stores. Methods of nutritional support in malnourishment may range from enteral routes such as oral or nasogastric, to parenteral nutrition. However, it must be remembered that parenteral nutrition is approximately 10 times more expensive than enteral and is associated with a higher incidence of serious side-effects. Nevertheless, it has an important role in the care of seriously ill patients.

Nurses can obtain details of nutritional sup-port regimens from specialist texts and experts such as dietitians with whom they should liaise closely. Patients' impaired physical mobility due directly to injury, to their condition or to pre-scribed therapy such as traction may further hinder nutritional support. It is often forgotten that failure to achieve the objectives of nutri-tional support may be due largely to the pa-tient's pain, which can cause anorexia, vomiting and a lack of interest in himself. Pain manage-ment by analgesic drugs can produce side-effects that further inhibit nutritional support.

Problems of self-image

The musculoskeletal system is an important and very visible component of the human body, and

Table 5.15 Metabolic changes due to starvation

Factor	Response/effect
Hormonal changes	early: small increase in catecholamines, glucagon, cortisol and growth hormone
	later: slow fall
	insulin decreased
Energy production	early: from protein and fat
	later: almost all from fat
Nitrogen	losses reduced
Weight loss	early: fast due to initial rapid losses of water and sodium
	later: slow
Metabolic rate	steady reduction

Table 5.16 Phases of metabolic response to injury

Phase	Duration	Role
Ebb	6–18 h	catecholamine secretion and maintenance of blood volume; allows escape to safety by mobilizing glycogen for immediate energy production
Flow (catabolic)	5–60 days; depends on type and extent of injury	maintenance of energy production
Anabolic	up to 30 days	replacement of lost tissue used in flow phase of metabolic response

Table 5.17 Flow phase metabolic changes

Factor	Response/effect
Metabolic rate	increased
Hormonal changes	Increased:
	catecholamines
	glucagon
	cortisol
	growth hormone
	insulin
Energy production	from protein and fat
Nitrogen	losses increased
Water and sodium	retention

Table 5.18 Examples of aetiology of body changes in orthopaedic patients

Aetiology	Example of body change
Congenital	muscular dystrophy, spina bifida
Hereditary	osteogenesis imperfecta
Medical/disease	arthritis
Trauma	spinal injury
Surgery	amputation

ily impair an individual's mobility significantly. But the individual's perception of how his body appears may give rise to significant problems. He may not be pleased with what he perceives as himself and may not accept the alteration in his body image, whether real or apparent. Disturbances to this self-image may make it very difficult for an individual to feel good about himself, and may thus reduce the extent to which self-empowerment (and hence his ability to overcome or accept his altered body image) can be achieved. These difficulties are compounded in our present society because, as Salter (1988) suggests, the mass media appears continually to confront society with the suggestion that it is essential to have a healthy, pleasant appearance. An inability to achieve this leads to dissatisfaction, a poor self-image and low self-esteem.

Court (1990) explains that body image loss in orthopaedic patients can be due to a combination of a change in appearance and impaired physical ability. How an individual responds to his altered body image will also be affected by society's response to and acceptance of the individual. The stigma that is sometimes attached to disabled people can affect their social identity and social encounters. For sufferers of chronic orthopaedic diseases, the disabilities experienced often accelerate their adaptation to ageing and diminishing function (Maycock 1988). 'Feeling older than one's years' is a phrase often used by these individuals and applies to their perceived physical, social and psychological age, but bears little relationship to their chronological age.

Many authors see the process of adjusting to altered body image as a grieving process. The fact that a patient advances through certain stages when experiencing a change such as an

many of the patients with orthopaedic problems have noticeable body changes due to a variety of causes and origins (see Table 5.18). However, physical changes to the body may not necessar-

alteration in body image is a useful framework on which patients and nurses can build. It enables the patient to realize that he is not the only individual who feels and reacts in these ways, and provides an end goal of acceptance or adjustment to the loss.

The nurse's involvement with individuals who have an altered body and self-image is discussed in depth in Chapter 17 with respect to the amputee. Crowther's article (1982) on new perspectives in nursing lower limb amputees reveals some interesting insights on limb loss and altered body image from the amputee's view.

CONCLUSION

An examination of the concepts of mobility and mobilizing provides an indication of why these activities are fundamental to people's health. But it is more important for nurses to understand the effects of impaired physical mobility and activity intolerance so that they can make a nursing diagnosis (that is identify patient problems, both actual and potential, that respond to nursing care) and then plan the care. From this a high standard of care may be provided, as demonstrated through evaluation.

Nurses are becoming increasingly more assertive and empowered. This serves to improve their professional status and clarify their roles and responsibilities within a multidisciplinary team without alienating their health care colleagues. With this increased sense of professional worth and self-esteem, the orthopaedic nurse is in a better position to empower patients to make their own decisions and take action related to their health and illness.

REFERENCES

Adam K, Oswald I 1984 Sleep helps healing. British Medical Journal 289: 1400–1401

Aggleton P J, Chalmers H 1989 Next year's models. Nursing Times 85(51): 24–27

Anderson E 1978 The bedpan and the commode. Nursing Times 74(16): 684

Barratt E 1987 Pressure sores. Nursing Times 83(7): 65–70

Barton A, Barton M 1981 The management and prevention of pressure sores. Faber & Faber, London

Boore J R P, Champion R, Ferguson M C 1987 Nursing the physically ill adult. Churchill Livingstone, Edinburgh

Boylan A, Brown P 1985 Respiration. Nursing Times 81(11): 35–38

Closs J 1988 Patient's sleep–wake rhythms in hospital, part 1 & 2. Nursing Times 84(1 & 2): 48–50, 54–55

Court G 1990 Image loss in orthopaedics. Unpublished paper

Creason N S, Pogue N J, Nelson A A, Hoyt C A 1985 Validating the nursing diagnosis of impaired physical mobility. Nursing Clinics of North America 20(4): 669–683

Crewe R 1987 Problems of rubber ring nursing cushions and a clinical survey of alternative cushions for ill patients. Care: Science & Practice 5: 9–11

Crow R 1988 The challenge of pressure sores. Nursing Times 84(38): 68, 71, 73

Crowther H 1982 New perspectives on nursing lower limb amputees. Journal of Advanced Nursing 7: 453–460

David J A 1986 Additions to the bed. Nursing 3(3): 112–114

Downie A, Kennedy P 1980 Lifting, handling and helping patients. Faber & Faber, London

Fenton M, Hughes P 1989 Passivity to empowerment. Royal Association for Disability and Rehabilitation, London

Ford R D 1987 Patient teaching manual 1. Springhouse, Pennsylvania

Gardner A M N, Fox R H 1983 The venous pump of the foot – preliminary report. Bristol Medico-Chirurgical Journal July: 109–112

Gardner A M N et al 1990 Reduction of post-traumatic swelling and compartment pressure by impulse compression on the foot. Journal of Bone & Joint Surgery 72-B(5): 810–815

Gott M, O'Brien M 1990 The role of the nurse in health promotion. Paper presented at Royal College of Nursing research conference, Surrey University

Henley A 1987 Caring in a multiracial society. Bloomsbury Health Authority, London

Hibbert D L 1980 A sore point at home. Nursing Mirror 151(6): 40–41

Horne J A 1983 Human sleep & tissue restitution. Clinical Science 65(6): 569–578

Judd M 1989 Mobility. Heinemann Nursing, London

Kendall & Co 1986 Prophylaxis of deep vein thrombosis. Kendall & Co, London

Kim M J, Aromoro-Seritella R, Gulanick M et al 1984 In: Kim M J, McFarland G K, McLane A M (eds) Classification of nursing diagnosis. C V Mosby, St Louis

Kirk L W 1986 Framework. In: Hurley M E. Classification of Nursing Diagnosis. C V Mosby, St Louis

Krause M V, Mahan L K 1984 Nutritional care in conditions of overweight and underweight. In: Food, nutrition and diet therapy, 7th edn. Saunders, Philadelphia

Locket B 1983 Prevalence and incidence in pressure sore disease. Symposium at the Royal Hospital and Home for the Incurables, London

Love C 1990 Deep vein thrombosis. Nursing Times 86(5 & 6): 40–43, 52–55

Lowthian P 1979 Turning clocks system to prevent pressure sores. Nursing Mirror 148(21): 30–31

Lowthian P 1987 The classification and grading of pressure sores. Care: Science & Practice 5(1): 5–9

Lowthian P 1989 Letter. Care: Science & Practice 7(27)

Mandelstam M 1990 How to get equipment for disability. Jessica Kingsley Publishers & Kogan Page, London

Maslow A H 1954 Motivation and personality. Harper, New York

Maycock J 1988 The image of rheumatic disease. In: Salter M (ed) Altered body image. The nurse's role. John Wiley, Chichester

Miller E 1989 How to make nursing diagnosis work. Appleton & Lange, Connecticut

National Dairy Council 1990 Our daily calcium. National Dairy Council, London

Nordin B E C, Heaney R P 1990 Calcium supplementation of diet justified by present evidence. British Medical Journal 300: 56–60

Office of Health Economics 1990 Osteoporosis and risk of fracture. Office of Health Economics

Open University 1984 Health choices, study package. Open University, Milton Keynes

Oswald I, Adam K 1983 Get a better night's sleep. Martin Dunitz, London

Powell M 1986 Orthopaedic nursing and rehabilitation, 9th edn. Churchill Livingstone, Edinburgh

Pritchard A P, David J A 1988 Manual of clinical nursing procedures, 2nd edn. Harper & Row, London

Reihl J, Roy C 1980 Conceptual models for nursing practice. Appleton-Century-Crofts, Connecticut

Roper N 1988 Principles of nursing in process context, 4th edn. Churchill Livingstone, Edinburgh

Roper N, Logan W 1985 The Roper/Logan/Tierney model. Senior Nurse. 3(2): 20–26

Roper N, Logan W W, Tierney A J 1990 The elements of nursing. Churchill Livingstone, Edinburgh, Ch 4, p 22

Royal College of Physicians 1983 Obesity. Royal College of Physicians 17: 3–58

Royal College of Physicians 1986 Physical disability in 1986 and beyond. Journal of the Royal College of Physicians of London 20(3): 161–194

Salter M 1988 Altered body image. The nurse's role. John Wiley, Chichester

Scales J 1982 Pressure sore prevention. Care: Science & Practice 1(2): 9–17

Scottish Health Services Council 1972 Medical rehabilitation. HMSO, Edinburgh

Seal D V, Borriello S P 1983 Management and treatment in control of hospital-acquired infections. Update Publications, London

Seedhouse D 1986 Health. The foundation for achievement. John Wiley, Chichester

Silk D B A 1983 Nutritional support in hospital practice. Blackwell Scientific, Oxford

Stamatakis J D, Sagar S, Nairn D et al 1977 Femoral vein thrombosis and total hip replacement. British Medical Journal 2(6081): 223–225

Torrance C 1981 The perennial pressure sore, part 3 & 4. Nursing Times 77(12): 9–12, 77(16): 13–16

Versluysen M 1986 Pressure sores in patients admitted for hip operations. Geriatric Nursing 6(2): 20–22

Wainwright H 1978 Feeding problems in elderly disabled patients. Nursing Times 74(13): 542–543

Webster R A, Thompson D R 1986 Sleep in hospital. Journal of Advanced Nursing, 11: 447–457

Woolley N 1990 Nursing diagnosis: exploring the factors which may influence the reasoning process. Journal of Advanced Nursing 15: 110–117

World Health Organization 1980 International classification of impairments, disabilities and handicaps. WHO

Wright L 1990 Bathing by towel. Nursing Times 86(4): 36–39

6

Why restrict movement?

Peter S. Davis

It may be necessary to restrict or limit movement for reasons of health, therapy or safety. It is no coincidence that we have to be able to move freely for reasons of health and safety. The art and science of orthopaedic nursing is based on understanding why an individual's mobility should be controlled and acquiring the skills to achieve this.

This chapter explores the need to restrict movement, both when the individual chooses to limit his own movement and when he is restricted due to the recommendations or prescription of others such as health care professionals. A person may choose to limit his movement if he has backache by lying flat and not lifting or bending until the pain diminishes. Most of this chapter describes the methods of restricting movement for therapeutic reasons, the effects this may have on the patient or client and the related nursing care.

IMMOBILITY

Murray (1976) describes immobilization as 'any prescribed or unavoidable restriction of movement in an area of a person's life. The source of immobilization may be physical, emotional, intellectual or social'. Murray reinforces one of the principal assumptions of immobility when it is due to therapeutic requirements: that generally the patient or client cannot choose or control the extent of his own immobility. The prescription of restricted movement is common in orthopaedic nursing, and it is often the nurse who enforces prescribed restrictions of movement made by the doctor – for example, bedrest, the wearing of a surgical collar or bilateral skin traction to lower limbs.

RESTRICTING MOVEMENT

An individual's freedom of movement is usually restricted for either protective or therapeutic reasons; the whole or part of an individual may be affected.

Protective restrictions

Protective restrictions prevent injury or damage from occurring and are related to aspects of safety. Generally, individuals accept imposed or recommended limitations to their movement. On a global scale, movement from one country to another is restricted for reasons of national security; a recognized document such as a passport is usually necessary to facilitate leaving and entering. The speed at which people travel by road is limited, with penalties imposed if the limits are exceeded. Similarly, the manner in which people travel and the condition of the vehicle in which they travel are monitored: vehicles are tested to ensure brakes and tyres are adequate and that passengers are restrained with seat belts or harnesses to minimize or prevent injury in accidents. (See Ch. 9 for statistical evidence of the number and nature of injuries due to accidents.) In many sports and leisure pursuits participants use strapping, supportive braces and similar appliances to limit the movement of joints, for example, the boots worn by mountain walkers to prevent excessive movement and thus injury to the ankle should they lose their footing.

Therapeutic restrictions

Therapeutic restrictions promote healing and prevent further damage or injury from occurring. In both protective and therapeutic restrictions of movement, it is important to establish who controls the restrictions, as this has implications for nursing care, particularly in the case of therapeutic restrictions.

Intrinsic choice

Restrictions that are chosen and controlled by the patient or client may be considered intrinsic; when making such choices the individual should be well-informed and offered an appropriate selection of alternatives. However, health education and promotion strategies have shown that, in addition to telling the individual why it is necessary to restrict his mobility, the health care professional must be aware of his feelings, values and beliefs if she wants to help him make a suitable decision. For example, a nurse may ask a patient suffering from a localized acute inflammatory condition of the tendons of the wrist, such as tenosynovitis, to rest the wrist for several weeks and explain the reasons for this to him. She may provide him with a wrist splint to be worn 24 hours a day except when he is attending to personal hygiene needs. However, the patient may feel conspicuous when wearing the splint and believe that if he does not rest and wear the splint all the time this will not significantly affect his progress. Also, he may value the activities of living he can carry out when not wearing the splint more than the speedy uneventful recovery that resting and wearing the splint offers. Therapeutic restrictions of movement can be inconvenient and impose major changes on an individual's lifestyle.

To enable or empower an individual to make these intrinsic choices about restrictions to his mobility, the nurse must be aware of all the factors influencing him as outlined above. It is to be hoped that, with knowledge and empowerment, the patient himself will make the decision that will promote a better and speedier recovery, and will be more likely to maintain the restrictions himself. (See Ch. 5 for a discussion of self-empowerment.)

Extrinsic prescription

Those restrictions of movement that are directed and controlled by the health care professional may be considered extrinsic; here, the locus of control is outside the patient or client. It should also be remembered that these prescribed restrictions of movement may not necessarily be in the patient's best interest. Extrinsic control of patient choice may not be deliberate but may be inherent within the health care system; an example of this is the use of technical or jargon terminology in discussing a patient's care and progress in front of him. This approach excludes the patient from the communication process and ensures that information about him remains the exclusive property of health care professionals.

Whenever approaches that ensure that patients receive little or no information about their health care or therapy are used, and patients' questions are discouraged, health care professionals are able to maintain a position of power and control. Patients and clients are often quickly discouraged from taking control of their own care (see, for example, Stockwell's (1972) descriptive research of the unpopular patient). In situations where therapeutic restrictions of movement are necessary, the relationship between patient and nurse must be an equal partnership in which restrictions of movement are prescribed but the patient or client makes his own intrinsic choice. The patient who is restricted to complete bed rest may understand that the more he gets up the slower his recovery will be, but may choose to get up for hygiene and toilet needs only, as slower progress is more acceptable to him than the embarrassment and unacceptability of fulfilling these needs while in bed.

METHODS OF RESTRICTING MOVEMENT

There are many ways of restricting movement for therapeutic reasons. These are usually prescribed by the doctor, but are often applied, maintained, altered and removed by nurses. The orthopaedic nurse, therefore, must have an in-depth understanding of the methods of restricting movement and must be able to relate this to relevant nursing care. A number of methods exist, and at different hospitals there might be slight variations of these, giving rise to wide variation in practice. The remainder of this chapter will describe these methods, discussing general principles rather than providing local detail,

and focusing on those areas that are related to nursing care.

Methods of restricting movement may be considered with reference to:

- drawing (i.e. traction)
- positioning (e.g. elevation of limbs, special beds and slings)
- casting
- splinting
- bandaging and strapping.

Traction

Traction is the act of pulling or drawing. More specifically, orthopaedic traction occurs when 'a pulling force is exerted on a part or parts of the body' (Davis 1989).

To be able to pull there must be something to pull against; that is, something which is pulling in the opposite direction. This is known as counter-traction and occurs when a pulling force is exerted that opposes the direct pull of traction. Hippocrates, in 350 BC, when describing the use of traction in the reduction (realignment of the bones) of a fractured leg, gave the example of two strong men pulling in opposite directions: the pull in one direction was traction, and that in the opposite direction, counter-traction. In this example, the surgeon applies the traction manually and the weight of the injured person with the fractured femur is the counter-traction.

Uses of traction

1. Traction can be used to reduce or hold, as in dislocations and fractures.

2. Traction, when applied to an injured limb, can overcome the effect of the original deforming force and thus reduce a fracture or dislocation of a joint.

3. Traction controls movement of an injured part of the body, thus facilitating the healing of bone.

4. Traction is able to lessen the muscle spasm that always occurs following fractures and dislocations.

5. Traction can be used to prevent or correct

deformity, as in contractures. For example, it can prevent or correct flexion deformity that may occur following inflammation of the hip joint due to infection.

6. Traction overcomes the inevitable muscle spasm and prevents or corrects soft tissue contracture which would reduce the range of movement in the joint.

7. For the same reason traction can be used to prevent contraction of healing soft tissues following joint surgery.

8. Finally, traction may be used to rest joints, as in disease or injury. It can lessen the muscle spasm, as in back pain, or reduce the movement of diseased joints, such as in tuberculosis, and thus minimize pain and facilitate initial healing.

Methods of applying traction

To apply traction a satisfactory grip must be obtained on a part of the patient's body. This may be achieved through the skin or bone and may be for short or long periods of time:

- Manual traction is applied by the hands, as, for example, when a doctor reduces a fracture or holds an alignment whilst a cast or more permanent form of traction is being applied.
- Skin traction is the application of the traction force over a large area of skin and this is then transmitted via the soft tissues to the bone; the maximum pull should not exceed that recommended by the manufacturers of the traction appliance, usually 10–15 lb (4.5–6.7 kg). Two common methods of applying this traction are the adhesive and non-adhesive forms. The adhesive type is not recommended for patients with friable or damaged skin, as the adhesive used and the removal of the adhesive strips may cause further damage. Non-adhesive types are preferred if the traction has to be on for only a short period of time; for example, when used to reduce muscle spasm due to a fractured neck of femur in the few hours prior to surgery.
- Skeletal traction is the application of the traction force directly to a bone, commonly through metal pins or wires.

Counter-traction

In any traction set-up, the whole body tends to be pulled in the direction of the traction force if counter-traction is not present. Counter-traction may be achieved in two main ways:

1. Fixed traction is the application of counter-traction acting through an appliance which obtains purchase on a part of the body. To apply a force against a fixed point on the body, an appliance such as a Thomas' splint is used (see Fig. 6.1). The ring of the splint snugly encircles the root of the limb, i.e. the groin and hip. Traction cords are tied to the distal end of the splint and the counter-traction force passes along the side bars of the splint to the ring, as indicated by the arrows. The grip on the leg is achieved by adhesive skin traction.

2. Sliding or balanced traction utilizes the weight of all or part of the body, acting under the influence of gravity, to provide counter-traction (Stewart & Hallett 1983) (see Fig. 6.2): for instance, the bed is tilted so that the patient tends to 'slide' or move in the opposite direction to that of the traction force. In reality, the pull of gravity should equal that of the traction so that the two are 'balanced' and hence the patient re-

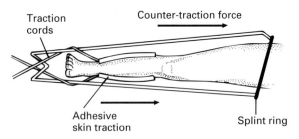

Fig. 6.1 Fixed skin traction using a Thomas' splint.

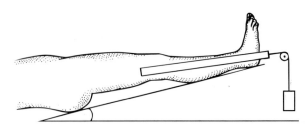

Fig. 6.2 Sliding traction using skin traction and weights.

mains stationary. The traction force is produced by weights and may be applied through a cord passing over a pulley.

Suspension is not traction, as no counter-traction is necessary; it occurs when part or all of the body is suspended to increase the mobility of the patient. It may be used on its own or as part of a traction/suspension system. It is sometimes confused with traction as the same types of equipment may be used to achieve both suspension and traction, and both may be carried out at the same time as part of the patient's treatment.

The nursing care of patients in traction

The nurse must have a clear understanding of how different types of traction work, and realize that although maintenance of a safe, efficient traction system is important, the patient must not be forgotten; for example, when the nurse is setting up or attending to a traction system.

The patient in traction has social and psychological needs as well as physical ones; most of these relate to maintaining a safe environment, and in helping to meet them the nurse should consider the following:

- The traction system should be thoroughly checked at least daily and always after interventions such as physiotherapy and radiographic examination, as the system may be inadvertently altered.

- The cords must be attached securely by standard knots that will not move or come undone – for example, a clove hitch or two half hitches (see Figs 6.3–6.6 and Taylor (1987) for further details).
- The ends of the cords should be short (5 cm) and bound back onto themselves with adhesive tape. This prevents fraying of the cord end and thus possible slipping and accidental disruption of traction. The knot itself should not be covered. It is a misconception that the tape reinforces the knot; the knot should be secure enough by itself.
- Short cords should not be joined by knots as they would not run freely through pulleys, and if incorrectly tied would slip and come undone.
- Cords should be checked daily for fraying, particularly where they pass over pulleys, or for rubbing against each other. Otherwise the system's efficiency is reduced or the cord may break.
- The line of pull of the cords should be correct and regularly checked. This ensures that the appropriate pulling force is applied for optimal therapeutic effect at all times.
- Pulleys must be free-running and oiled as necessary to prevent squeaking. Friction is thus minimized and efficiency maintained, and the patient is not disturbed by the noise. Many pulleys today have plastic components and thus need minimal maintenance.

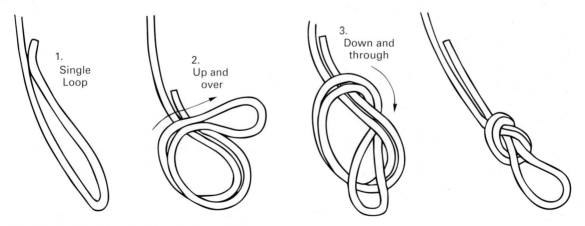

Fig. 6.3 Overhand loop knot, for attaching weights.

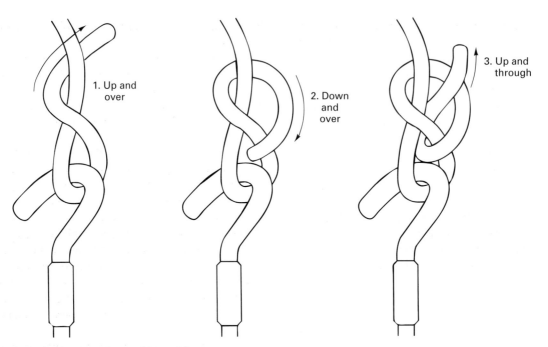

1. Up and over

2. Down and over

3. Up and through

Fig. 6.4 Slip knot, for attaching weights.

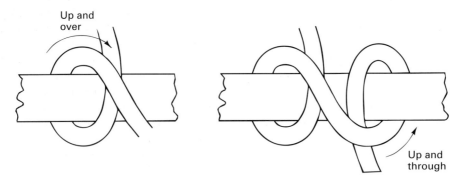

Up and over

Up and through

Fig. 6.5 Clove hitch, for attaching to an appliance such as a Thomas' splint (will not slip).

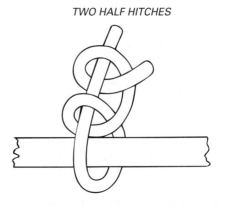

TWO HALF HITCHES

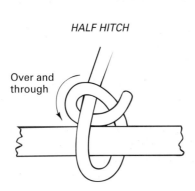

HALF HITCH

Over and through

Fig. 6.6 Half hitches, for reinforcing.

- The cords must rest comfortably in the pulley, one cord to each pulley wheel. This reduces friction and fraying of the cord.
- The weight(s) used must be known and recorded in the nursing documentation, as the required pulling forces of a traction system are often changed during the course of treatment and members of the caring team need this information.
- The weight(s) must hang free and not rest on the floor; otherwise, the efficiency of the system is not maintained.
- To minimize discomfort for the patient, the weight(s) should not catch or jam, particularly on the bed ends, when the patient moves.
- Weight(s) should not be hung over the patient; however, if this is necessary, an extra safety cord should be used.
- Weight(s) should be securely attached by a fish hook (S hook), where available. This aids safe but easy removal of the weight(s) if necessary, for example during physiotherapy.
- Pointed ends of pins or wires, used in skeletal traction, should be covered to prevent injury to the patient and staff.
- The patient should be on a firm-based bed to give full support and comfort and allow efficient action of the traction system.
- Bed aids, such as cradles, should be used to keep bedclothes away from the patient as necessary, for comfort and to ensure free running of the traction cord(s).

The patient in traction will have problems and needs due to reduced mobility and as a direct result of the traction system, such as:

- The traction system itself may apply pressure to certain parts of the patient's body and thus potentially cause pressure sores. These areas – for example, the area in contact with the ring of the Thomas' splint – should be checked 2–4-hourly and the patients themselves taught how to relieve this pressure.
- Skin covered by the traction system should be assessed daily for signs of dryness or allergic reaction. This ensures early detection in, for instance, those patients who are allergic to the adhesives in adhesive skin traction appliances.

- The part of the patient's body which is in the traction system must be correctly aligned and the patient's whole body must be correctly positioned. In this way the efficiency of the system is maintained.
- Any parts of the body not affected by the traction should be moved, using active exercises, to prevent muscle atrophy and joint stiffness, which occur quickly in situations of reduced mobility. For the same reasons the parts of the body in traction should be moved, if possible, using passive and/or active exercises.
- Neurovascular observations – i.e. movement, sensation, colour, warmth and swelling – of the affected limb(s) should be carried out at least 2–4-hourly. The traction equipment, injury or surgery may all, through increased pressure on nerves and blood vessels, cause temporary or permanent damage to nerves and blood vessels.
- Inspection for looseness of the pins or wires and infection at the sites of insertion of skeletal traction should be performed daily or more often, and prevented where possible. Infection at the site of insertion can easily spread to the bone itself, leading to osteomyelitis (Morris et al 1988).

As the most effective way of preventing infection is a controversial issue, agreement should be reached between nurses and medical staff within a unit as to the methods used (see Wallis 1991). After the initial oozing from the site has ceased, the site may be covered with an occlusive or gauze dressing or may be left exposed. Covering the wound may prevent possible contamination and touching by the patient; however, leaving it exposed allows easy observation of the site. Cleaning the site to remove crusts and clots is not recommended for single skeletal pins as the crust provides a barrier to the outside environment. As yet there is no conclusive research to suggest that any one solution is better than another for cleaning pin site wounds (Sproles 1985, Wallis 1991). The site is often sprayed with povidone iodine or covered with a povidone iodine-soaked gauze, both daily, to prevent infection. However, it is suggested that this practice may cause corrosion of the pins and possibly increase the risk of infection.

Bandaging and strapping

The term bandaging will be used to refer to the application of extensible bandages for the purpose of compression or support of an injury, to prevent oedema or to retain other dressings in place. The term strapping will be used to refer to the application of non-extensible strapping for the purpose of support and protection of an injury, to retain dressings in place and to hold lacerated skin edges together.

Uses of bandaging

A common use of bandaging for orthopaedic nurses is to provide compression in order to either control or prevent oedema. For example, a stump bandage applied after amputation will control oedema; a Robert Jones bandage applied immediately after surgery or injury to the knee will prevent oedema (Brodell et al 1986). Whatever the reason for bandaging, it must be remembered that, if applied incorrectly or inappropriately, bandages can easily and quickly cause further injury to the patient. By understanding and putting into practice the basic principles of application and care the nurse is able to minimize risk to the patient and promote rapid healing and recovery.

Tension and pressure

The pressure of a bandage must not exceed the intravascular hydrostatic pressure, if bandaging is to reduce oedema formation without increasing vascular resistance to the detriment of the blood flow. The orthopaedic nurse should understand the purpose of the bandage as different amounts of tension are required depending on the function of the bandage. For example, Chant (1972) showed that the pressure in the lower limb of a recumbent patient is usually exceeded by a pressure of 15–22 mmHg applied externally. However, the pressure beneath a variety of stump bandages was found to average 30–50 mmHg, although some were as high as 170 mmHg (Isherwood et al 1975), thus exceeding the intravascular hydrostatic pressure.

Provided that the tension in the bandage remains constant, then the pressure exerted on the body surface will increase as the radius of curvature or diameter of the limb decreases, according to Laplace's law which states that:

$$Pressure = \frac{tension}{radius}.$$

This means that if a bandage is applied at constant tension to the lower leg of an adult, the pressure will be highest at the ankle where the leg is narrowest and lowest at the top of the calf. This is useful, as a beneficial pressure gradient promoting blood flow back to the heart is naturally achieved from the shape of the leg. Thomas and colleagues (1980) warn that a tension which is acceptable in a bandage applied to a large adult would be potentially hazardous if applied to the decreased diameter of a child's arm or leg due to the increased pressure impeding blood flow.

Surface pressure is also related to the number of layers of bandage applied. The degree of overlap between successive turns will affect the final pressure; every effort should be made to ensure each turn overlaps the one before it by an equal amount to avoid local oedema, caused by tight bands.

Thomas and co-workers (1980) demonstrated that nurses learn to obtain the right amount of tension when bandaging through practice. To develop skills in gauging pressure and tension when applying bandages it is useful for the nurse to practise on a colleague or herself. She can do this by using a sphygmomanometer; for moderate pressure the cuff is put on her ankle and inflated to about 40 mmHg and on her calf it is inflated to 20 mmHg. It should feel pleasantly firm and supportive but not tight. She can then practise applying a bandage to achieve the same effect.

The nurse should always read the manufacturer's instructions when gauging tension to find out how much the bandage should be stretched in application. She can practise stretching the bandage by unrolling about 2 m of new bandage and marking it with a pen, across its width, at 10 cm intervals. She then applies the bandage and measures the distance between the marks. If, for example, the distance between the marks is now 13 cm the bandage has been stretched by 30%. Uniformity of the increased intervals will indicate that the tension has been applied evenly.

Elasticity

The elastic properties of a bandage determine:

- how much tension is necessary to achieve the required pressure
- how well it maintains pressure
- how comfortable it is to wear (Dale 1985).

There is considerable variation in the properties of different types of bandages. For example, cotton stretch bandages require less force to produce a particular extension than crepe or cotton crepe. All bandages tend to lose their tension over a period of time from application. This 'relaxation' can be as much as 50% in less than 20 minutes from application, but again there is a marked variation in the rate of relaxation of different bandage types (Thomas et al 1980).

Types of bandage

The choice of bandage type will depend on how and for what it is being used. The required amount of pressure or compression is a key factor in its selection (see Fig. 6.7). Moderate pressure will improve or increase circulation, thus aiding healing. High compression is most frequently used to prevent oedema and increase venous return, but may also be useful in protecting injured areas and preventing injury by limiting joint movements.

Common types of bandage are listed below in order of their potential to apply increasing pressure.

Conforming bandages These are used primarily for dressing retention (see Orford 1989). They tend to be light and absorbent and have two-way stretch. Common types are cotton BPC and equivalents made from viscose or rayon.

Tubular bandages Tubular bandages have a wide variety of uses and are popular because of their ease of application (see Love 1989). The simple sizing charts enable the user to select the size of dressing most appropriate to the patient's needs with a choice of high, medium or low pressure on application. Thomas and colleagues (1980) recommend Tubigrip-type bandages in situations where low to moderate pressures are desirable.

Low pressure	Moderate pressure	High compression
5–20 mmHg	20–35 mmHg	35–50 mmHg
Dressing fingers	Shoulder spica	Joint injuries involving damage to either muscles or ligaments
Limb dressing retention	Minor sprains and strains	
Securing backslabs in acute injuries	Control of oedema	Major sprains or soft tissue injuries
	Speciality dressing e.g. splinting	Minor fractures
	Robert Jones bandaging	Amputation stumps
		Tenosynovitis
		Corrective bandaging e.g. club foot

Fig. 6.7 Bandage type and possible use.

Lightweight stretch bandages These are probably the most widely used type of bandage (see Love 1989). They may be employed to achieve a moderate pressure. There are two main types: those with twisted cotton, wool or rayon threads, e.g. crepe bandages, and those containing elastomer, such as Lycra or rubber.

Heavy compression bandages These bandages contain varying amounts of elastomeric thread. They are used to apply moderate to high compression over long time periods for support and the prevention of oedema. Usually they are removed at night.

Bandaging techniques

There are many ways to bandage; the choice of technique will depend on the purpose, the area of the body to be bandaged and personal preference. Some techniques may be quite complex. As yet, little research has been carried out on the effectiveness of bandaging in specific situations, which makes it difficult for the nurse to decide whether to bandage or not and which techniques and type of bandage to use.

The nurse may use three basic turns when bandaging (see Fig. 6.8):

1. A circular turn to anchor a bandage
2. A spiral turn used to bandage a long straight part of the body or a part of the body of increasing circumference
3. A figure-of-eight turn to bandage a part of the body of increasing or decreasing circumference.

Dale and associates (1983) found that the figure-of-eight technique appeared to give better graduated pressure than the simple spiral when applied above the ankle for moderate pressure bandaging.

Principles of bandaging

The nurse should remember the following principles when bandaging:

- Select a bandage of appropriate type, width and length.
- Where possible use new bandages; elastic bandages, in particular, lose their elasticity after use or washing.
- Ensure that the patient's skin is clean and dry.
- Cover any wounds before bandaging the injured area.
- Check for pulses, if relevant.
- If appropriate, add padding to pressure risk areas.
- Seek assistance if the part of the body affected needs to be supported during the bandaging process.
- Bandage the part of the body in the position you want it maintained.
- Bandage from smaller to larger circumferences for closer shaping of the bandage to the affected body part.
- If possible, bandage in the direction of venous blood return to prevent blood pooling.
- Keep an even tension on the bandage. This is helped by ensuring that the unrolled part of the bandage is kept close to the body surface.
- Ensure that overlaps of the bandage are even and that the bandage has no creases or wrinkles.
- Be sure to bandage the body part well above and below the affected area, but leave the fingers or toes exposed so that neurovascular observations may be performed.
- Cut the bandage if it is too long; never 'use up' the bandage by applying extra turns when finishing.
- Secure the ends of the bandage, ensuring that the patient cannot injure himself.
- If the bandage is likely to slip, secure it with extra strapping across all the turns.
- Instruct the patient in the care of the bandage and observation of the affected part.

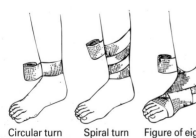

Circular turn   Spiral turn   Figure of eight turn

Fig. 6.8 Basic bandaging turns.

- The skin beneath the bandage should be inspected carefully each time the bandage is removed for signs of damage due to pressure. Remember that sores or nerve damage can occur very rapidly if the bandage is too tight.
- Ensure that the skin is washed each time the bandage is removed.
- Record the details of the bandaging in the patient's documentation.

Uses of strapping

In acute injuries, strapping may be used with compression bandaging to control bleeding, effusion or post-traumatic oedema. The use of strapping on its own to control swelling is not advised as with further swelling the circulation and peripheral nerves may be compromised (Adams 1985). Strapping may be used to prevent the patient making the injury more severe, or for protecting a joint against injury in the first instance.

Types of strapping

Common types of strapping are as follows.

Elastic cohesive strappings These possess a limited amount of elasticity and stick only to themselves and not to skin or hair (see Jamieson 1989). They are an alternative to adhesive strapping as they do not cause allergic reactions or skin trauma on removal.

Adhesive strappings Adhesive strappings are coated on one side with an adhesive (see Jamieson 1989). They possess little elasticity. Skin preparation is usually necessary prior to application, or the bandage may be applied over stockinette, Opsite or conforming bandage.

Principles of strapping

The nurse should follow the guidelines listed below when carrying out strapping:

1. Select strapping of appropriate type and width. The more irregular the surface and the more acute the angles, the narrower the strapping should be; for example, for hands use ½- or

1-in strapping, and for ankles use 1½- or 2-in strapping.

2. Ensure that the patient's skin is clean and dry.

3. If adhesive strapping is applied directly onto the skin, remove hair from the affected part to prevent discomfort on removal of the strapping.

4. Check for pulses, if relevant.

5. Strap the affected part of the body in the position required for support.

6. Avoid encircling turns, if possible, as further swelling may occur.

7. Overlap strapping by at least half its width; otherwise, the strapping may separate during activity and damage the skin trapped between the edges.

8. Instruct the patient in the care of the strapping and in observation of the affected part.

9. Inspect the skin carefully each time the strapping is removed.

10. Record the details of the strapping in the patient's documentation.

Adams (1985) suggests that the average ankle strapping applied in an Accident and Emergency Department performs badly biomechanically due to poor application and inappropriate selection of bandage and technique. However, in some cases, such as neighbour strapping – strapping an injured finger to a sound one to act as a splint – there is real benefit from the procedure. (For other examples of some common bandaging and strapping techniques, see Barrett 1980.)

Casting and plaster casts

For several hundred years, casting in many different materials has been used to immobilize fractured limbs due to injury. Hippocrates in about 350 BC used cloth stiffened by waxes and resins for fractures. In the 16th century, Cheselden, an English surgeon, used bandages soaked in egg white and flour to form a cast. Matthysen, a Dutch military surgeon, was the first to record the use of plaster of Paris bandages in 1852. The bandages were made by rubbing dry plaster of Paris into coarsely woven cotton bandages; these were then soaked in water before application. It is only in the recent past that a range of materials with different properties to suit specific purposes has been developed and produced commercially.

Use of casts

To make a cast, the casting material is applied to the patient's limb or trunk and held in position until it hardens sufficiently. Materials are chosen which can be moulded to fit closely to the bone contours. The functions of casts in therapy and following traumatic injury and orthopaedic surgery may be summarized as follows (Stewart & Hallett 1983):

1. To support fractured bones, controlling movement of the fragments and resting the damaged soft tissues
2. To stabilize and rest joints in which there has been ligamentous injury
3. To support and immobilize joints and limbs postoperatively until healing has occurred, e.g. after nerve or tendon repair
4. To correct deformity by wedging the cast or by the application of serial casts
5. To ensure that infected tissues rest
6. To make a removable splint to aid progressive mobility programmes or prevent deformity
7. To render it difficult for a patient, such as a child, to remove dressings or tamper with the wound
8. To make a negative mould of a body part, as a preliminary step in the accurate construction of orthotic or prosthetic appliances.

Materials used for casts

There are an increasing number of materials available for casting, either on their own or in combination. These fall into the following categories (Stewart & Hallett 1983):

- Plaster of Paris (Gypsone BP)
- Plaster of Paris with melamine resins
- Materials which undergo polymerization, i.e.:
  — Water-activated
  — Non-water-activated
- Low-temperature thermoplastics.

Plaster of Paris　Plaster of Paris bandages are manufactured by heating gypsum powder and suspending it in a solvent. The slurry is used to coat gauze cloth and the solvent is then removed by drying the cloth in an oven. The bandages are cut, rolled and wrapped in moisture-resistant packets. They will last for about 2–3 years if stored appropriately. Plaster of Paris consists of the compound calcium sulphate.

When the bandage is immersed in water and then removed, heat is given off and quickly growing solid crystals of mouldable gypsum are produced:

$$2(CaSO_4{\tfrac{1}{2}}H_2O) + 3H_2O \Leftrightarrow 2(CaSO_4 2H_2O) + heat$$

Plaster of Paris　　water　　gypsum

This reversible reaction explains the properties of plaster of Paris. The patient must be warned that the plaster will feel warm when first applied. Additional heat, usually from the patient's body and surrounding air, drives off water from the gypsum, producing plaster of Paris. The patient must therefore be advised that the plaster will feel cold during the drying process and that he must not cover the cast, to allow for evaporation of the water.

Plaster of Paris with melamine resins　The addition of melamine resin, which sets after being in contact with water, reinforces the plaster of Paris bandage; this produces a lighter and more X-ray-translucent cast than those made only from plaster of Paris.

Materials which undergo polymerization　When the smaller molecules of the resin link to form long-chain polymers (polymerization), the resin's properties change from a mouldable form to a rigid state. This process is usually activated by water, but some resins may be polymerized by other agents. Resins are used to coat fabrics such as polyester, cotton or even fibreglass.

Low-temperature thermoplastics　These materials are plastic and have properties which change with temperature. They become soft and mouldable when heated and harden when cooled. Providing that they are dry when applied to the patient they will not burn at the temperatures required to make them soft; the increased conductivity of water would cause rapid transfer of heat to the skin and lead to burning.

Selection of appropriate casting material

For further details of available casting materials, their trade names, relative costs, advantages and disadvantages and methods of application, see Stewart and Hallett (1983), Smith and Nephew Medical Ltd (1991) and Wytch and Mitchell (1986). There is, at present, much debate about which casting material is most appropriate for which purpose. Wytch and Mitchell (1986) argue that, despite the popularity of plaster of Paris, it is not an ideal splinting material as it has a poor strength-to-weight ratio and loses strength rapidly when wetted. It can affect adversely the definition of X-rays, is messy and takes days to dry. Conversely, Loder (1986) suggests that plaster of Paris is preferred by patients as it is slightly supple at its edges, whereas synthetic casts have ragged edges which may easily damage delicate skin. Plaster of Paris can be split if tension increases due to swelling or if it is windowed for dressings or bivalved for splints. Furthermore, it is significantly cheaper than synthetic casting materials.

It is an important principle that a synthetic cast should not be put on anyone with a history of allergic reactions. Gloves should be worn by the person applying the cast and by the assistant when using synthetic materials.

Ideally, a casting material should be:

- Able to be applied directly to the patient
- Easy to mould to the body contours
- Non-toxic to the patient and user during application, while it is worn and when it is removed
- Unaffected by fluids such as water
- Transparent to X-rays
- Easy to alter and modify
- Quick-setting
- Easy and safe to remove
- Permeable to air, odour, water and pus
- Light but strong
- Non-inflammable

- Clean to use and remove
- Cheap and easily available in a variety of sizes.

Principles of applying a cast

Many different techniques are used in applying a cast but the basic principles remain the same whether the cast is made from plaster of Paris or synthetics (Miles & Barr 1991).

Preparation of equipment and materials All equipment and materials should be prepared and assembled before application commences. The basic casting trolley should contain the following (Miles & Barr 1991):

- Stockinette, if required
- Synthetic padding and / or felt
- Plaster of Paris bandages and slabs if necessary
- Plaster strips to finish
- Marking pencil
- Knife
- Scissors
- Elbow or knee rest
- Protective plastic sheeting
- Plastic aprons
- Plastic-covered pillows
- Bucket or bowl of water
- Bowl of water for washing the patient's skin
- Towel
- Rubbish bag
- Patient information leaflet.

Preparation of patient The person applying the cast and the assistants should not forget the patient in the effort to ensure that an appropriate and good quality cast is applied. The following guidelines illustrate those areas of patient care that are of particular importance:

1. Pain and anxiety should be relieved as much as possible prior to application. Appropriate analgesia and correct positioning of the patient and affected part of the body will alleviate the pain. Reassurance and an explanation of the process throughout the procedure will reduce anxiety.
2. The nurse should:
   a. check the patient's documentation for relevant information, treatment details and casting instructions

b. seek the patient's permission to proceed
c. maintain privacy while removing relevant patient clothing
d. remove and store safely any relevant rings or jewellery; remember some cultures wear rings on toes and chains around ankles
e. check the skin on the affected body part for sores, abrasions and bruising; clean, wash or dress as appropriate
f. ensure that the patient is in a comfortable position and that the affected part can be maintained in the same position during application; this can be achieved either with supports such as knee rests and pillows or with an assistant(s)
g. protect the patient with plastic sheeting.

Applying the cast   When the patient and equipment have been prepared, application may commence. Stockinette should be fitted only if there is no likelihood of any swelling, as stockinette is difficult to cut through and may crease causing further localized pressure. Fitting a cast is a highly skilled task and should not be undertaken lightly as a poor cast rapidly causes temporary or permanent injury to the patient. The average orthopaedic nurse should:

- understand the principles of casting
- be able to recognize a good and bad cast
- be able to identify and prevent potential problems
- be able to act swiftly and appropriately if problems do occur.

However, she should not be expected to apply the 'occasional' cast once or twice a year without supervision or guidance. All nurses who are regularly applying casts should seek to maintain and improve their skills as part of their professional development through courses and skills training.

The following guidelines on fitting a plaster of Paris cast apply to any type of casting material. The nurse should:

1. Apply wool padding, usually as a single layer but with extra layers around bony prominences; this allows for swelling of the body part, reduces friction of the cast against the skin and acts as a protective barrier when shears and saws are used to remove the cast
2. Soak the bandage in lukewarm water, 25–30°C; cold water slows and hot water quickens the setting process
3. Remove the bandage when bubbles stop, squeezing very gently; only soak one bandage at a time
4. Roll the bandages on, maintaining contact between the roll of the bandage and the body part
5. Start from one end of the affected part, covering approximately one-third of the previous turn; tension on the bandage is not required
6. Allow the bandage to form tucks to fit the contours of the body; never twist the bandage as ridges will be formed
7. Apply all the bandages successively, continuously smoothing and rubbing to enable the cast to bond and laminate
8. Trim the edges when the cast is complete and has set, to allow all joints not encased to move freely; this should be carried out on a pillow with a waterproof cover so that the cast is not indented
9. Handle the cast at all times during setting and drying with the palms of the hands and not fingers; otherwise, indentations will be formed with the risk of pressure sore development
10. Turn back the stockinette, if used, over the edges of the cast and hold it in place with strips of plaster of Paris bandage
11. Clean the patient's skin and supply any necessary supports or walking aids such as arm slings, collar and cuff or crutches.

Drying the cast   A plaster of Paris cast takes minutes to set firmly enough to maintain the affected part of the body in the required position. However, the cast will take from 24 hours for a small arm cast to 96 hours for a total body cast to dry and reach its full strength. As the cast dries it will change from a matt grey colour with a musty smell, to a shiny white colour with no odour. The nurse should take the same care when drying a cast as when applying one. The following principles should be understood:

1. The cast should be well supported, to prevent sagging; a fracture board can be used for large casts such as hip spicas.
2. To prevent pressure on bony prominences, the affected part should be rested on pillows with waterproof coverings.
3. To aid drying:
   a. The pillows should be covered by towelling or similar absorbent material, which should be changed every few hours.
   b. The cast must be exposed to the air in a warm dry atmosphere and not covered by clothing or bed clothes; the rest of the patient should be kept well covered so that he does not feel cold.
   c. The use of artificial heat, such as that obtained from lamps or hairdryers, is not recommended as the cast may crack if it dries too rapidly; there is also a danger of burning the patient as the cast stores heat and transmits it only slowly through to the body surface, which means that the wet skin surface may be at a high temperature even after the heat source is removed.
   d. Patients in large casts should change position by turning every few hours so that all of the cast is dried. This may require the assistance of a nurse(s).
4. Limbs in casts should be elevated using pillows, foot rests or slings to aid venous return and, if trauma has occurred, to prevent or reduce oedema.
5. The cast should be observed regularly for cracking, softening and breakdown at the edges and acute angles. These observations should be continued by the nurse and patient once the cast is dry.

The nursing care of a patient in a cast

There are two main complications which may occur: the development of pressure sores under the cast, and circulatory impairment due to the constriction of the cast. Both of these problems are more prevalent immediately after surgery, trauma or therapy, when the affected body part may swell or become oedematous. Greater vigilance is therefore required when the cast is first applied, and for a few days following application. A swelling limb within a rigid cast rapidly leads to an increase in pressure which affects circulation and impedes nerve conduction, and therefore action must be taken promptly before irreversible damage occurs. It is essential that, whenever possible, the patient is involved in his own care to detect and respond appropriately to problems that may arise.

The guidelines outlined below on the nursing care of patients in a cast are listed under the potential complication to which they refer. The nurse should make the relevant observations every 30 minutes initially, reducing these to daily as the patient's condition dictates and when the cast has dried.

Circulatory and nerve impairment

1. To detect arterial compression, the nurse should observe the extremities of the limb for whiteness/pallor or blueness. The toes or finger nails will remain white, or be slow to return to pink when pressed. The movement of the digits will also be limited and painful. If accessible, peripheral pulses should be felt for.
2. To detect venous compression, the nurse should observe the extremities of the limb for excessive redness, pain and, sometimes, swelling.
3. To detect nerve compression, the nurse should be attentive to complaints of pins and needles, which if not acted upon may lead to numbness, limitation of movement and pain in the limb.
4. To detect compartment syndrome, the nurse should be alert to pain on passive movement of the digits or limb, as well as the signs of circulatory and nerve compression (Farrell 1986). A compartment consists of a muscle group surrounded by a tough inelastic fascial tissue. There is little room for swelling to occur and

pressure quickly builds up, impeding circulation and compressing nerves. The muscle group then rapidly becomes ischaemic. Medical staff should be informed immediately. If problems are detected, all or some of the following actions should be taken:

a. The limb should be elevated.
b. The cast should be split right down to the skin as even a few threads of padding left uncut could impair circulation.
c. If there is local pressure on a nerve, a window may be cut.
d. Compartment syndrome may require immediate surgery – a fasciotomy – to relieve the pressure built up in the muscle compartment before irreversible damage occurs to the ischaemic muscle.

Pressure/cast sores

1. To detect pressure/cast sores the nurse should observe for the following (Powell 1986):
a. itching beneath the plaster
b. a characteristic burning pain; this should not be ignored as the tissues quickly become ischaemic leading to numbness and disappearance of the pain
c. disturbed sleep, restlessness and fretfulness in children
d. local areas of heat on the plaster
e. swelling of the fingers or toes once immediate swelling has subsided
f. a characteristic offensive smell due to tissue necrosis
g. the appearance of discharge.

2. Edges of casts can be eased or trimmed, but should not have extra padding inserted as this will only increase the pressure or the padding could fall further down into the cast. Cotton wool should not be used for padding as it tends to be compressed into hard small pellets which cause further problems when the pellets fall into the cast and become lodged.

3. A window should be carefully cut and removed as a whole piece for inspection of a potential sore site. To prevent local oedema the window must be replaced.

4. Foreign objects inside the cast (see Fig. 6.9) can be detected by radiography and the cast may have to be removed.

5. No objects, such as knitting needles, must be pushed down the cast to scratch itching areas as skin damage can easily occur.

Stiffness of joints and allergic reactions

Stiffness will occur in those joints held in the cast; the patient can overcome this by undertaking progressive exercise programmes when the cast is removed. However, joints outside of the cast may also become stiff if the patient is unwilling to move them or does not understand that they can and should be moved.

Plaster of Paris itself or other synthetic casting material rarely produces an allergic reaction but the padding may. The possibility of an allergic reaction may be anticipated from the patient's past history, and the patient should be instructed in what to observe for.

The nurse should follow the principles of care

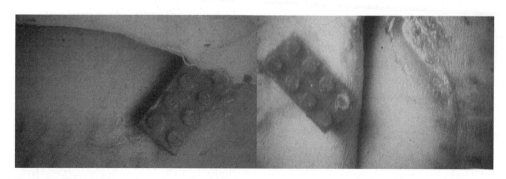

Fig. 6.9 Plaster sores.

listed below to reduce the effects of joint stiffness and a possible allergic reaction in the patient.

1. To prevent joint stiffness, the patient should be given verbal and written instructions on specific exercises to be carried out.

2. To detect allergic reactions, the nurse should observe for complaints of itching, a non-localized burning pain, rashes and blistering of the skin. The medical officer should be informed and the cast will need to be removed. The skin is cleaned and treated and a new cast applied using other materials.

Instructions to patients

During the period of wearing a cast, the patient must always be sufficiently well-informed to take control of his own care by looking after himself and the cast and checking for and responding to any problems that may arise. This should apply whether the person is in hospital or in the community. Any information given should be reinforced and supported by written instructions, which should contain information similar to that in Figure 6.10. Whenever necessary, these instructions should be given to any other relevant carers, such as parents and relatives.

Footner (1987) describes the patient's fears of not being able to move or perform daily living activities when a cast has been applied. She emphasizes that with gentle explanation and reassurance these worries can be alleviated. Some patients report feeling anxious and agitated as a result of being partially enclosed, which is similar to a claustrophobic reaction. However irrational this may appear, the patient must be comforted, and in some cases relaxation exercises or the prescription of a mild tranquillizer may be necessary.

A quick and simple means of determining whether a patient is having problems with his cast is to observe the following elements (see Fig. 6.10) in relation to the affected limb:

- colour
- warmth
- sensation
- movement
- swelling.

Report back to the hospital if at any time you experience any of these:

- Toes or fingers become blue, swollen or difficult and painful to move
- The limb becomes painful
- You feel 'pins and needles' or numbness
- You have 'blister-like' or 'burning' pain
- You see any discharge or wetness or detect an unpleasant smell from the cast
- If you drop anything under the cast
- If the cast becomes cracked, soft or loose
- If you are worried at all about yourself or your cast

THE TELEPHONE NUMBER TO RING IS: ....

- Keep the cast dry and allow it to dry out naturally, leaving it uncovered
- Do not apply external heat such as a hairdryer or by sitting in front of a fire
- If an irritation occurs under the cast, never poke anything down the cast
- Wash the skin around the cast daily, checking for redness or sores
- Never try to pad the edges of the cast if it is rubbing, but seek advice
- Do not let the limb hang down, especially in the first few days
- Carry out the exercises you have been shown for your fingers or toes and other joints of your body, for 5 minutes every hour during the day
- Do not misuse your cast, for instance by weight-bearing before you have been instructed to do so

Fig. 6.10 Instructions for patients.

It is also useful to compare the affected limb with the unaffected limb, if it is available. For example, the fingers of a person wearing an arm cast may feel cold to an active busy nurse, but when compared to that person's other hand they may be at the same temperature.

When observing casts that are stained by oozing of blood or pus, the nurse may find it useful to mark the edges of the stain with a pen and put a time next to it. When subsequent observations are made, then a comparison with any further oozing that has occurred can be made.

Coping with a cast

Pearson (1987) found that patients wearing below-knee casts had difficulty in carrying out activities of living, which had not been anticipated by nurses. Most patients experienced at least some difficulty with those activities related to hygiene. Over 90% of those not given specific information about how to take a bath were unable to do so. However, of those given information on how to prevent the cast getting wet, 90% were able to take a bath. Empowering patients to make decisions and take control of their care in this way is an essential element of the nurse's role but, as Pearson showed, it is not often carried out by nurses.

Removing a cast

The removal of a cast is a skilled task and is usually achieved by bivalving it, i.e. deliberately cutting it in half, and not by hacking it off the body or limb. The following principles should be applied:

1. Clear instructions should be obtained from the medical staff.
2. The patient should be positioned appropriately, for example lying supine using a knee rest for the removal of a lower leg cast.
3. A clear explanation and, if necessary, a demonstration of the procedure and how the equipment is used should be given to the patient.
4. Equipment and techniques used should not damage the patient's skin.
5. The patient should be comfortable and not subjected to any pain.
6. The bivalved cast should be kept on to support the limb until it is decided by medical staff that it can be discarded.

Casts may be cut with shears or oscillating electric saws. Synthetic casts require special shears and saws with tungsten hardened blades. Generally, shears are used for casts on children, small casts and upper limb casts. Oscillating saws must not be used on unpadded casts as the skin beneath will be cut.

Bivalving casts The technique and equipment used to remove casts should at all times be safe for patient and operator. The lines along which the cast is to be cut should be marked with a pen or pencil. The lines should avoid bony promi-

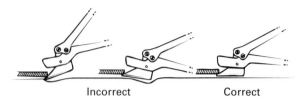

Incorrect   Correct

Fig. 6.11 Bivalving with plaster shears.

nences to reduce the risk of skin damage; for example, a lower leg cast should be marked down either side with lines passing in front of the lateral malleolus and behind the medial malleolus.

Using shears The blade of the shears passes between the cast and the padding and should be kept parallel to the limb. This prevents the point of the heel of the shears digging into the patient's skin and pinching it (see Fig. 6.11). After both sides have been cut, the plaster is eased open with spreaders and the padding cut with bandage scissors.

Using an oscillating saw The saw has an oscillating circular blade; the blade does not rotate but vibrates back and forth at high speed, rubbing its way through the cast. It should be used only on dry padded casts. The blade is held at right angles to the cast and applied with light pressure to make a cut. The blade is then removed and reapplied slightly higher or lower down the cast along the line to be cut (see Fig. 6.12). The blade must not be dragged along the cast as the skin may be cut. As with all electrical appliances, the saw should not be handled by someone with wet hands. The blade may become very hot and burn the skin if it is used continuously for long periods of time, particularly on synthetic materials. To reduce the risk of inhalation of fine dust particles, and to comply with safety regulations, a vacuum removal system should be used with the saw.

To allay the patient's anxiety, the nurse can demonstrate the use of the saw by placing it on the palm of her hand to show that it will not cut. She must remember not to move it across the hand as it will cut if dragged in this way.

Skin care

When a cast is worn for any length of time the

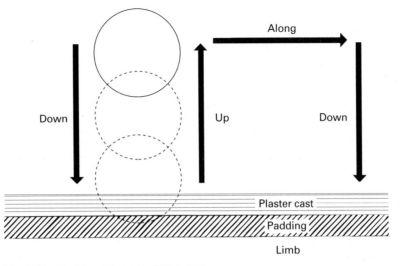

Fig. 6.12 Bivalving with an oscillating saw.

upper layers of skin cannot be shed as normal and so collect as flaky yellow scales. In addition, the muscles lose tone and bulk because of disuse. Before the nurse finally removes any part of the cast she must warn the patient of this scaly, withered appearance.

The skin can be washed gently and patted dry. The skin flakes should not be picked off. Oil or cream should be applied if the skin is dry. Some support, such as bandages or shaped support stockings may be necessary to control swelling, particularly for lower limbs. The patient then begins a progressive, gentle exercise programme.

Splinting and appliances

The term 'orthosis' is gradually replacing words such as splint, appliance and brace (Footner 1987). An orthosis is a device which is added externally to the patient, to enable him to get better use of the part of the body to which it is fitted. This should not be confused with a prosthesis, which replaces a missing part of the body such as an amputated limb.

Use of orthoses

Powell (1986) proposes that orthoses can be used for the following purposes:

- To provide immobilization and local rest by limiting movement of the limb
- To provide fixed traction
- To provide a cradle for the limb in a balanced traction system
- To prevent deformity, correct mild deformity or retain correction when this has been achieved
- To relieve weight
- To stabilize joints and protect weak muscles
- To maintain extension of the spine or hips and knees for maintenance of the correct posture when the individual is weight-bearing.

The nursing care of a patient with an orthosis

Many of the principles of nursing care for a patient with an orthosis are similar to those for a patient in a cast. In particular, there is the potential problem of pressure sore development due to an ill-fitting splint. For patients with a neurological deficit whose skin is anaesthetic, the problem is more serious as they are unable to feel the development of a sore. It is essential for the nurse to teach the patient to apply, use and maintain the orthosis so that he can care for himself and detect any problems at an early stage. Any information given by the nurse should be reinforced and supported with written instructions, as with casts.

Pressure sores

In addition to being aware of the causation and prevention of pressure sores in patients with casts, as described on page 118, the nurse should take note of the following additional points:

• The skin should be kept clean and dry, as dampness, usually due to sweating, is a contributory cause of pressure sores.
• Talcum powder should be used only in moderation.
• When the splint is applied initially, the areas of skin beneath it which are subjected to pressure should be observed every 2 hours. Once the skin has hardened and got used to pressure, the number of observations and amount of care may be reduced.

Orthotic designs are continually changing as new materials and techniques are developed and expertise increases. Simpson and Greig (1984) describe the full range of materials in use and their applications for orthoses. The continued increasing development of dynamic splints for limbs and hands has led to a dramatic improvement in the range of movement of joints following trauma or surgery (Swan 1984, Levins & Stuttle 1984).

An orthosis is made by an orthotist but it is the patient, doctor, orthotist and nurse, functioning as a team, who ensure that the patient continues to wear the orthosis correctly and safely. An orthosis can make a substantial difference to the quality of life of an individual, giving him a greater independence and functional ability. However, even though aesthetically acceptable orthoses can now be made, wearing an orthosis can affect an individual's body image and self-esteem. The nurse's empathy and support are necessary to help the patient adjust to and accept the situation.

Instructions to patients

Patients must be instructed in caring for an orthosis (and themselves) (see Fig. 6.13) to ensure that it functions properly.

Report back to the hospital if at any time you experience any difficulties:

THE TELEPHONE NUMBER TO RING IS: ....

• Always handle the orthosis with care and avoid dropping it or leaving it where it may get damaged.
• Examine your skin at least twice daily for signs of pressure or damage due to the orthosis. Get these seen to immediately.
• Keep up the simple maintenance schedule given to you, e.g. clean locks and oil joints weekly.
• Inspect all moving parts regularly for wear and tear.
• Clean the orthosis and your skin as directed.
• Keep the heels and soles of footwear in good condition to prevent falls.

Fig. 6.13 Instructions for patients.

WALKING AIDS

Most people at some time in their life will depend on or require an aid to help them walk. Toddlers require adults or push-walkers to help them balance as they begin to learn to walk, and the same support is often required when people's coordination and muscle strength diminish with age.

The patient's safety, when using walking aids, is essential. He should be well-informed, instructed correctly and monitored to ensure that they are used properly; this applies to all aids. There are many types of walking aids, some of which have been discussed in Chapter 5 (see also Mandlestam 1990 for information on the full range of aids to ambulation and where they may be obtained). The rate and extent of the development of these aids is demonstrated in Broadhurst's (1990) description of the total support walking frame. This frame is intended for people who do not have sufficient balance to use a normal wheeled walker, as it is virtually impossible to tip over and yet small enough to fit through a 26-inch doorway.

Crutches and walking sticks are commonly used when walking restrictions are prescribed, as for example when a lower limb cast is applied and the patient has to be non-weight-bearing, or when the stresses through a joint need to be reduced due to diseases such as osteoarthritis.

Stewart and Hallett (1983) identify four criteria which should be considered each time a walking aid is selected:

1. The stability of the patient
2. The strength of the patient's upper and lower limbs
3. The degree of coordination of movement of the upper and lower limbs
4. The degree of relief of weight-bearing required.

Crutch walking

Sykes (1985) and Kay (1990), both student nurses, independently describe the problems they encountered when they started walking with crutches. They relate feelings such as: 'For the first time in my adult life, I was completely dependent on others. I could no longer go where I wished'. Previously unconsidered restrictions were encountered: 'Somebody had to stay with me to carry my handbag'.

Axillary crutches are the most commonly used type in the UK, whereas elbow crutches are favoured on the Continent. However, recent work by Hall and Clark (1990) has led to the recommendation that open-cuff elbow crutches should be withdrawn as they have been shown to be unsafe and do not conform to British Standard Specification 4988.

Measurement for crutches

The length of the crutch for each patient may be measured in several ways:

- Subtract 16 inches (40 cm) from the patient's height.
- With the patient lying supine, measure the distance from the axilla to the bottom edge of the heel of the shoe.

If the patient is standing with feet together and with the crutches placed under the arms and resting on the floor by the patient's feet, there should be a 1–2-inch gap between the top of the crutch and the axilla.

The position of the handgrip should be such that the elbow is at 30° of flexion when the person is standing.

Standing position

When first using the crutches the patient should be allowed time to feel stable in the upright position. With the crutches, a balanced or tripod position is achieved with the foot of the crutch about 4 inches (10 cm) in front and 6 inches (15 cm) to the side of the outside edge of each foot. All walking starts from this position. The weight must rest on the hands and not the axilla, as pressure on the axilla will press on the nerve plexus leading to possible crutch paralysis or palsy. Indications of this are complaints of pins and needles or paraesthesia, inability to make a fist and wristdrop.

Walking

Lane and Leblanc (1990) and Stewart and Hallett (1983) identify and describe several types of gaits that may be used for crutch walking. These provide varying speeds of movement for the crutch walker and require varying balancing abilities as a prerequisite:

- Swinging crutch gait; fast, needs good balance
- Four-point crutch gait; slow, for poor balance
- Three-point crutch gait; fairly fast, needs reasonable balance
- Two-point crutch gait; fairly fast, needs good balance.

Which gait to use will also depend on the amount of weight the person can put through each or both feet. This may range from non-weight-bearing to partial weight-bearing to full weight-bearing.

Three-point crutch gait The commonest gait used by a patient needing to be partial or non-weight-bearing on one leg is the three-point gait, as the weight will be supported by the stronger leg and the two crutches; for example, after unilateral surgery or injury to the lower limb.

Starting from the balanced or tripod position the crutches are simultaneously moved forward a short distance, about 12 inches (30 cms). The patient must be advised not to attempt large distances at each movement. The affected leg is then swung forward to the crutches, then the patient steps forward with the unaffected leg, and so on (see Fig. 6.14).

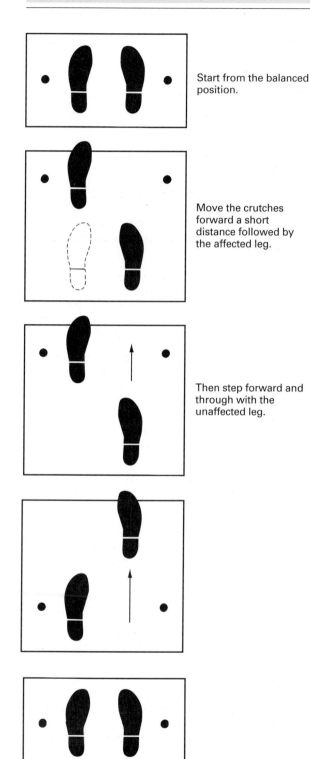

Start from the balanced position.

Move the crutches forward a short distance followed by the affected leg.

Then step forward and through with the unaffected leg.

Fig. 6.14 The three-point crutch gait.

Sitting and standing

There are several ways for a patient to sit and get out of a chair safely. The simplest way to sit down is for the patient to position himself so that he stands with his back to the chair and the unaffected leg just touching the seat of the chair. Both crutches are then transferred to the hand on the affected limb's side and the other hand is used to grasp the arm rest and sit down (see Fig. 6.15). The crutches are then placed within reach in a safe position. The reverse procedure is carried out when standing.

Going up and down stairs

To go up stairs the patient positions himself at the bottom of the stairs. Both crutches are then transferred to the hand opposite the wall or handrail. Pushing down on the crutches and supported by the wall or handrail the patient lifts the unaffected leg onto the first step (see Fig. 6.16). Remember, 'up with the good' leg first. The affected leg and crutches are then lifted onto the first step and the process repeated.

To go down stairs the same procedure is followed except the affected leg and crutches are the first to be moved onto the first step down, followed by the unaffected leg (see Fig. 6.17). Remember, 'down with the bad' leg first.

In going up and down stairs the crutches are moved with the affected leg.

Care of the crutches: instructions to patients

Written instructions to patients should contain

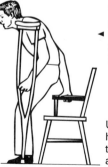
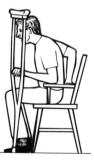

Transfer both crutches to the hand on the affected limb's side

Use the other hand to grasp the arm rest and sit down

Fig. 6.15 Sitting in a chair.

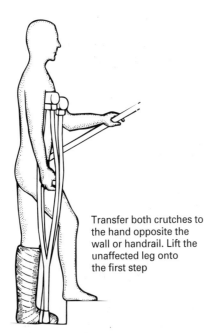

Transfer both crutches to the hand opposite the wall or handrail. Lift the unaffected leg onto the first step

Fig. 6.16   Going up stairs.

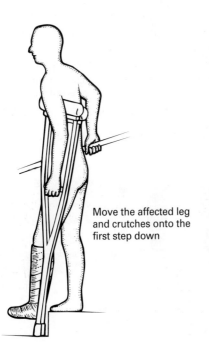

Move the affected leg and crutches onto the first step down

Fig. 6.17   Going down stairs.

information similar to that in Figure 6.18. To promote safety the crutches must be checked regularly to:

- Ensure the wood or metal is not cracked
- Tighten all adjusting nuts and ensure any

Report back to the hospital if at any time you experience any difficulties:

THE TELEPHONE NUMBER TO RING IS: ....

Generally:
- Stand with the crutches about 4 inches to the side of your feet and 6 inches in front, making a triangle
- Always take small steps
- Be careful on slippery or wet floors
- Wear tie shoes with low heels
- Check the rubber tips for wear twice a week
- Do not rest your armpit on the top of the crutch
- Your hands should take the weight on the hand grips
- You should be able to put two fingers between your armpit and the top of the crutch
- Your elbows should be slightly bent

Walking:
- Move both crutches in front of you
- Move the affected leg forward
- Move the unaffected leg through

Sitting in a chair:
- Stand with your back to the chair
- Put both crutches into the hand on the side of the affected leg
- Use the other hand to grasp the arm rest and sit down
- Place the crutches safely and within reach
- Reverse the procedure to stand up

Going up stairs:
- Move to the bottom of the stairs
- Put both crutches into the hand opposite the wall or handrail
- Lift the unaffected leg onto the first step
- Move the crutches and your affected leg onto the same step

Going down stairs:
- Move to the top of the stairs
- Put both crutches into the hand opposite the wall or handrail
- Move the affected leg and crutches onto the first step down
- Move the unaffected leg down onto the same step

Fig. 6.18   Instructions for patients using crutches.

spring-loaded double-ball catches are working properly

- Determine that rubber tips are in good condition and change them if badly worn
- Ensure hand grips and axillary pads are in good condition.

Stick walking

The walking-stick is usually made of wood with a C-curved handle and a rubber tip on the lower end. Adjustable sticks made from aluminium alloy tubing are also available. Walking sticks are lighter and more easily stored than crutches, but are only able to assist balance slightly and to provide moderate support for the lower limb. They cannot be used unless the person can partial or full weight-bear on the affected limb. They can be used to decrease the amount of body weight taken through the lower limb, compensating for weakness and providing pain relief.

Once a lower limb is able to partial weight-bear, two sticks may be substituted for crutches.

Measurement for sticks

The length of the walking stick may be measured by placing the handle of the stick on the floor. With the patient standing upright, and wearing walking shoes, the lower end of the stick should be level with the wrist when adjusted. To check, reverse the walking stick and ensure the patient's elbow is flexed to 30° when standing in the stable position.

Walking

Walking with two sticks using a three-point gait requires the same technique as when using two crutches. Using a single walking stick needs the stick to be carried in the hand opposite to the affected lower limb. However, some patients may find holding the stick on the same side gives more relief in knee or ankle injuries. Again, the technique is similar to the three-point gait used with crutches (see Fig. 6.19).

The role of the nurse in any situations where individuals require restrictions to their movement for therapeutic reasons is changing rapidly.

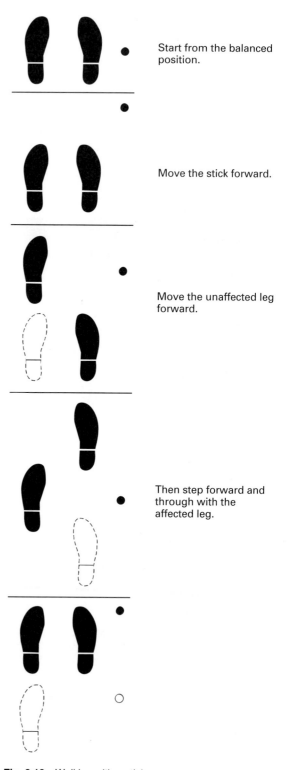

Start from the balanced position.

Move the stick forward.

Move the unaffected leg forward.

Then step forward and through with the affected leg.

Fig. 6.19 Walking with a stick.

The patient or client needs to be given more control of his care and treatment. To enable this to happen, the nurse must have in-depth knowledge and good communication skills, and the confidence that derives from the former. In this way the nurse is able to ensure the patient selects appropriately, understands and becomes skilled in his own care when movement is restricted.

REFERENCES

Adams I 1985 Strapping in sport. Nursing, 2nd edn suppl. Bailliere Tindall, London, p 5–6

Barrett J 1980 Bandaging techniques. Nursing Times 76(26): 1127–1132

Broadhurst M 1990 Total support walking frame. Physiotherapy 76(5): 300

Brodell J D, Axon D L, Evarts C M 1986 The Robert Jones bandage. Journal of Bone & Joint Surgery 68B(5): 776–779

Chant A D B 1972 Editorial. British Journal of Surgery 59: 552–555

Dale J J, Callam M J, Ruckley C V 1983 How efficient is a compression bandage? Nursing Times 79(46): 49–51

Dale J J 1985 Compression bandaging of the leg. Nursing, 2nd edn suppl. Bailliere Tindall, London, p 6–7

Davis P S 1989 The principles of traction. Nursing (Oxford) 3(34): 5–8

Farrell J 1986 Illustrated guide to orthopaedic nursing, 3rd edn. J B Lippincott, London

Footner A 1987 Orthopaedic nursing. Bailliere Tindall, London

Hall J, Clarke A K 1990 Open-cuff crutches. Physiotherapy 76(5): 271

Isherwood P A, Robertson J C, Rossi A 1975 British Journal of Surgery 62: 982–986

Jamieson E 1989 Strength and stability. Nursing Times Supplement 85(27): 13–15

Kay J 1990 Trying to keep a balance. Nursing Times 86(19): 37

Lane P L, Leblanc R 1990 Crutch walking. Orthopaedic Nursing 9(5): 31–38

Levins D, Stuttle W 1984 Dynamic splinting for the unstable elbow. Physiotherapy 70(9): 348–350

Loder J 1986 The case of combination casts. Nursing Times 82(45): 49

Love C 1989 The light touch. Nursing Times Supplement 85(27): 9 12

Mandlestam M 1990 How to get equipment for disability. Jessica Kingsley & Kogan Paul, London

Miles S, Barr L 1991 Principles of casting. In: A practical guide to casting. Smith & Nephew Medical, Hull

Morris L, Kraft S, Tessem S, Reinisch S 1988 Special care for skeletal traction. Registered Nurse 24–29

Murray M 1976 Fundamentals of nursing. Prentice Hall, New Jersey

Orford J 1989 Keeping things in place. Nursing Times Supplement 85(27): 4–8

Pearson A 1987 Living in a plaster cast. Royal College of Nursing, London

Powell M 1986 Orthopaedic nursing and rehabilitation, 9th edn. Churchill Livingstone, Edinburgh

Simpson D, Greig R 1984 Orthotic application of plastic materials. Physiotherapy 70(9): 332–340

Smith & Nephew 1991 A practical guide to casting. Smith & Nephew Medical, Hull

Sproles K 1985 Nursing care of skeletal pins: a closer look. Orthopaedic Nursing 4(1): 11–19

Stewart J D M, Hallett J P (1983) Traction and Orthopaedic Appliances, 2nd end. Churchill Livingstone, London

Stockwell F 1972 The unpopular patient. Royal College of Nursing, London

Swan D 1984 Low temperature hand splinting with thermoplastic materials. Physiotherapy 70(9): 341–345

Sykes J 1985 A night out on the crutches. Nursing Times 81(48): 32–33

Taylor I 1987 Ward manual of orthopaedic traction. Churchill Livingstone, Edinburgh

Thomas S, Dawes C, Hay P 1980 A critical evaluation of some extensible bandages in current use. Nursing Times 76(26): 1123–1126

Wallis S 1991 An agenda to promote self-care, nursing care of skeletal pin sites. Professional Nurse 6(12): 715–720

Wytch R, Mitchell C 1986 Getting plastered. Nursing Times 82(36): 48–50

7

Reducing pain

Peter S. Davis   Carol Horrigan

Everyone experiences pain at some stage in his life; very often it is an integral part of being ill. Pain is the commonest complaint of patients with orthopaedic problems, as it is particularly associated with movement. Orthopaedic nurses must therefore have a comprehensive understanding of pain and how it can be relieved in order to care for these patients effectively.

'Freedom from pain should be a basic human right limited only by our knowledge to achieve it' (Liebeskind & Melzack 1987). Research has demonstrated that pain relief in adults and children is often inadequate (Marks & Sachar 1973, Cohen 1980, Weis et al 1983, Mather & Mackie 1983, Donovan et al 1987, Seers 1989a). In both the hospital and primary care setting, large numbers of people continue to suffer from poorly controlled pain. Nurses appear to lack knowledge about pain and its relief (Cohen 1980, Watt-Watson 1987) and do not accurately assess it (Hunt et al 1977, Seers 1989b, Choiniere et al 1990). Despite the evidence that pain is not well controlled, new studies indicate that the situation is changing only slowly and much unnecessary pain is still suffered by people in hospital care.

This chapter will explore ways of helping nurses alleviate a person's pain by:

- increasing nurses' knowledge and understanding of pain and its management
- introducing complementary methods of pain control
- considering the more subjective meaning of pain to the sufferer.

DEFINING PAIN

The pain experience is often so complex that it is impossible to define. Merskey and colleagues (1979) define it as 'an unpleasant sensory and emotional experience associated with actual or potential tissue damage, or described in terms of such damage'. However, nurses are more familiar with McCaffery's (1983) definition: 'Pain is whatever the experiencing person says it is, existing whenever the experiencing person says it does.' All definitions must assume that the patient's complaints and descriptions of pain are believed. Although a precise definition of pain is not possible, the attempt to define it provides a starting point for debate and illustrates the complexities and contexts of the pain experience. Often it makes the nurse realize how little she knows and is able to do.

TYPES OF PAIN

Pain can be classified according to whether it is acute or chronic. This classification provides an initial framework for understanding the patient's pain experience and selecting appropriate interventions in order to reduce the patient's suffering. Other classifications may also be useful, for example to help distinguish between malignant and non-malignant causes of the pain.

Acute pain

Acute pain has a brief duration – that is, less than 6 months; it subsides as healing takes place and, importantly, has a predictable end; examples are postoperative pain and pain from a fractured bone. Acute pain is nearly always related to movement of the patient, or his operated limb, during nursing manoeuvres. With the availability of a range of analgesics and sophisticated equipment, it is possible to control acute pain to a level acceptable to the patient. However, this does not often occur: the Royal College of Surgeons and Anaesthetists report (1990) makes clear that patients still suffer from unnecessary pain.

Spence (1991) suggests that doctors and nurses must take most of the blame for the lack of progress in this fundamental area of patient care. Patients unfamiliar with hospital procedures may spend hours waiting and hoping for pain relief from the drugs they have been given after surgery, too frightened to trouble the staff with their pain. They are left wondering if relief will ever come at all.

Chronic pain

Chronic pain is prolonged: the same pain experienced continuously or intermittently for 6 months or more. Depending on its origin and the patient's prognosis, chronic pain can be further categorized:

1. Ongoing time-limited pain has the potential for lasting months, perhaps years, but has a probability of ending. Examples include cancer or burn pain, e.g. osteosarcoma. The pain disappears only when the condition is controlled or cured or the patient dies.

2. Chronic non-malignant pain, due to non-life-threatening causes, is not responsive to currently available methods of pain relief and may continue for the remainder of the patient's life (McCaffery & Beebe 1989). Chronic non-malignant pain sufferers include those with low back pain, rheumatoid arthritis, osteoarthritis, phantom limb pain and neck pain such as whiplash. These sufferers form a large proportion of the patients for whom orthopaedic nurses care, especially in the community or day care setting.

THE MEANING OF PAIN

The meaning of pain to an individual is subjective and multifaceted. To the sufferer it brings recognition of a world which was previously only seen as a distant possibility or as the plight of another. Bury's (1982) research describes lucidly how rheumatoid arthritis can disrupt the lives of those suffering from it.

Society's perception of the nature and functions of pain has changed over the ages and will continue to do so: some existing beliefs will continue to be valid, while others will be altered or dropped altogether as new ideas take their place.

2. Pain as a necessary warning; this hypothesis suggests that pain alerts the sufferer to the fact that something is wrong. Even today many nurses believe that to alleviate pain in people following trauma may mask diagnosis. This belief exists despite the fact that diagnosis based on subjective symptoms is rare and is always confirmed by radiographic and laboratory evidence.

3. Pain as emotion; this view attempts to separate the psychogenic aspects of pain from the somatic. It originates from Aristotle, in the 4th century BC, who thought that pain was experienced by the heart rather than the brain. Today this is reflected in therapies such as relaxation.

4. Pain as neurotransmission; pain is held to be the transmission of an impulse from one nerve to another. This idea has led to the development of neurosurgical procedures to stop these transmissions. This has often resulted in significant damage to the individual with little pain relief: for example, after the amputation of painful limbs the patient may continue to suffer phantom limb pain.

5. Pain as a challenge to science; this perspective sees pain as a challenge, something to be beaten and mastered, but when pain's subjective nature is identified it is quickly discounted or ignored as it cannot be explained or abolished.

6. Pain as a complex interaction; the belief that mind and body interact indivisibly when pain is perceived by an individual is now widely accepted.

One or more of these beliefs may be held by patients and carers, and will affect the meaning of pain to them as individuals. Davis (1988) showed that the attitudes of nurses had a crucial effect on the quality of care given to patients with acute postoperative pain due to orthopaedic surgery. These attitudes are difficult to change but respond to education and role modelling over a period of time; they can be assessed using the scale illustrated in Figure 7.1.

GATE CONTROL THEORY

In 1965 Melzack and Wall (1982) developed a theory of pain that included both physiological and psychological components which interacted, and called it the 'gate control theory'. According to the theory, information concerning pain stimuli is transmitted along nerve fibres to the spinal cord and thus to the brain. The site of control is believed to be in the substantia gelatinosa, which caps the grey matter of the dorsal horn in the spinal cord (Fig. 7.2). The control mechanism is referred to as a 'gate' and is operated by external (ascending) and internal (descending) influences. For example, rubbing or massaging a painful area is thought to relieve pain by stimulating the flow of impulses in large sensory nerve fibres; these impulses stimulate activity in the substantia gelatinosa cells. High activity in the substantia gelatinosa cells opposes the relay of nerve impulses of any kind to the transmission cells (T cells), which convey information about pain to the brain. It is as though a gate has been closed that stops or controls input from the thinner pain-transmitting fibres from the same area that has been massaged. The opposition of the substantia gelatinosa cells in this instance is an example of negative feedback.

When a volley of pain impulses arrives at the spinal cord in small nerve fibres, the substantia gelatinosa cells are not stimulated, the gate stays open and impulses are transmitted to the T cells. Suppression of activity of the cells in the substantia gelatinosa seems to increase the effect of the impulses arriving in the small fibres; this is positive feedback. Each succeeding volley entering the pathway makes the T cells produce an increasingly prolonged burst of impulses, which are interpreted as pain (Fig. 7.3). This explains

	strongly agree	agree	unsure	disagree	strongly disagree
1. Patients should expect to suffer some pain.					
2. Anxiety increases the perception of pain.					
3. Nurses are better qualified and more experienced to determine the existence and nature of the patient's pain than the patient himself.					
4. The patient who uses his pain to obtain benefits or preferential treatment does not hurt as much as he says he does and may not hurt at all.					
5. Talking and listening to patients can reduce their pain.					
6. Patient's pain can always be detected by their behaviour and physiological signs.					
7. Some ethnic groups can tolerate more pain than others.					
8. All real pain has an identifiable physical cause.					
9. Nurses always make accurate inferences about the severity and existence of the patient's pain.					
10. Care should be taken when giving controlled drugs postoperatively as patients easily become addicted.					
11. It is best that patients should not know what is happening to them as this may cause anxiety.					
12. All patients can and should be encouraged to have a high tolerance for pain.					
13. What the patient says about his pain is always true.					
14. Nurses can determine accurately the amount of pain a patient will suffer from knowledge of the surgery.					
15. Analgesics are always the best way of reducing pain.					
16. Nurses most often underestimate the severity and existence of the patient's pain.					

Fig. 7.1 Attitude to pain control scale.

why many niggling aches and pains, producing low-key input in the small fibres, keep the gate open and are self-perpetuating.

Current research of the internal influences on pain explains some of the so-called psychological aspects of pain. It has been shown that pain impulses are suppressed or modified at the substantia gelatinosa by descending influences from the brain. For example, if someone picks up a hot plate his first impulse is to drop it; but he may decide to put it down. At the time he may not have felt the full intensity of the pain because, while he was carrying the plate, internal descending influences closed the gate. After the plate is put down, the pain will be felt in all its intensity. But now external influences may be used: by blowing on his hands, the gate may again be closed and thus the pain reduced.

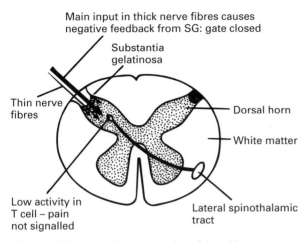

Fig. 7.2   Diagrammatic cross-section of dorsal horn.

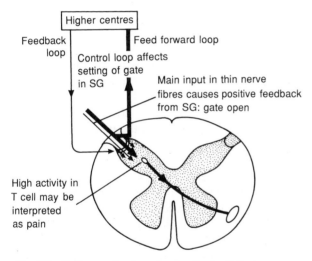

Fig. 7.3   Gating mechanism showing feedback loop.

It is thought that in order to close the gate at the moment when we are about to receive potentially painful information, and thus keep one step ahead, impulses are relayed to the higher centres through side branches of the fast-conducting thick nerve fibres in the dorsal columns of the spinal cord. These impulses set up what is known as a 'feed forward loop', and are followed by descending impulses in a feedback loop from the brain, which alter the setting of the gate.

The gate control theory has provided a theoretical basis for many holistic practices. Examples of those having an ascending action, i.e. those providing external influences, are transcutaneous electrical nerve stimulation (TENS), acupuncture, acupressure, reflexology, Shiatsu and massage. Examples having a descending action, i.e. those providing internal influences, are meditation, relaxation techniques, hypnosis, imagery and music. Many of these therapies will be described later in this chapter but TENS needs further explanation as it is used on a large number and variety of orthopaedic patients.

Transcutaneous electrical nerve stimulation

There are stone carvings in tombs dating back to 2500 BC which show that a species of electrical fish found in the Nile was used to treat different pain conditions. Roman literature of about 46 AD describes how gout pain could be treated: 'For all types of gout, when pain begins, a living electrical ray should be placed under the foot of the patient, who should stand on a moistened floor and should remain there until his whole foot and leg up to the knee has dozed away. This takes away the present pain and prevents pain from occurring if it hasn't already' (Sjölund & Eriksson 1985).

Over the past decade TENS has become accepted as an effective method of relieving chronic pain in pain clinics and physiotherapy departments. The pulses of electrical energy generated from the stimulator unit are transmitted to the skin through conductive electrodes. Controls are provided to vary the amplitude and frequency of stimulation. Two distinctly different means of achieving pain relief can be utilized:

1. If high-frequency TENS (15–150 Hz) is used, stimulation of the large diameter fibres occurs, thus blocking the gate.
2. If low frequency 'burst' stimulation (2 Hz) is used, commonly known as acupuncture-like TENS, an increase in endogenous opiates is produced.

The opiate antagonist naloxone has been shown to reduce the pain-relieving effect of acupuncture-like TENS. When naloxone is given to conventional TENS users it has no effect. This suggests that acupuncture-like TENS does not use the gate control mechanism of conventional TENS, but probably utilizes areas of the spinal cord associated with pain, such as the dorsal horn, where concentrations of the endogenous opiates may be found.

Because TENS can be effective in relieving chronic pain, it would seem sensible to give each patient with this type of pain an adequate trial with TENS. This may be quite time-consuming as it is often necessary to experiment with different electrode placements and stimulators.

Although many studies now indicate that TENS has a marked effect on acute pain it is still used very little for this purpose in this country. This is surprising, as in postoperative pain, electrode placement and predictability of success are far easier and simpler than for chronic pain.

Endogenous opiates

The gate control theory has been given further validity by the discovery in the 1970s of endogenous opiates; these are substances, produced by the body, with properties similar to those of morphine.

This discovery was preceded by the discovery of opiate receptor sites in those areas of the central nervous system that are believed to mediate the motivational–affective components of pain; that is, the thalamus, hypothalamus, prefrontal lobe and limbic lobe. The question was then raised as to why a receptor had evolved for which the only known binding particles were poppy plant alkaloids; this led to the search and eventual discovery of the endogenous opiates.

Encephalins were the first of these substances to be discovered at these sites; because of their site and duration of action they are now believed to be neurotransmitters. Endorphins, another form of internal opiate, have since been discovered; they are produced predominantly in the pituitary gland.

These endogenous opiates can be closely related to the gate control theory since the dorsal horn and the originating sites of the descending pathways are rich in encephalins. It is thought that encephalins may be inhibitory neurotransmitters which are capable of modulating pain impulses at the spinal gate, and that this is achieved by the inhibitory effect of encephalins on substance P, which itself is concerned with sensory impulse transmission.

ASSESSING PAIN

Nurses have a professional responsibility to assess patients' pain and make decisions on appropriate nursing interventions (Mooney 1991). Several studies (Bondestam et al 1987, Seers 1989b, Willetts 1989) have compared patients' own ratings of their pain with those of the nurses caring for them. The results show that in the majority of assessments, nurses underestimate patients' pain.

Pain may be assessed from the patient's verbal report, but the orthopaedic nurse should be aware that many patients wait for the nurse to ask them if they are in pain rather than volunteer the information (Carr 1990). Often a situation occurs where the nurse is waiting for the patient to tell her he is in pain and the patient is waiting to be asked, resulting in unnecessary delay and suffering.

The type of pain, its position, severity and, importantly for the orthopaedic nurse, what movements exacerbate the pain should all be considered in pain assessment. The effects of the pain on the patient's ability to carry out the activities of living are also important elements of the assessment. For example, sleep pattern disturbance is common in patients suffering from both acute and chronic pain.

Pain management tools

Pain management tools have many advantages:

- They enable accurate pain assessment.
- They improve the nurse/patient relationship.
- They aid evaluation of any pain-relieving interventions.
- They help to ensure that the nurse acts on the outcome of the assessment.
- They promote better understanding of the pain for the patient and the nurse.

- The patient is able to assess, communicate and control his own pain with the support of the nurse.
- The patient feels that his complaints of pain are being believed.
- The pattern of the pain can be seen.
- The charts are quick and easy to use, providing an unambiguous record of the patient's pain management.

Crocker (1986) suggests that pain assessment tools should be multidimensional, accurate, brief, quick to complete, easy for the patient to use and applicable in a variety of settings.

There are several types of pain rating scales that may be used by orthopaedic nurses. The commoner ones will be described.

Visual analogue scale

The scale consists of a straight line, usually 10 cm in length, with one end marked 'no pain' and the other 'worst pain suffered' (see Fig. 7.4). The patient makes a mark on the line at right angles to a point which represents the level of pain at that time. The line can be measured to give a pain score. Some patients have difficulty in using this type of scale and it also consumes large amounts of paper if frequent recordings are made.

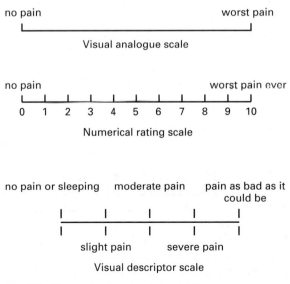

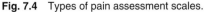

Fig. 7.4   Types of pain assessment scales.

Numerical rating scale

The scale consists of a continuum of numbers, usually 0–5 or 0–10. Zero signifies 'no pain' and 5 or 10 signifies 'worst pain ever' (see Fig. 7.4). The patient gives a number to his pain at that time. Some patients have difficulty conceptualizing pain in numbers. However, many researchers (Crocker 1986, Bondestam et al 1987, McCormick Vandenbosch 1988) are finding the numerical rating scale a useful tool.

Verbal descriptor scale

The scale contains words describing different levels of pain at equal intervals on a continuum (see Fig. 7.4). The patient uses the words to describe his pain at that time. Some researchers suggest that the descriptors are too limiting to give accurate assessments. However, the scales are popular and easy to use and may produce a more valid assessment of the pain.

The above rating scales are becoming more widely used, as they can be adapted easily to particular clinical settings. Often they form part of a pain management tool which uses other data-gathering methods in the assessment process, such as locating the site of the pain(s), and provide a means to plan and then record the nursing intervention and its evaluation. Different pain tools are required for different types of pains; for example, postoperative acute pain requires a different tool to the chronic non-malignant pain of rheumatoid arthritis that is present day after day.

Davis (1988) developed a chart, which is still in use, for assessing postoperative pain caused by orthopaedic surgery. The chart assesses pain on a five-point verbal descriptor scale. The recommendations given below on how to use the charts are derived from experience gained during a trial period.

The nurse should not duplicate information by entering pain chart information in the normal nursing documentation. The charts are used to make an assessment whenever the patient and/or nurse feels it appropriate to do so, but are also used when other postoperative observations are made, for example every 30 minutes or every 4 hours. However, if the nurse has intervened to attempt to reduce the patient's pain – for example by giving analgesia or changing the patient's position – she must return to the patient within a reasonable period, i.e. 5–30 minutes, and not wait until the next postoperative observations.

Johnson (1976) classifies the distress and physical elements of the pain experience as 'response' and 'sensory', respectively; this suggests that it is possible to pin-point and assess the sensory component in terms of location, quality, intensity, etc. However, the response component can vary markedly among individuals, and is dependent on psychosocial factors such as personality and cultural background. The response component may also vary in the same individual as it is related to a person's ability to tolerate pain at any one time. For example, during the day a patient with many distractions may assess his pain as severe with respect to its physical ele-

ment, but only slightly distressing, and therefore may require only minimal intervention. However, the same patient awakened by his pain in the night may assess the physical element as slight but may find it severely distressing and thus require a more radical intervention. The information gained from assessing both physical and distress elements thus enables a more appropriate and sensitive control of a person's pain to be achieved. Figure 7.5 is an example of the type of chart that may be used to assess these elements of the pain experience, and thus enable a patient to receive more appropriate intervention.

NURSING DIAGNOSIS AND PAIN

Chapter 5 describes the nursing diagnoses related to mobility, impaired physical mobility and activity intolerance. These diagnoses are particularly appropriate for patients with pain. McCaffery and Beebe (1989) list the nursing di-

PAIN CHART

WARD .... PATIENT'S NAME ....

		Tick for how painful Cross for how distressing					
Date	Time	Not or asleep	Slight	Moderate	Severe	Worst ever	Site

Fig. 7.5 Postoperative pain chart.

agnoses that are related to patients in pain. For the orthopaedic patient some of these are:

- Anxiety
- Impaired physical mobility
- Activity intolerance
- Constipation
- Fatigue
- Knowledge deficit
- Powerlessness
- Feeding self-care deficit
- Dressing/grooming self-care deficit
- Sexual dysfunction
- Sleep pattern disturbance
- Social isolation.

Using the components of the model of orthopaedic nursing that are described in Chapter 3 and elsewhere in this book, the orthopaedic nurse should be able to identify patient problems (i.e. make nursing diagnoses) and plan care with the patient. For example, sleep pattern disturbance may result from the pain experienced by the patient when he moves during the night. In this instance analgesia would be a more appropriate intervention than sleep inducing drugs.

PHARMACOLOGICAL CONTROL OF PAIN

The orthopaedic nurse should be able to choose the appropriate analgesia, if and when to give it, evaluate its effectiveness and obtain a change in analgesic prescription if required. McCaffery and Beebe (1989) stress that how an analgesic is used is probably more important than which one is used.

Pain should be prevented whenever possible and kept under control. Once the patient is in pain it is often more difficult to bring it under control again and more analgesia may be required. In situations where prolonged pain, such as that due to surgery or cancer, can be predicted, analgesia should be given regularly and before pain occurs or increases. This may mean

Comment and/or action	Analgesia given				
	Name	Dose	Route	Time	Signature

waking the patient at night to give him analgesia if pain usually causes sleep pattern disturbance. Analgesia on a p.r.n. (pro re nata or as required) basis may be useful if pain is not predictable or prior to treatment such as physiotherapy if this is painful. If ongoing pain can be predicted to be continuous or frequent, p.r.n. analgesia should be given 24 hours a day.

Analgesia should be adjusted to each individual patient, so that it produces the desired pain relief with minimal side-effects. Pain assessment tools are essential in this process.

Whenever possible, the patient should control the treatment of his pain. Patient-controlled analgesia may be defined as the patient's self-administration of all forms of pain control by safe methods. It involves the patient's ability and desire to choose to exercise control; some patients do not want to have control and choose to leave it to the health care professionals. With respect to analgesia, this may be as simple as the nurse providing the patient with the knowledge and understanding of the analgesic and allowing him to self-administer. Many orthopaedic patients with conditions such as osteoarthritis are able to control their pain in their own homes by taking oral analgesia, but it does not necessarily follow that they are well educated about the effects, administration and potential side-effects of their drugs.

Types of pharmacological interventions

Analgesics may be peripheral or central in their action. Peripherally-acting analgesics are often termed non-steroidal anti-inflammatory drugs (NSAIDs).

Peripherally-acting analgesics (NSAIDs)

These drugs help to relieve orthopaedic patients' pain in the following situations:

- Inflammatory conditions, e.g. rheumatoid arthritis
- Mild to moderate pain of peripheral origin such as low back pain
- When a baseline of non-narcotic analgesia is needed in severe, acute or chronic pain requiring narcotics

- Conditions associated with excessive prostaglandin at the site of pain, such as certain malignant tumours, bone metastases and postoperative pain
- When the patient wants to avoid drugs, such as the narcotics, that affect thinking, alertness or emotions.

NSAIDs have three effects:

1. Anti-inflammatory
2. Analgesic
3. Antipyretic.

The degree of these effects varies from one NSAID to another.

Examples of common peripherally-acting analgesics used by orthopaedic patients are:

- Aspirin
- Ibuprofen
- Indomethacin
- Naproxen
- Phenylbutazone.

Generally these drugs are taken orally and should be swallowed with or immediately after a meal. This is because they are gastric irritants, and patients should be educated to detect signs of gastric bleeding and irritation when these drugs are used long-term, as in the treatment of rheumatoid arthritis. Other side-effects include dizziness, headache, blurred vision, ringing in the ears, urticaria and unusual bleeding, as the drugs affect blood platelets.

Centrally-acting analgesics

Centrally-acting analgesics include the opioids; they help to relieve the following types of pain:

- Moderate to severe acute pain such as that caused by fractures and surgery
- Prolonged time-limited pain such as in bone cancer pain and terminal illness
- Sudden, severe pain such as in trauma – rapid relief is provided.

There are two main types of narcotics:

1. Narcotic agonists, such as codeine and morphine

2. Narcotic agonists–antagonists, such as buprenorphine and pentazocine.

These drugs act at the level of the central nervous system by attaching to opioid receptor sites in the brain and spinal cord. They are very effective if used correctly. It is estimated that about 90% of patients with acute or chronic pain due to end-stage disease could be comfortable if narcotics on their own were given in the correct way and amount. The principal reason why narcotics are not used is a lack of knowledge of their use and safety. Nurses, doctors and patients still hold ungrounded fears about narcotics in this situation causing addiction, dependence, tolerance and respiratory depression. Jaffe (1985) has found this fear of addiction to be irrational and misplaced.

These narcotics can now be taken via many routes and under various regimens and forms of control. Ideally, the patient should be allowed to control his pain, if he desires to do so, even if this is achieved through intravenous, subcutaneous or spinal routes with patient-controlled pumps. These pumps can be used safely to administer a continuous infusion, and in addition allow self-administration of a bolus dose if the patient has a sudden increase of pain.

Other pharmacological interventions

Drugs that are not normally given as analgesics may be used to relieve pain. Antidepressants can be used to affect the patient's perception of pain and his mood. For example, individuals suffering from rheumatoid arthritis often become depressed; if their depression is relieved, they are better able to cope with chronic pain as their perception of the pain is altered through increased tolerance. Muscle relaxants, such as baclofen and diazepam, may be useful in relieving the muscle spasm caused by arthritis, vertebral disc protrusion or bone metastasis.

INTERVENTIONS FOR CHRONIC NON-MALIGNANT PAIN

'They told me they couldn't do any more about my fingers. The doctor said it (rheumatoid arthritis) was out of control and there wasn't anything they could do. I'm really tired I'm just tired of the pain . . . just five minutes to be without the pain.' These are the words of a 76-year-old lady who had suffered from rheumatoid arthritis for many years. The National Health Service tends to encourage a patient's complaints due to the adoption of a scientific perspective of disease, i.e. that cure is possible and that all pains are relievable. Extensive efforts are made to explore and treat conditions but when there is no effective line of approach to managing pain, patients and doctors may come into conflict and the frustrations of the patient often lead to an unsatisfactory doctor/patient relationship. Fisher (1988) attributes this to the fact that pain consists of perceptual and emotional variables as well as physical ones, and that the present approach does not deal effectively with the behavioural and cognitive aspects of the pain. A holistic approach using the whole multidisciplinary team and family would be more effective.

Orthopaedic nurses frequently have to care for patients who are significantly disabled by pain, but for whom there is no effective surgical or medical treatment. When it is not possible to eliminate pain, interventions are aimed at increasing the patient's ability to cope. Many of the problems encountered by nurses caring for these patients arise from their misunderstanding of and attitude toward the patients (see Fig. 7.3 for an indication of how nurses' attitudes may affect their nursing care). These patients do not 'get used' to their pain; in fact, over time they may feel worse because of their fear of pain and their inability to control it. Depression does not cause pain: chronic pain causes depression. This can sometimes confuse the carer, as the symptoms of chronic pain are similar to those of depression. However, this is not surprising as both are forms of suffering.

The nurse must be knowledgeable about the behavioural and cognitive aspects of this type of chronic pain to be in a position to alleviate it. For example she should:

- Always believe the patient
- Be sure that the patient receives what he considers an acceptable explanation of why he has the pain

- Review the effects of his analgesics regularly even though the patient may have been on them for a long period of time
- Decrease the severity of chronic sleep pattern disturbance
- Help the patient to use coping strategies, especially relaxation
- Help the patient to set goals and to achieve them.

Fisher (1988) describes a multidisciplinary pain management programme for orthopaedic patients with chronic non-malignant pain which is based on many of the concepts discussed above. The patients on the programme have to make the transition from seeing the pain as the doctor's responsibility to seeing it as a problem which they will have to learn to manage. This may involve learning new approaches which are independent of medical intervention and traditional methods.

Low back pain is the commonest condition to be treated on this programme. The patients are admitted to the unit for 4 weeks; a set programme is followed which contains:

1. Assessment
2. Personal goal-setting
3. Activities to get fit and swimming
4. Relaxation, auto-hypnosis and Alexander technique
5. Lectures from psychologists, nurses, doctors, pharmacists and physiotherapists.

Progress on the programme is indicated by the degree of achievement of personal targets. This approach has been shown to produce significant improvements in general disability ratings and activity tolerance. Many of the principles applied in such programmes are transferable to the management of patients suffering from chronic non-malignant pain.

COMPLEMENTARY THERAPIES

Orthopaedic nurses are in an ideal position to inform patients about lifestyle changes which will not only help them through a period of acute stress caused by pain, but will also enable them to feel more in control during any future episodes. The patient's ability and enthusiasm for learning pain and stress reduction techniques can be assessed by an orthopaedic nurse soon after his admission.

Contrary to popular belief, it is very easy to include massage or any other complementary therapy into a patient's daily care; the day can be planned by the patient, his nurse and the complementary therapist.

The patient's interaction with his environment is the first consideration: a peaceful, calming atmosphere is the aim of all complementary therapists. When a patient is in pain and under stress from orthodox treatment such as chemotherapy, his sympathetic nervous system is in a constant state of arousal. It may take only a further small increase in this state of arousal to carry the patient to the point where his coping mechanisms are seriously affected (Nixon 1988).

Planning care that includes periods of non-orthodox treatment calls for diplomacy and tact if the idea is new to a ward. Evenings and weekends are often the most suitable times to carry out this treatment. Therapies that are most useful for chronic pain relief require a calm and, if possible, quiet atmosphere. But success in obtaining this will depend upon the nurses' duty rota, the therapist carrying out the treatment and, most importantly, how the therapy fits in with the patient's overall plan of care. Acute pain would obviously be treated immediately.

The alleviation of pain by complementary therapies can be carried out before, during or after painful procedures, and can be nurse- or patient-controlled. If the doctor, physiotherapist or other health care worker is unfamiliar with the therapy, a few minutes of explanation is usually all that is required before the procedure can go ahead.

Obviously, the patient is the most important member of the 'team'; his cooperation and enthusiasm are fundamental to the success of self-help techniques, and highly desirable although not essential for those therapies that involve touch. Relatives can derive great satisfaction from supporting patients through their orthodox treatments by using complementary therapies. When a patient is experiencing pain that is all-consuming, he sometimes cannot see an end to it;

but if it is a shared, supported experience, it can be enriching for both participants (Fisher 1990).

At the present time, the following therapies are most frequently used by nurses:

- Massage
- Aromatherapy
- Reflex zone therapy
- Shiatsu
- Guided imagery
- Visualization
- Relaxation.

Each of the therapies has guidelines and treatment schedules that have been developed over many (sometimes thousands of) years, and there are instructive textbooks and courses available for the aspiring therapist. The following overview will give the reader some indication of the background, modalities and potential value of each therapy, although it must be appreciated that the information given here is an outline and should not replace comprehensive training and study of the subject.

Massage

Massage can be slow, gentle and relaxing or vigorous and stimulating. The patient may wish to have the deeper tissues manipulated or he may be able to tolerate only the lightest touch. Pain can be alleviated by either method; which is chosen will depend upon the patient's physical stamina, the type of pain and the patient's perception of the fragility of his own body.

Acute pain which has been caused by trauma, such as a sports injury, will respond to moderately deep massage, but patients with chronic pain or with terminal cancer pain will appreciate a gentler method. Receptors for pain and touch in the skin transmit both sensations at once, but it has been found that a caring touch of less than 1 second has the power to make a person feel better (Doerhing 1989).

Oil, talc or even the soapy water during a bed bath can be used as a lubricant for massage; the only criteria for choice are the condition of the patient's skin and his preference for the texture of the preparation used.

Aromatherapy

Aromatherapy is fast becoming the most popular and widely practised complementary therapy in hospitals and hospices. Aromatic essences have been known to have beneficial effects for thousands of years; some doctors were investigating their antibacterial properties in the last century. However, over the last 40 years there has been a rapid increase in the use of essential oils, at first by French aromatherapists, and now all over the world.

Aromatherapy centres recommend the use of essential oils which are distilled or obtained by other natural methods from plants. They are not only pleasant to use because of their fragrance, but many have specific therapeutic actions. These include relief from several types of pain, as each has an affinity to a specific body site.

Most aromatherapy oils are safe to use and are available from reputable suppliers by post or through retail shops. However, it should be noted that some are of better quality than others, and some are very costly. Occasionally patients are sensitive to these oils, even when they are correctly diluted. Nurses who wish to practise aromatherapy are advised to consult a qualified aromatherapist before purchasing or using oils for the first time.

Aromatherapy can alleviate pain if the appropriate oil is used. Some oils are effective because they are relaxing and evoke memories (rose, lavender and jasmine); others have a local warming effect (black pepper, rosemary – with caution, and juniper), and are useful for muscle pain.

Aromatherapy oils can be mixed into a carrier oil, such as sunflower oil, and used for massage, or in vaporized form, they can relieve sinusitis, bronchitis, (eucalyptus, benzoin, ti-tree) and insomnia (neroli, sandalwood). Patients who are deprived of sleep are less able to tolerate pain, but aromatherapy affects the limbic system, and encourages relaxation.

Essential oil will evaporate when dropped onto hankies or pillows, put into hot water or diluted in water and used in a room spray (e.g. rose geranium, bergamot and lavender create a 'garden' fragrance). The use of electric or candle heaters which also vaporize the essential oil may not be permitted by fire officers, and they should be consulted before the heaters are used. The addition of a judicious amount to the bath water can ease aching joints and muscles (rosemary, bergamot, camomile); gentle massage and warm compresses applied to the abdomen can ease dysmenorrhoea or constipation (camomile, marjoram – with caution, and lavender). Cold compresses can be used for headache (lavender and peppermint), or for sprains and bruises (lavender and camomile).

As a general rule, essential oils should be used as follows:

1. Massage oil: mix 25–50 drops of essential oil with 50 ml of carrier oil. Aromatherapists often use costly base oils, but sunflower oil is quite suitable, inexpensive and is the least likely to cause an allergic reaction. Olive oil has a strong unpleasant smell of its own, and baby oil is unsuitable as essential oils will not mix with it.

2. Bath oil: add 2–6 drops of essential oil after the bath has been filled to the correct temperature. If the oil is added when the water is hot it will quickly evaporate and its benefits will be lost. The essential oil is less likely to irritate the perineum if mixed with a dessertspoonful of milk first.

3. Inhalation: put no more than 6 drops of essential oil in a bowl of very hot water. Take all precautions against the patient being scalded.

4. Slow evaporation: put 2–3 drops of essential oil onto a tissue or bed linen. Tissues are not suitable for children or confused patients.

5. Compresses: add 6–8 drops of essential oil to cold or warm water as required; wring out a thick cloth in it and apply it to the appropriate area.

Aromatherapy is both a science and an art; if it is treated with respect many patients will benefit from its myriad uses. However, as some essential oils are not suitable for use with pregnant, hypertensive or epileptic patients, the nurse should check before treating them.

Reflex zone therapy

Reflex zone therapy is known as reflexology when the practitioners are not trained in ortho-dox medicine. Based on an ancient skill that has been developed by several cultures simultaneously, it has been formalized and used as a therapy in the West since the 1950s.

The reflexes referred to in the name are responses elicited by the therapy. Every part of the body has a reflex point on the foot, and by sedating or stimulating the reflex points a balance of the body's functions is restored. The patient experiences a sense of well-being and relaxation which can be pain-relieving in itself; or it can prelude a session of manipulation by physiotherapy or osteopathy – for example, for patients with sports injuries and long-term back problems. The effect of this technique is similar to that achieved by acupuncture without needles; many of the pressure points used are the same. But it is not invasive, and with suitable training it is a safe method for nurses to use.

Treatments take the form of a detailed progression of thumb and fingers across the feet or hands of the patient. The practitioner is trained to feel for changes in texture and tone in the tissues of the feet. These changes coincide with sensations experienced by the patient, ranging from normal awareness of being touched to exquisite tenderness, with the feet being withdrawn from the therapist. When an area of tenderness is found, the therapist concentrates on that area by applying pressure in a specific manner so that stimulation or sedation of the reflex is obtained.

Reflex zone therapy can be used to encourage normal functioning of organs and glands and thus relieve pain in dysmenorrhoea, constipation, irritable bowel syndrome and retention of urine. It can also be used to induce relaxation and control pain in muscle spasm. This can take the form of a series of treatments, during which the number and intensity of the painful points diminishes. Finally, it can be used as a first aid measure to calm muscles and nerves which have been damaged by sports injuries.

Relaxation

One method of relaxation is for the patient to become aware of and to control his breathing. Another method is to contract and relax muscle groups in sequence. The technique concentrates the mind on a specific physical function and by so doing distracts him from his pain. The exercises can be performed in any comfortable position, but the patient will be able to relax more muscle groups if he lies on a soft but supportive surface. Painful or weak joints and muscles should always be supported with pillows before the patient begins the exercises (Levin et al 1987, Sims 1987, McCaffery & Beebe 1989).

The patient may wish to use additional methods such as visualization, music (Fisher 1990), or a particular configuration and colour of light. Quiet, non-vocal classical music and low, pink- or peach-coloured light is very comforting.

Guided imagery

Guided imagery and, to a lesser extent, visualization are methods of distraction with which most small children are familiar, but which adults fail to develop. These methods are now used extensively for cancer patients to help alleviate the pain caused by investigations and terminal pain (Simonton et al 1978, Sims 1987, Moorey & Greer 1989).

Initially, guided imagery has to be nurse-led, but before long many patients take themselves on imaginary journeys to their favourite real or fictional places. In this method the patient not only concentrates on breathing and relaxing his muscles, but also distracts his mind through memory or imagination. A suitable mixture of photographs, music, sounds (such as birdsong), and aromas can help stir the patient's imagination to produce images.

Sometimes patients have happy, peaceful memories that they want to dwell on. These evoke the most powerful and useful images, which can be repeated at will by memory or by using the 'props' mentioned above.

The main advantage of this method is that the memories can be manipulated to be totally positive whereas some distractions, such as television, books or radio, can inadvertently interject poignant or unhappy memories which would destroy the pain-relieving effect. (Hendricks & Willis 1975, Keable 1989, Moorey & Greer 1989).

Visualization

This is the most difficult of all the therapies described to practise because, although it is initially nurse-led, the power of the patient's imagination is the most important factor and it is his belief in the method that will dictate its efficacy. It is a controversial method and should not be used for patients who also have serious psychiatric problems such as schizophrenia or manic depressive psychosis. The patient should not be led to believe that he will be 'cured' of his disease (Moorey & Greer 1989).

Visualization can be used in two ways. One way is for the nurse to ask the patient to describe his disease in his own imagination; the patient then describes how he sees his orthodox therapy and his natural body defences fighting the disease. Some proponents believe that the more bizarre the images, the more powerful the effect (Simonton et al 1978). Children, and some adults, find it useful to draw or paint their images.

The second style, which is more useful for patients with pain, is for the nurse to ask patients to imagine that the pain has a colour. When they have described the 'colour' of their pain, they imagine the colour fading or changing to another colour that they feel is less painful. Finally, they imagine that it moves to another part of their body, usually from a central organ or a joint out to the periphery, and that it changes colour to the 'less painful' colour as it moves. Pain is usually perceived to be less important and threatening when it is less central. If the patient is very skilled at using his imagination he will even be able to visualize the pain 'flowing out' of his fingers or toes.

Experience with this method has shown that it is enhanced by the added distraction of massage of the feet or hands any by the use of quiet music.

Shiatsu

Shiatsu is a traditional Japanese therapy based upon promoting the body's own powers of healing. Pressure points are used, but in this case pressure is applied with the fingers, elbows, knees and feet. There are many levels of skill, ranging from everyday first aid to high levels of

Oriental diagnosis and healing. It is a powerful relaxation and pain-reducing therapy that can be utilized in any situation. The patient remains clothed; no oils are used and the patient can be treated while lying in bed or on a carpeted floor.

Nurses should feel confident when practising

complementary therapies. In order that their concentration is at an optimal level, they should undertake some form of relaxation themselves, and never practise when they are feeling stressed; the practitioner must feel at ease with the therapy and with herself.

REFERENCES

Bondestam E, Hovgren K, Johansson F et al 1987 Pain assessment by patients and nurses in the early phase of acute myocardial infarction. Journal of Advanced Nursing 12(6): 677–682

Bury M 1982 Chronic illness as biographical disruption. Sociology of Health and Illness 4(2): 167–182

Carr E 1990 Postoperative pain: patients' expectations and experiences. Journal of Advanced Nursing 15(1): 89–100

Choiniere M, Melzack R, Girard N, Rondeau J, Paquin M J 1990 Comparisons between patients' and nurses' assessment of pain and medication efficacy in severe burn injuries. Pain 40: 143–152

Cohen F 1980 Postsurgical pain relief: patients' status and nurses' medication choices. Pain 9: 265–274

Crocker C 1986 Acute postoperative pain: causes and control. Orthopaedic Nursing 5(2): 11–15

Davis P S 1988 Changing nursing practice for more effective control of postoperative pain through a staff initiated educational programme. Nurse Education Today 8: 325–331

Doehring K M 1989 Relieving pain through touch. Advancing Clinical Care Sep/Oct: 32–33

Donovan M I 1989 An historical view of pain management. Cancer Nursing. 12(4): 257–261

Donovan M, Dillon P, McGuire L 1987 Incidence and characteristics of pain in a sample of medical–surgical inpatients. Pain 30: 69–78

Fisher E 1990 Behavioural sciences for nurses – towards project 2000. G Duckworth, London

Fisher K 1988 Early experiences of a multidisciplinary pain management programme. Holistic Medicine 3(1): 47–56

Hendricks G, Willis R 1975 The centering book – awareness activities for children and adults to relax the body and mind. Prentice Hall, New York

Hunt J M, Stollar T D, Littlejohns D W, Twycross R G, Vere D W 1977 Patients with protracted pain: a survey conducted at the London Hospital. Journal of Medical Ethics 3: 61–73

Jaffe J H 1985 Drug addiction and drug abuse. In: Gillman A G et al (eds) The pharmacological basis of therapeutics, 7th, edn. Macmillan Publishing, New York

Johnson M 1976 Pain. How do you know it's there and what do you do? Nursing 76(6): 48–50

Keable D 1989 The management of anxiety. Churchill Livingstone, Edinburgh

Levin R F et al 1987 Nursing management of post-operative pain: use of relaxation techniques with cholecystectomy patients. Journal of Advanced Nursing 12: 463–472

Liebeskind J C, Melzack R 1987 The international pain foundation: meeting a need for education in pain management (editorial). Pain 30: 1–2

McCaffery M (1983) Nursing the patient in pain. Harper & Row, London

McCaffery M, Beebe A 1989 Pain. Clinical manual for nursing practice. C V Mosby, St Louis

McCormick Vandenbosch T 1988 How to use a pain flow sheet effectively. Nursing 18(8): 50–51

Marks R M, Sachar E J 1973 Undertreatment of medical inpatients with narcotic analgesics. Annals of Internal Medicine 78: 173–181

Mather L, Mackie J 1983 The incidence of postoperative pain in children. Pain 15: 271–282

Melzack R, Wall P D 1982 The challenge of pain. Penguin, London

Merskey H, Albe-Fessard D G, Bonica J J et al 1979 Pain terms: a list with definitions and notes on usage. Pain 6: 249–252

Mooney N E 1991 Pain management in the orthopaedic patient. Nursing Clinics of North America 26(1): 73–87

Moorey S, Greer 1989 Psychological therapy for patients with cancer: a new approach. Heinemann Medical, Oxford

Nixon P G F 1988 Human functions and the heart. In: Seedhouse D, Cribb A (eds) Changing ideas in health care. John Wiley, Chichester

Royal College of Surgeons & Anaesthetists 1990 Pain after surgery. Royal College of Surgeons of England, London

Seers K 1989a Patients' perceptions of acute pain. In: Wilson-Barnett J, Robinson S (eds) Directions in nursing research: ten years of progress at London University. Scutari, London ch 12 p 107–116

Seers K 1989b Assessing pain. Nursing Standard 15(3): 33–35

Simonton S et al 1978 Getting well again. Bantam Books, New York

Sims S E R 1987 Relaxation training as a technique for helping patients cope with the experience of cancer: a selective review of the literature. Journal of Advanced Nursing 12: 583–591

Sjölund B, Eriksson M 1985 Relief of pain by TENS. John Wiley & Sons, Chichester

Spence A A 1991 Pain after surgery. Journal of Bone & Joint Surgery 73-B(2): 189–190

Watt-Watson J 1987 Nurses' knowledge of pain issues: a survey. Journal of Pain and Symptom Management 2: 207–211

Weis O F, Sriwatanakul K, Allozoa J L, Weintraub M, Lasagna L 1983 Attitudes of patients, housestaff, and nurses toward postoperative analgesic care. Anaesthesia and Analgesia 62: 70–74

Willetts K 1989 Assessing cardiac pain. Nursing Times 85(47): 52–54

8

Preventing infection, promoting healing

Dinah Gould

Patients are at risk of infection following traumatic injury if they have sustained contaminated wounds. Once admitted, orthopaedic patients are even more susceptible to the hazards of nosocomial (hospital-acquired) infection than the average patient, because they undergo longer and more complex operative procedures, increasing the risk of contamination when the deep tissues are exposed. Nosocomial infections are notorious for the manner in which they complicate the course of the original illness or operation and delay recovery, but in the field of orthopaedics, where prosthetic implants are widely used, the consequences are particularly damaging. Any nurse who works in the orthopaedic department must have a good understanding of the nature, consequences and prevention of infection in order to plan and deliver care of a high standard.

BODY DEFENCES

In order to prevent and control infection the nurse needs to appreciate how the healthy human body defends itself against invasion by microorganisms, through mechanical arrangements of the tissues and physiologically by bactericidal secretions (see Fig. 8.1). Disease and trauma often breach these defences, increasing the risk of infection. The greater the number of invasive procedures (injections, catheterization, endoscopy etc.) that the patient is required to undergo, the greater is the risk of contaminating tissues usually free of microorganisms.

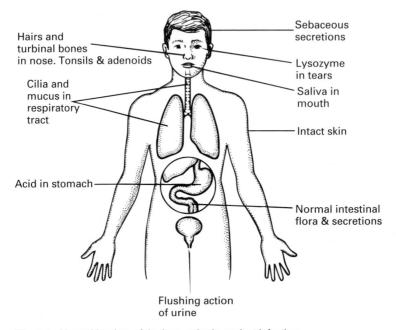

Hairs and
turbinal bones
in nose. Tonsils & adenoids

Cilia and
mucus in
respiratory
tract

Acid in stomach

Sebaceous
secretions

Lysozyme
in tears

Saliva in
mouth

Intact skin

Normal intestinal
flora & secretions

Flushing action
of urine

Fig. 8.1 Natural barriers of the human body against infection.

Skin

The skin provides a mechanical barrier against microorganisms when intact. Sebaceous secretions are mildly bactericidal and the normal skin flora, consisting of harmless bacteria living on the body surface, compete with pathogenic bacteria (those able to cause disease), keeping them at bay. However, if these commensal bacteria gain access to the deeper tissues via a wound or injection site they may cause infection. *Staphylococcus aureus* is carried asymptomatically on the skin of 10–30% of the general population, but can cause boils and abscesses if it enters the tissues. It is responsible for most orthopaedic postoperative wound infections developing in hospital (Sanderson 1988), and is carried more often on the skin of hospital personnel. Common sites of carriage include the nose, pharynx, forehead, webs of fingers and toes and the perineum.

Gastrointestinal system

Many of the gastrointestinal secretions are able to destroy bacteria. Saliva contains lysozyme, an antimicrobial enzyme, and removes microorganisms mechanically by its flushing action. These effects are lost when the patient develops a dry mouth through fear, dehydration or the use of drugs in premedication to suppress secretion. Patients undergoing surgery are therefore at risk of developing oral infections.

Mucus secreted throughout the gastrointestinal system also appears to act as a mechanical barrier against infection, while secretions such as hydrochloric acid in the stomach and bile in the duodenum destroy many bacteria. Enteric infection is more likely to occur when secretion is suppressed (Horan 1984). The large bowel contains a normal flora (mostly gram-negative rods such as *E. coli*) which is destroyed when the patient receives large doses of antibiotics, allowing superinfection with resistant hospital strains and pathogenic organisms to supervene. Diarrhoea is very common among patients affected in this way. Orthopaedic patients often receive large doses of antibiotics prophylactically because of the dramatic consequences of wound sepsis, and so are particularly likely to be affected.

Outbreaks of infective diarrhoea have been reported on orthopaedic units among patients receiving large doses of antibiotics (Degl' Innocenti et al 1989).

Respiratory tract

The entire respiratory tree, except for the alveoli, is lined with ciliated mucous membrane. Inhaled particles become trapped in the mucus and are carried up the airways by the beating cilia, where they are swallowed. About 100 ml of mucus are secreted daily in health. Coarse hairs in the nostrils and the arrangement of the turbinal bones in the nasal cavity, acting as 'baffles', keep large foreign particles out of the respiratory system, while lymphoid tissue in the pharynx (tonsils and adenoids) helps prevent infection.

Cigarette smoke is an irritant, paralysing ciliary action and increasing the secretion of mucus, which stagnates in the air passages. Patients admitted for planned surgery should be advised to avoid or reduce smoking for several weeks before their operation to reduce risks of postoperative chest infection. Anaesthetic agents further depress the protective action of cilia.

Genitourinary system

The adult vagina has a pH of 4.5, unfavourable to most bacteria, owing to its resident population of lactobacilli which metabolize glycogen in cervical secretions, forming lactic acid. Vaginal infections are more common in young girls and postmenopausal women who lack oestrogen which is necessary to maintain cervical secretion.

Two sexually transmitted infections may occasionally be encountered in the orthopaedic patient. Gonorrhoea is sometimes responsible for septic arthritis. Reiter's disease is a late sequel to this infection, a poorly understood syndrome combining arthritis, urethritis and conjunctivitis. Gonorrhoea is still a very common infection in the UK, but between 1976 and 1985 its incidence declined for the first time since the 1940s. Syphilis is a very chronic sexually transmitted infection, which, if untreated, may cause progressive widespread damage to tissues and bones. Good contact tracing and effective treatment with penicillin have made this infection uncommon in the UK today.

The tip of the urethra is colonized by the same species of microorganism present on the skin, but in health the bladder is sterile. During catheterization, a procedure still very commonly performed in hospital, bacteria may be carried directly into the bladder, which seems to have few natural defences against invading pathogens. Urinary infections are, not surprisingly, the most common hospital-acquired infections. They occur almost exclusively in patients with indwelling urethral catheters. Risks of developing infection increase with the length of time the catheter remains in situ, as bacteria can gain access to the catheter via the outlet if it is handled by contaminated hands, if it drags on the floor, or if the catheter and drainage bag become disconnected for any reason, accidental or otherwise (see Fig. 8.2).

A small but significant proportion of hospital patients develop ascending infections of the urinary tract every year as a consequence of catheterization. Renal infection may lead to septicaemia (active bacterial multiplication in the blood), a life-threatening condition which is often fatal (Clifford 1982).

Other invasive procedures

All invasive procedures bypassing the body's natural defence mechanisms are accompanied by a high risk of sepsis. Those performed most often have been examined in most detail. Next to catheterization, most research has been conducted with intravenous lines. Figure 8.3 shows how microorganisms may contaminate and enter the system.

FACTORS AFFECTING INDIVIDUAL SUSCEPTIBILITY TO INFECTION

Patients in hospital share a number of common risk factors increasing the threat of infection. Facilities such as bathrooms and items concerned with personal hygiene (wash bowls, bedpans, urinals) are shared to a much greater extent than at home. If they are not properly decontaminated between one person and the next, the potential for cross-infection is considerable. Objects carrying microorganisms between one person and another are described as fomites. Most

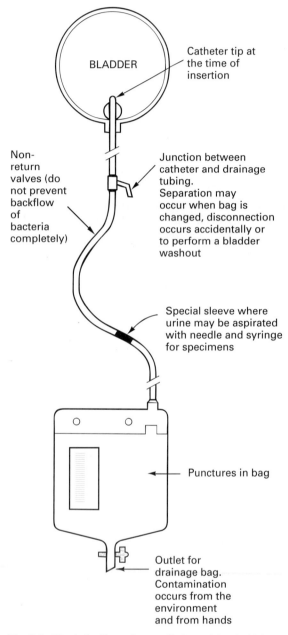

Fig. 8.2 The indwelling urinary catheter: points at which microorganisms may enter.

BLADDER

Catheter tip at the time of insertion

Non-return valves (do not prevent backflow of bacteria completely)

Junction between catheter and drainage tubing. Separation may occur when bag is changed, disconnection occurs accidentally or to perform a bladder washout

Special sleeve where urine may be aspirated with needle and syringe for specimens

Punctures in bag

Outlet for drainage bag. Contamination occurs from the environment and from hands

cross-infection in hospital occurs via the hands of personnel, especially if washing and drying are inadequate, as is often the case (Taylor 1978). The more often a patient is touched by nursing and medical staff, the greater the risk of cross-infection; and the more unwell or incapacitated the individual, the more he or she will require physical nursing care. The physical and psychological stress experienced by the very sick increases their risks of sepsis (Boore 1978), a hazard which can be reduced by allaying anxiety and providing information in terms the patient can understand. Finally, people in hospital eat mass-produced food which, in recent years, has been recognized as a possible source of nosocomial infection.

For individual patients, nurses must anticipate specific risks of infection in order to prescribe appropriate care rather than adopt blanket routines. A number of factors may influence individual susceptibility to infection, although, in general, the more unwell the patient, the more at risk he or she will be.

Age

Both the very young and very old are particularly susceptible to infection, a reflection of the state of development of the immune defences which mature throughout childhood and show some decline with advancing years. In practical terms, this means that the young man who has sustained an open fracture may well escape infection if the wound is adequately cleansed, but the elderly patient with a closed fracture may still fall prey to a hospital-acquired infection.

Nutrition

Optimal nutrition reduces susceptibility to infection. Sadly, many elderly people admitted to hospital are already undernourished, especially if shopping is difficult through reduced mobility which an operation is planned to relieve. People who live alone may feel little incentive to cook for themselves. Once in hospital, pre- and post-operative fasting and a period of anorexia through pain and enforced dependence may further reduce appetite. Even more alarmingly, hospital food itself has been shown in many studies to be nutritionally deficient in protein, calories and vitamin C, all essential for tissue repair.

Obesity, a common condition in the Western

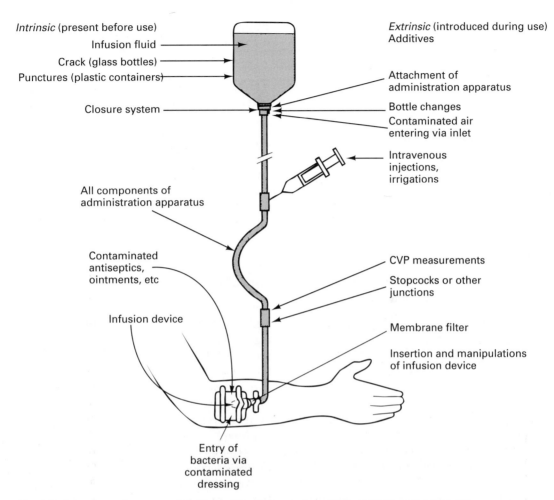

Fig. 8.3 Intravenous therapy: portals of entry for microorganisms; CVP = central venous pressure.

world, also increases susceptibility to infection. Obese patients are unable to expectorate and expand their lungs fully, increasing the risks of respiratory stasis. Immobility, which often accompanies obesity, increases the risk of pressure sore formation. This is more likely to occur in areas such as the sacrum which is readily subject to contamination. Adipose tissue has a poor vascular supply, hence healing is slow.

Dehydration

Dehyrated patients pass little urine and the loss of its mechanical flushing action places them at risk of urinary stasis and urinary infection. Mouth care is essential to prevent a foul mouth containing large numbers of bacteria in patients who are unable to take oral fluids.

Immobility

This patient problem, so commonly encountered on orthopaedic units, increases risks of infection through urinary stasis, stagnation of respiratory secretion and pressure sores. Degrees of mobility vary. The patient who spends a great many hours sitting in a chair every day is not mobile, although secretions will drain to a different segment of the lungs than if he were lying supine, and pressure sores are likely to develop at a different anatomical location (see Ch. 5).

Metabolic disorders

Disturbance of normal metabolic function increases the risk of infection, although the reasons are not always clearly understood:

1. Malignancy is commonly accompanied by infection, which may result from general debility compounded by the effects of radiotherapy and chemotherapy.

2. Diabetes mellitus is an extremely common metabolic disorder, especially among the elderly who are so often admitted to orthopaedic units. High levels of blood sugar and glycosuria may contribute to infection.

3. Peripheral vascular disease, which frequently affects diabetics, commonly results in infection of the extremities, usually the toes. Meticulous care of the feet is necessary for these patients and should be emphasized when they leave hospital, as neglect may lead to necrosis which may eventually involve the whole limb, with tragic consequences. In severe cases, amputation of an infected, gangrenous limb may be the only treatment option.

Even in healthy people, healing can be impaired at sites of the body which receive a poor blood supply. Only slight trauma may result in a wound both slow to heal and easily infected. Tissue covering the front of the tibia, for example, is poorly vascularized, so varicose ulcers commonly develop in this region.

Drugs

Antibiotic therapy and replacement of the normal body flora by foreign microorganisms has already been discussed. Destruction of bacteria which normally live in the mouth and vagina can lead to a fungal infection, *Candida* ('thrush'). *Candida* also causes urinary infections among severely debilitated patients taking antibiotics.

Steroids depress the normal inflammatory response which helps to protect the body against trauma and infection, and they reduce the number of white cells, impairing phagocytosis. Like antibiotics, steroids are widely prescribed and many patients may already be taking these

drugs for some condition not connected to their orthopaedic problem.

TRANSMISSION OF MICROORGANISMS

In hospital and the community microorganisms are spread by direct and indirect contact. Dissemination can occur by the airborne route, via contaminated food and water, and parenterally, i.e. from one host to the next in infected blood and body fluids derived from blood, on needles and other sharp instruments. Some organisms are also transmitted in breast milk (e.g. HIV).

Direct contact

Spread by direct contact between one individual and the next is particularly common in hospital, especially when very ill and debilitated people receive physical care from many different members of staff. The advantage of individual patient care (where the same nurse looks after the same group of patients) in minimizing the spread of infection is obvious. Nursing staff may be deployed so that a highly susceptible patient does not receive care from a nurse also attending a very infectious patient.

Crowded wards and understaffing increase the risk of infection by direct contact, especially when there is inadequate time for thorough handwashing. On orthopaedic units, infection may develop after exposure to contaminated water in a hydrotherapy pool. Continuous chlorination is necessary to ensure that a sufficiently high level of free chlorine is maintained to kill bacteria. The filters of the plant need checking and regular maintenance by the hospital engineer to ensure that they are in correct working order.

Indirect contact

Indirect transmission of microorganisms via fomites is particularly likely to occur on orthopaedic units where may patients are bedfast for long periods of time and therefore reliant on washbowls, bedpans, urinals etc. Bacteria require warmth, moisture and a supply of nutrients before they will grow and multiply. Consequently they are more likely to flourish in warm, damp bedclothes than on the cold, metallic surface of a bedcradle. Clearly, objects near the patient are more likely to be contaminated than distant ones, i.e. a book will probably carry more bacteria than the television on the patient's locker. And obviously, prevention of infection depends on keeping all equipment as clean and dry as possible. The water in humidifiers, tubing of all kinds and flower vases can act as a reservoir of bacteria, as may buckets used for soaking plaster bandages.

Airborne spread

Infection is transmitted by respiratory and salivary droplets which dry, leaving airborne particles as dust. Early research by Duguid (1946) demonstrated that on average 39 000 bacteria-containing droplets are released by a single, unstifled sneeze, 710 from a cough and only 36 during loud speech. The fate of these droplets depends on their size, as this will influence drying and settling. Gravity will force a large droplet to fall rapidly before drying, so any bacteria will still be viable. Smaller droplets dry, and the solid materials they contain pass into the air circulation of the room, where they represent a source of infection.

Most infections in the community affect the upper or lower respiratory tract (e.g. colds, influenza, measles) and are transmitted as airborne droplets. In theatre, this is a major route for postoperative wound infections, especially those caused by staphylococci, which are often carried in the nose and throat of hospital personnel as well as on the hands. It is generally accepted that a significant reduction in the incidence of deep sepsis complicating total hip and knee replacement operations can be achieved by an ultra-clean air environment in theatre (Jalovaara & Puranen 1989). Masks and gowns made of non-woven synthetic fabric reduce airborne dispersal of particles, and laminar flow (rapid filtration of the air in the operating room) reduces the risk

further. Numbers of airborne particles increase with the number of people in theatre and the degree of activity taking place in theatre and on the ward.

Faecal–oral route

Faeces contain large numbers of bacteria, which can contaminate the environment and be transmitted to food and water. Organisms which form spores resistant to drying can remain infectious for long periods outside the body. An example is the disease tetanus (causative organism, *Clostridium tetani*). The organism is shed in the faeces of farm animals and may cause infection following a deep cut or puncture sustained by gardeners or agricultural labourers.

In recent years, large outbreaks of food poisoning have been reported in hospitals. Perhaps the most notorious culprit is *Salmonella*, but numerous other bacteria are associated with food poisoning and it is always worth considering the food brought into hospital by well-meaning relatives when a case occurs. The young man supplied with a Chinese takeaway meal might develop a mild form of food poisoning caused by *Bacillus cereus*. Spores of this bacteria are sometimes found in rice, and they survive initial boiling. Freshly cooked rice is safe, as the bacteria remain inactive, but if the rice is left in a warm atmosphere spores germinate and bacteria multiply. They are not destroyed by gentle frying so food poisoning results.

Parenteral spread

The risk of infection on contaminated needles and other sharp instruments is very high in hospital. Two virus infections are transmitted in this way: HIV and hepatitis B. Of the two, hepatitis B is by far the most virulent, but neither virus survives long outside the body. The rate of carriage is particularly high among the promiscuous, especially active homosexuals who have had large numbers of different sexual contacts, and intravenous drug abusers. People from certain parts of the world have a high rate of carriage for one or the other of these viruses. HIV is widespread in Africa, while carriage of hepatitis B occurs very commonly in people from the Middle East. Nurses therefore need to be familiar with the community outside their hospital. Those who work in an area known for its high incidence of African immigrants or drug abusers can expect to encounter a correspondingly high incidence of HIV in hospital. This is not the same as 'labelling' individual patients as likely to carry HIV or hepatitis B. As recent health education campaigns emphasize, these viruses are not discriminating: anyone can become infected. Good practice when handling all blood and disposing of all sharps is essential. Immunization against hepatitis B is now available, but not against HIV.

PATHOGENESIS OF INFECTIOUS DISEASE

The pathogenicity of a microorganism is its ability to cause disease. Most bacteria are not pathogenic, but live freely in the environment, mainly in soil and water, where they decompose dead animal and plant material. Some live on the skin and in the gut of man and other animals, where they are beneficial by competing with foreign bacteria, keeping them at bay in return for shelter. Bacteria in the human large intestine synthesize vitamin K which the body requires but is unable to make.

These beneficial bacteria are said to be commensals. Relatively few bacteria behave as active pathogens.

A pathogenic species establishes disease through the following sequence of events:

1. Invasion of the tissues, overcoming the body's normal defences
2. Evading phagocytosis and the activities of the immune system once within the host
3. Multiplication
4. Destruction of host tissues; this is often achieved by enzyme secretion
5. Release of toxins. These are potent poisons, usually responsible for the specific signs and symptoms of disease. In the example given above of tetanus, it is the toxin released by *C.*

tetani that causes muscle paralysis resulting in spasm.

A virulent pathogen has greater capacities of invasion, destruction and toxin production than a less virulent species. Another type of bacteria responsible for many orthopaedic wound infections, *Staphylococcus aureus*, owes its pathogenicity to an enzyme, coagulase, which converts the plasma protein fibrinogen to fibrin. Release causes a mesh of fibrin to develop around the bacteria, protecting them from phagocytosis. *Staph. epidermidis* is a commensal species forming part of the normal skin flora. It is unable to release coagulase and is therefore of low-grade pathogenicity. However, it is capable of active infection in severely debilitated patients whose host defences are poor, and is frequently associated with sepsis of catheters and intravenous lines. Today *Staph. epidermidis* is recorded as an increasingly common cause of severe, deep-seated orthopaedic infections after prosthetic implants (Lidwell et al 1983), apparently through its ability to colonize plastic and metal inserts.

Bacteria able to cause low-grade infections among the severely debilitated are described as opportunists. They represent a major source of nosocomial infection as their growth requirements are extremely simple, allowing them to flourish wherever there is moisture and simple environmental contamination, conditions met all too frequently in hospitals.

Another important factor contributory to pathogenicity is size of the infective dose. It is logical to suppose that a large inoculum of bacteria will be able to overcome host defences more effectively than a small number, but this may be a simplified view. Deep tissues such as bones and joints, which are usually sterile, have low resistance to bacteria because they would not normally encounter them, and only a small inoculum during surgery (as few as 15 organisms) can have devastating consequences. Nurses working on the ward need to remember that, under ideal conditions, bacilli such as *Escherichia coli* and *Pseudomonas* can replicate approximately once every 30 minutes. Urine stagnating in a catheter bag is readily subject to environmental contamination. If the bag is allowed to fill, a large infective dose may rapidly develop and gain access to the bladder.

Response of the body to infection

Pyrexia

Pyrexia (fever) is a systemic reaction of the body to infection, provoked by microorganisms and their toxins. Body temperature is controlled by the hypothalamus. The temperature-regulating centre is often compared to a thermostat, which in human beings is usually fixed at about 37°C. Control is by a negative feedback mechanism (see Fig. 8.4). When infection occurs, chemical groups called antigens, present on the bacterial cell walls, cause the thermostat to 'reset' at a higher temperature until they have been elimi-

nated from the body. A higher temperature appears to enhance phagocytosis, and it is the neutrophils (see Fig. 8.5) which release a protein, stimulating pyrexia. As far as the patient is concerned, fever has a number of disadvantages as it is accompanied by an increase in metabolic rate which can be exhausting. For every 1°C rise above 37°C, the adult pulse increases at a rate of about 20 beats per minute and respiratory rate by 7 breaths per minute. Body stores of glycogen become depleted, and if fever is prolonged, negative nitrogen balance will follow.

Pyrexia as a sign of infection is not infallible. Elderly people may not develop pyrexia, and often confusion and restlessness in a formerly lucid and cooperative individual are the first indications to the nurse that all is not well. Anaesthesia may leave patients disoriented for a few days postoperatively, especially elderly

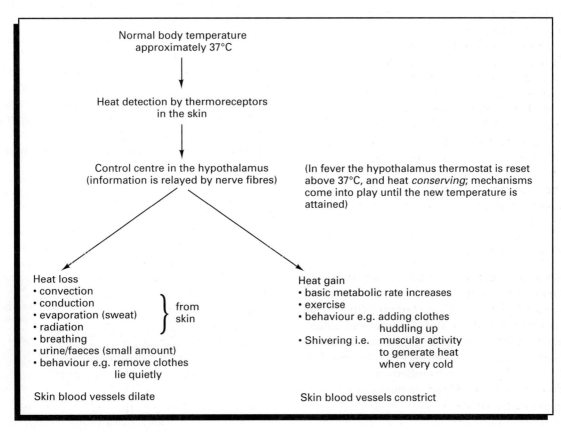

Fig. 8.4   Temperature control.

Neutrophil
10–14 µm

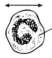

Cytoplasm containing 'granules'
— inclusions of enzymes able
to lyse bacteria

Macrophage
15–20 µm

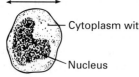

Cytoplasm with granules

Nucleus

Fig. 8.5 Neutrophils and macrophages. Neutrophils originate in the red bone marrow and are continually replaced throughout the lifespan of the individual as they survive only 1–3 days. Numbers increase in acute infections, e.g. acute osteomyelitis; they are the first white cells to appear at sites of acute inflammation. Macrophages originate in red bone marrow, enter the blood and migrate into the tissues. They are replaced throughout the lifespan, but are believed to survive for weeks or months. They appear at the site of inflammation after neutrophils, but, as they are larger, have a greater capacity for phagocytosis. They are also active in chronic infections, including tuberculosis.

people removed suddenly from familiar home surroundings. Often the general condition of the patient is the best indication of developing sepsis.

Inflammation

Inflammation is the reaction of living tissues to injury. Response occurs chiefly through activity of the vascular and connective tissues and is non-specific; physical trauma (excessive heat, cold and radiation) and chemicals evoke the inflammatory response, as does infection. This is an important point often overlooked by nurses, who equate the signs and symptoms of inflammation exclusively with infection. Following accidental trauma or surgery it is normal for damaged tissue to appear inflamed.

The classic signs and symptoms of acute inflammation are:

1. Redness
2. Heat
3. Swelling
4. Pain
5. Loss of function.

At the microscopic level these readily observable changes are explained by hyperaemia, exudation of plasma from blood to the extracellular spaces and migration of white cells from the capillaries to the damaged area. The white cells most important in inflammation and healing are shown in Figure 8.5.

Hyperaemia This is the initial response, beginning within seconds of injury when the local area becomes momentarily white due to vasoconstriction. A dull red flush follows as the vessels dilate, increasing local blood supply, and hence redness and heat. The mechanisms responsible for these changes interact (see Fig. 8.6).

Exudation Chemicals released from the injured cells combined with some damage to the endothelium of the local capillaries increase their permeability, allowing plasma proteins to escape from the vessels to the surrounding extracellular space. Water follows by osmotic attraction, leading to oedema. Pressure from oedema on nerve endings and the action of chemicals such as prostaglandins and kinins released by damaged cells, explain the pain associated with inflammation, leading to reduced function.

Vasodilation and exudation are valuable

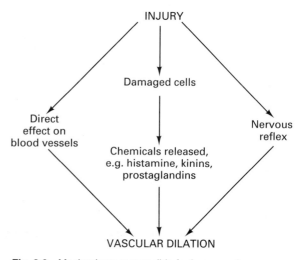

Fig. 8.6 Mechanisms responsible for hyperaemia.

defence mechanisms because they carry more white cells and antibodies to the damaged area to fight infection and more fibrinogen to produce blood clotting, i.e. to stem bleeding if physical trauma has occurred.

Migration Vasodilation reduces the speed at which the blood is flowing in capillaries immediately adjacent to the damaged area, causing neutrophils to congregate ('marginate') close to the vessel walls. Chemicals released by the damaged cells attract neutrophils, which have the property of amoeboid movement. They are able to squeeze through narrow slits between the capillary endothelial cells and migrate towards the wounded area (see Fig. 8.7). Attraction by chemical substances is called chemotaxis. Ability to squeeze between the capillary cells is known as diapedesis. Once in the damaged area, the neutrophils begin by phagocytosis to engulf and digest bacteria and foreign debris contaminating the wound. Only bacteria to which host antibodies have become attached can be phagocytosed, showing how the specific immune system and non-specific inflammation cooperate to destroy infection.

Antibodies are proteins produced by the body in response to foreign particles, including bacteria. The immune response is specific, as there are thousands of different antibodies, a different one produced in response to every different kind of foreign particle encountered by the tissues. During the course of his or her life everybody is challenged by slightly different microorganisms, so everyone contains a unique spectrum of antibodies. The field of immunology is rapidly expanding and a more detailed discussion is beyond

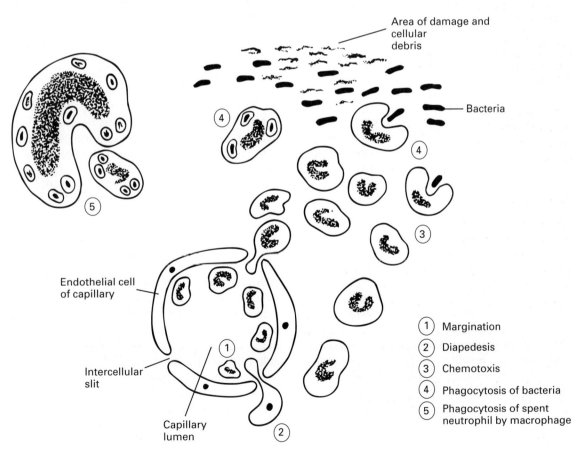

Fig. 8.7 Activities of neutrophils during acute inflammation.

the scope of this text. Suggestions for further reading are given at the end of the chapter.

Neutrophils have a short lifespan (1–3 days) and expire after successfully phagocytosing a given number of bacteria. They are later phagocytosed themselves by the much larger and longer-lived macrophages (see Fig. 8.5) which arrive at the site of damage a day or so after the acute inflammatory response develops. Sometimes, however, virulent bacteria resist attack by degradative enzymes within the neutrophil. Instead, they multiply inside it, causing the cell membrane of the neutrophil to burst open, allowing the bacteria to escape again.

Sequels to acute inflammation

If the inflammatory reaction proceeds successfully it is followed by resolution, a return to normal conditions which is possible under the following circumstances:

- minimal host cell death and damage
- rapid elimination of the causal agent
- local conditions favouring prompt removal of exudate and debris via the blood.

Inflammation and resolution proceed more swiftly in tissues which are well vascularized than in those which receive a poor blood supply.

If bacteria and other contaminants are not readily removed, suppuration will follow. As dead neutrophils, dead bacteria and other debris accumulate they form pus and an abscess develops, 'pointing' towards an internal or external body surface under the influence of gravity. If the contents of the abscess are discharged naturally or by a surgical incision, pain and swelling subside, the remaining cavity gradually heals and scar tissue forms. An abscess deep in the tissues may be overlooked. Gradually a long, tortuous track develops between the abscess and a body surface, resulting in the formation of a chronically discharging sinus, especially if contaminated matter is retained. Sinuses are extremely difficult to heal and may require surgical intervention. Deep cavity wounds must be packed to prevent superficial healing over a potentially infected underlying layer. The tradi-

tional approach with ribbon gauze is now being superseded by more effective modern preparations such as foam elastomer agents (e.g. silastic foam). The wound must be free of infection before these are applied.

WOUND HEALING

The acute inflammatory reaction continues for about 3 days and as it draws to a close, wound healing begins by first or second intention. Both processes involve collagen synthesis, repair of blood vessels and re-epithelialization of the damaged area.

Healing by first intention

This occurs in clean, incised wounds with good apposition of the tissue margins. Typical examples include cuts and surgical incisions. (see Fig. 8.8).

Towards the end of the inflammatory response macrophages in the wound attract fibroblast cells. These begin actively to synthesize a network of collagen fibres in the cleft of the wound, holding the two lips together. Collagen is a tough, fibrous protein forming the chief constituent of skin, fascia, tendons and ligaments. In the healing wound it forms granulation (scar) tissue.

In surgical wounds collagen synthesis becomes optimal between the 5th and 7th postoperative day. Collagen provides tensile strength to the wound, but damaged tissues never quite regain their original strength. Infected wounds are further weakened when collagen is digested by pathogenic bacteria able to release an enzyme, collagenase. Collagen formation depends on an adequate supply of nutrients and oxygen, for which bacteria compete, further delaying healing.

Fibroblast activity is stimulated in an acidic environment, rich in lactate and vitamin C. The pH is low deep within the tissues where the viable cells are metabolizing, releasing lactic acid; hence, collagen formation begins deep inside the wound and extends away from the damage.

Wounding severs local capillaries which undergo repair, a process known as angiogenesis. New capillary growth is stimulated by low oxygen levels, so repair proceeds from the healthy

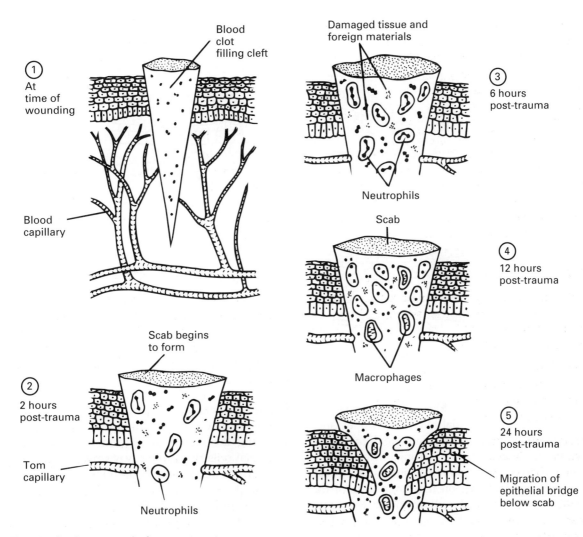

Fig. 8.8 Caption see overleaf.

margins of the wound into the centre of damage. Granulation tissue is highly vascular, causing it to appear pink, and the new vessels are easily traumatized. While it is forming, the surface of the wound is re-epithelialized, a process beginning less than 24 hours after a clean wound has been made and complete within 2 or 3 days. Once the surface of the wound has become covered with an intact epithelial bridge it is impermeable to bacteria and it is at this stage that the initial dressing applied in theatre is often removed to allow inspection of the healing tissues. Figure 8.8 shows that the new epithelial bridge develops beneath the scab left by bleeding. The scab provides mechanical protection and helps prevent desiccation. It should not be removed.

Wound healing has been the subject of considerable research and it has been determined beyond all doubt that re-epithelialization proceeds more readily in a moist environment; yet many old practices can still be observed today among nursing and medical personnel who remain convinced that a wound should appear clean (i.e. free of scab) and dry. Once re-epithelialization is complete the scab begins to slough away gradually without intervention.

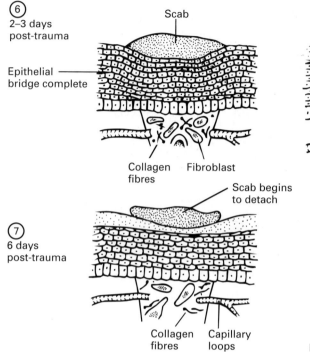

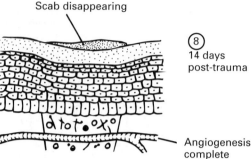

Fig. 8.8 Wound healing by first intention.

As inflammation subsides the wound begins to mature, losing its initial red, raised appearance as the collagen fibres gradually realign, lacing themselves together in a strong, three-dimensional weave. Maturation continues for weeks or months, depending on the magnitude of the injury, so the wound will continue to regain strength throughout convalescence. Maturation is accompanied by decreasing vascularity and shrinking of the fibroblasts as they become quiescent. The scar eventually becomes white and less pronounced. Patients often worry about the appearance of the wound and should be advised of these changes before they leave hospital.

Wound healing by second intention

This is the mechanism of healing in open wounds where there has been loss of tissue, necrosis or infection. Burns, ischaemic and varicose ulcers and pressure sores fall into this category. After tissue destruction the wound cavity is filled with blood and fibrin (see Fig. 8.9). Acute inflammation commences at the junction, with viable cells remaining at the base and around the edges of the cavity. Within a few days the scab covering the wound dries and newly forming epithelial cells thrust their way upwards between the surface debris and underlying tissue. Capillary loops grow into the new epithelium, bringing macrophages and fibroblasts. In time, the cavity fills with granulation tissue and the scab is shed. Epithelium covers the surface of the wound completely within approximately 2 weeks, although this depends on the size of the wound.

Second intention proceeds more slowly than primary intention, especially as wounds of this type are subject to recurring episodes of inflammation which may lead to excess, inappropriate collagen deposition and pronounced scarring. Contamination exacerbates this situation.

Contaminated wounds and wound closure

Nurses who have admitted victims of major trauma to the ward and those who work in the Accident and Emergency Department will be aware that patients may come into hospital with

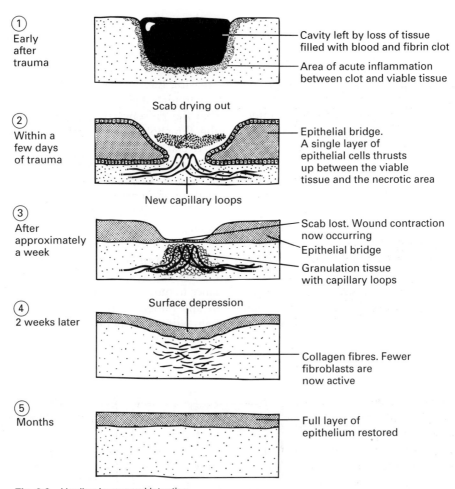

① Early after trauma
— Cavity left by loss of tissue filled with blood and fibrin clot
— Area of acute inflammation between clot and viable tissue

Scab drying out

② Within a few days of trauma
— Epithelial bridge. A single layer of epithelial cells thrusts up between the viable tissue and the necrotic area

New capillary loops

③ After approximately a week
— Scab lost. Wound contraction now occurring
— Epithelial bridge
— Granulation tissue with capillary loops

Surface depression

④ 2 weeks later
— Collagen fibres. Fewer fibroblasts are now active

⑤ Months
— Full layer of epithelium restored

Fig. 8.9   Healing by second intention.

wounds that are heavily contaminated (see Table 8.1). For many pathogenic microorganisms, it appears that an infective dose of 10^6 bacteria for every gram of tissue is necessary before infection supervenes in a healthy adult. Host defence mechanisms can usually cope with smaller doses, so many bacteria present in contaminated wounds will be destroyed. However, the local defence mechanisms may become overwhelmed when large amounts of necrotic tissue are present, for example following open compound fractures, and an ideal medium is provided for bacterial growth, especially species of clostridia which are responsible for tetanus (*C. tetani*) and gas gangrene (*C. perfringens*). Surgical debridement under general anaesthesia and large doses

Table 8.1   Wound classifications

Clean wounds: no evidence of inflammation, no lapse in aseptic technique during surgery and no entry into the respiratory and gastrointestinal tracts, e.g. total hip replacement.

Clean contaminated wounds: those generated by surgical procedures which involve entry into the respiratory or gastrointestinal tracts, but in which no significant spillage has occurred.

Contaminated wounds: those in which there is evidence of acute inflammation without the formation of pus; an otherwise clean operation in which there has been a major breach of aseptic technique, and recent traumatic wounds are considered to be contaminated.

Dirty wounds: those in which pus or a perforated internal organ are encountered. Traumatic wounds not of recent origin are also placed in this category, e.g. discharging sinus.

of broad spectrum antibiotics are required. As few as 15 bacteria may be sufficient to cause infection in joints and bones.

Minor wounds heal spontaneously but in the case of more severe trauma, surgical intervention is essential to speed tissue repair and help minimize deformity, as well as to avoid infection. The method of wound closure will depend on the amount of tissue lost. Direct suturing of the wound edges (primary closure, see Fig. 8.10A) is appropriate for clean wounds and contaminated wounds in which thorough debridement has been possible.

Delayed primary closure (see Fig. 8.10B) is the method of choice for heavily contaminated and dirty wounds. As damaged tissues reach the height of their immune response within 4–5 days of injury, suturing is delayed until this time, because natural resistance to infection is then at its maximum. Initially the wound is covered with sterile, non-adherent dressings and when wound closure ultimately takes place, the minimal amount of suture material is employed, as sutures operate as foreign bodies, greatly decreasing the threshold of infection necessary for any remaining bacteria. It has been estimated that the presence of one silk suture can reduce the threshold for clinical infection by a factor of 10 000.

Patients for whom a policy of delayed primary closure has been decided will require a great deal of supportive nursing care to allay the psychological fear of being left 'unintact' or 'cut open', and to relieve anxiety that they are being neglected. Physical nursing care is crucial to the prevention of urinary stasis, pressure sore formation and respiratory infection through reluctance to move. Pain control is of major importance in any patient with a traumatic injury because pain will probably be exacerbated by fear.

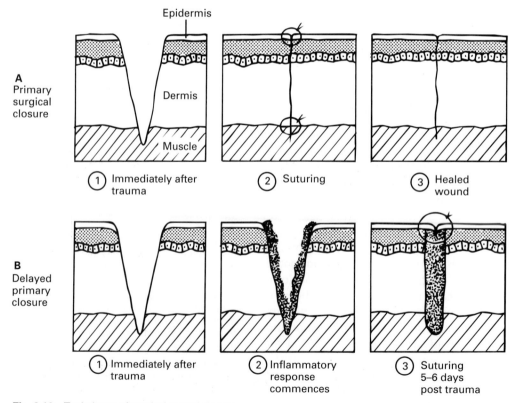

Fig. 8.10 Techniques of surgical wound closure.

Factors influencing surgical wound infection

For wounds created surgically, numerous factors interact to determine whether or not infection will supervene. Clearly, the patient's general condition and the site of the incision (degree of contamination, vascularization) will be of major importance but, particularly in orthopaedic surgery, much will also depend on the number of bacteria able to gain access to the open tissues.

Theatre clothing

Staphylococci are shed in large numbers from the nose, throat, perineum and on skin scales. A single skin scale may carry 100 individual bac-

teria, presenting a threat when the deep tissues are exposed. Contamination may occur via the airborne or contact route and the bacteria may originate from the patient or from the theatre team (see Fig. 8.11).

John Charnley was responsible in the early 1960s for the development of a mechanically satisfactory hip joint prosthesis, but the dramatic success of total hip replacement in the relief of pain and restoration of function was marred by a high rate of sepsis, often exceeding 10% in some centres. Infections sometimes developed months after surgery, representing a disaster for the patient who returned to a state of functioning worse than before the operation. Charnley concluded that the implanted prosthesis must be

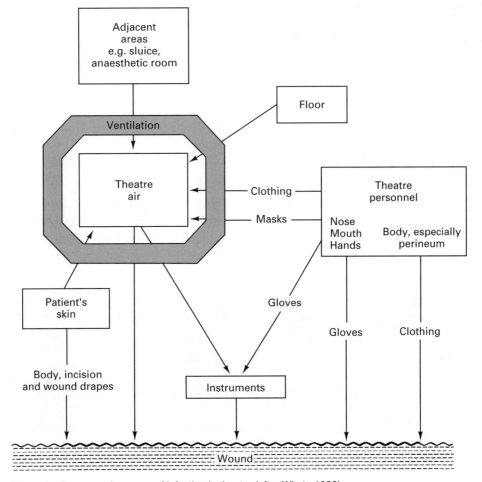

Fig. 8.11 Routes and sources of infection in theatre (after Whyte 1988).

particularly susceptible to infection, requiring only a small airborne inoculum for sepsis to develop. Between 1960 and 1970 he refined a system of theatre ventilation and clothing which reduced contamination of the ambient air in the theatre suite to less than 1% of that found in a conventional operating suite. Even without the use of prophylactic antibiotics, the rate of sepsis fell to below 1%.

Cotton is not suitable for use in orthopaedic theatres because bacteria can escape through its loose weave. Charnley advocated the use of a special non-woven fabric called 'ventile' in conjunction with a total body exhaust gown and helmet. Air is removed from the helmet and upward flow helps to keep the individual cool. Bacteria are dispersed beneath the gown, so the system is fully effective only if there is also uni-directional ultraclean airflow within the theatre. Unfortunately, many surgeons have found the total body exhaust system hot and claustropho-bic and the exhaust hose supplying the air can be restricting. The quest to find a comfortable non-woven fabric continues.

Filtered air systems

Filtered ventilation systems reduce the airborne bacterial count, but must be switched on before the operating list commences and checked at regular intervals by the hospital engineer to ensure that they are in correct working order. Air should flow from clean to dirty areas, never the reverse, by maintaining a higher pressure in the operating room than in sluices, etc. In high risk areas, such as the orthopaedic theatre, high speed laminar flow is effective in removing airborne particles swiftly from the patient's vicinity. Air moving at very high speed (ap-proximately 30 m/min) is passed through a bank of filters which replace a conventional wall or ceiling in the room, and is extracted through the opposite wall or floor.

Down-flow systems appear to have better per-formance than cross-flow, but both are rendered less effective by excessive movement of person-nel within theatre. The passage of airflow can be seriously disrupted by large obstacles – i.e. there

should be only essential furniture and fittings within the operating room; it is never a suitable place for equipment storage.

Masks

The efficiency of masks in reducing the airborne bacterial count has been studied by many authors. It appears that if the mask is made of a thin material (usually paper) or is ill-fitting because it is small and stiff, effectiveness can be as little as 50%. Most of the cheaper brands fall into this category. Loss of efficiency occurs through small particles escaping round the sides. Effec-tive masks are the more expensive types, manu-factured from one thick layer of fabric or from laminated material. They are soft and pleated, fitting the contours of the individual's face.

Experiments have shown that when theatre personnel have not worn masks, there is little difference in the number of bacteria growing on culture plates positioned beneath the operating table. This has led some authorities to question the routine use of masks. However, during ortho-paedic operations, the hazards are so great that there is no doubt as to whether masks should be worn.

Gloves

Although millions of bacteria are carried on the hands, these can be reduced substantially by scrubbing with a skin disinfectant, especially if this is followed by an alcohol rub. Most of the bacteria removed are those present from envi-ronmental contamination. Those remaining tend to be the resident flora which are often sheltered deep in the sweat glands. Gloves are essential during surgery to prevent these gaining access to the wound. Several studies have indicated that over 10% of gloves worn during general surgery become punctured. During orthopaedic opera-tions the rate may reach nearly 50%. The wearing of double gloves adopted by many orthopaedic surgeons appears a sensible precaution.

Duration of the operation

The risk of infection increases according to the

length of time the tissues are exposed. After the first hour, it has been estimated that the infection rate will double for every additional hour that the operation is prolonged. This is a major hazard during complicated, lengthy orthopaedic surgery.

Preoperative preparation

In most hospitals patients are advised to have a shower or bath before going to theatre, except in emergencies. Often, antiseptics containing chlorhexidine or povidone iodine are provided for use in the bath. The results of research studies investigating their effectiveness are conflicting. Chlorhexidine is an expensive preparation, but povidone iodine derivatives are much cheaper and have the added advantage of destroying spores as well as vegetative bacteria. Commercial preparations intended for use in the bath and shower do not stain the skin.

Shaving the site of the operation the day before surgery increases the risk of sepsis because it damages the epithelium, increasing the rate of growth and multiplication of bacteria already present. Orthopaedic surgery generally involves the limbs, where removal of hair in the region of the incision is essential. Shaving is best performed at the last possible minute before the operation. Trials with depilatory creams have been disappointing as they are not associated with any greater reduction in postoperative wound infection than shaving.

Wound site

The site of the wound is closely related to the likely degree of contamination and therefore to infection. A well-vascularized wound is capable of a more efficient inflammatory response, and more likely to heal while remaining free of infection. A sacral pressure sore is very likely to become contaminated. Surgical repair of a deep sore in this region may be problematic, especially as dressings are very difficult to hold in position. A high incidence of sepsis has been reported from leg wounds. The bacteria responsible often have been faecal in origin, suggesting that the legs should be regarded as a potentially contaminated site requiring meticulous preoperative skin preparation.

Length of pre- and postoperative stay

The longer the period spent in hospital before surgery, the greater the patient's risk of developing heavy skin contamination with multiple resistant hospital strains of bacteria. Thus, the risk of sepsis is increased and it is more difficult to provide effective antibiotic treatment.

In the past it has been argued that patients profit from hospital admission 1 or 2 days before the operation is scheduled in order to be prepared psychologically as well as physically for surgery. Cost-cutting and bed closures in the National Health Service now mean that hospital stay is curtailed as far as possible. Patients who are to undergo planned orthopaedic surgery will already have had time to consider the implications of the operation and the need to cope with temporary disability, as these points will have been broached during assessment in the outpatient clinic. Regrettably, many people wait far too long for othopaedic surgery owing to the length of waiting lists in some parts of the country.

Similarly, prompt discharge from hospital reduces the length of exposure to hospital populations of microorganisms.

Mechanical cleansing

The purpose of mechanical cleansing is to remove heavy contamination from a wound. This can take place in theatre before the wound is closed or before going to theatre if a method of delayed primary closure has been selected. In the ward a stream of sterile, antiseptic fluid is driven over the wound under hydrostatic pressure. The solution does not remain in contact with the tissues for long; its main effect is to dislodge contaminants.

Some authorities believe that the high pressure necessary may damage tissue defences, and advocate a compromise in which the wound is intermittently irrigated from a conventional syringe. Although this method is less traumatic it is also less efficient.

Antibiotic therapy

Indiscriminate use of antibiotics is associated with a high risk of bacterial resistance, especially among staphylococci. In the 1950s large outbreaks of staphylococcal cross-infection led to the closure of many hospital wards. These outbreaks were intensively investigated and research led to the development of many of the hospital policies which have since helped reduce the spread of infection in wards and theatre. During the 1980s it became apparent that staphylococci were developing multiple resistance to a wide range of antibiotics. Many hospitals have now instituted strict 'antibiotic policies'; a number of broad-spectrum antibiotics are withheld from routine use, so hospital strains have little opportunity to become resistant. These drugs provide a valuable reserve if a patient is admitted carrying a multi-resistant strain. Such patients often have sustained injury when travelling in countries where antibiotic prescription is less carefully monitored than in the UK, sometimes drugs can be purchased over the counter.

Patients undergoing orthopaedic procedures are placed in such jeopardy that prophylactic antibiotic treatment is justified. Hughes (1988) advocates high doses of antibiotics given over a short period closely related to the time of surgery. The aim should be always to protect a particular patient from bacteria known to represent a specific threat. Cement primed with antibiotics may be used to fix implants in patients undergoing arthroplasty.

Gram-negative bacilli (*E. coli, Proteus, Klebsiella, Pseudomonas*), which are spread by the contact route, have been found in deep-seated orthopaedic wounds as well as being responsible for other problematic nosocomial infections, especially those involving the urinary tract. Few antibiotics are effective against these species; this emphasizes the need for strict implementation of prophylactic antibiotic treatment.

Anaesthetic equipment

Like all equipment in theatre, anaesthetic machines must be thoroughly cleaned and decontaminated after use, as the warm, moist tubing can harbour bacteria, especially gram-negative bacilli. Spread to the wound is often by contact.

Wound drainage

Drains are inserted after surgery or trauma when fluid is expected to accumulate in the tissues, where it will serve as a focus for bacterial infection. Following orthopaedic surgery, there may be seepage of serous and serosanguinous fluid unless it is removed via closed suction drainage systems under pressure. Usually two drains are inserted, one to draw fluid from deep in the wound and the other to drain the superficial tissues. Closed suction drainage significantly reduces the incidence of postoperative sepsis, providing the drain is inserted through a stab wound separate from the main incision. However, the drainage system must be handled with aseptic technique.

Surgical technique

The technique of the individual surgeon undoubtedly contributes towards the postoperative infection rate, as the beneficial effects of inflammation depend on a good blood supply which can be impaired through rough handling or excessive use of diathermy, or by knotting ligatures so tightly that the tissue held between them becomes 'strangled' and necrosis results. The choice of suture material is also known to be influential. Bulky, braided materials are more often implicated with episodes of sepsis than monofilamentous ones because microorganisms can evade host defences through concealment in the weave. Surgeons tend to be conservative in their choice, and often prefer traditional products to the many new varieties now appearing on the market.

Wound management

Events in theatre are usually beyond the control of the individual nurse although the nursing voice may be represented at management level, as hospitals commonly include a senior nurse on panels such as the infection control and theatre users' committees. However, all nurses need to know the rationale behind infection prevention in theatre, as most surgical infections originate when the tissues are exposed but do not manifest until the patient has returned to the ward. In contrast, wound management is clearly a nursing responsibility, especially in the realms of problematic, slowly-healing wounds. Surgeons commonly prescribe policies of care for uncomplicated, technically clean wounds created under highly controlled conditions in theatre which will heal by first intention. It is left to the nurse to cope with pressure sores and varicose ulcers which heal slowly and unpredictably and which are frequently contaminated. Often patients' surgical wounds fail to heal or they develop chronic lesions because of poor underlying health. Tissue repair will not proceed satisfactorily until the patient's general condition has been improved by supportive nursing care. The choice of dressing materials is now bewildering and as many are expensive and all require detailed knowledge of their properties and performance, the nurse must appreciate factors influencing healing.

Humidity

The inflammatory response produces exudate, but there is a critical balance between optimal wound humidity and the amount of fluid present. A wound allowed to become too dry will develop a hard, impermeable scab, while migration of the epithelial bridge will be impaired. Intensive research in the 1960s and 1970s demonstrated that occlusion beneath a dressing designed to retain moisture will promote re-epithelialization, angiogenesis and granulation.

Polyurethane dressings (e.g. Opsite) and hydrocolloids (e.g. Granuflex) fall into this category. The differences between a wound that has been covered and one that has been exposed are shown in Figure 8.12. Occasionally nurses voice anxiety about the excessive amount of exudate which sometimes appears beneath polyurethane dressings, believing that an ideal growth medium is provided for bacteria. However, this exudate is bactericidal, as it contains large numbers of active neutrophils. Provided the edges of the dressing do not lift from the skin, no bacteria from outside can reach the wound. Excess exudate can be aspirated via a sterile needle and syringe.

Gaseous exchange

An adequate oxygen supply is essential to metabolically active tissue in a healing wound and is

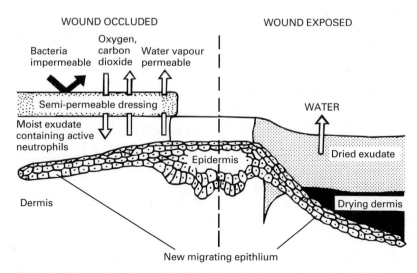

Fig. 8.12 Comparison of wound healing with and without an occlusive covering.

supplied mainly via the blood. Hyperbaric oxygen has been shown experimentally to increase the rate of epithelial migration in wounds covered by occlusive dressings, but it is effective chiefly because it increases oxygen tension in the blood supplying the wound. High levels of oxygen destroy anaerobic bacteria such as clostridia which cause gangrene but, as dead cells are no longer metabolically active, they have no action on necrotic tissue.

pH

Outside a very narrow pH range, living tissues lose metabolic function because enzyme activity is disrupted. Alterations in pH rapidly have a deleterious effect on re-epithelialization and phagocytosis. Eusol, with a pH of 8, is not, therefore, a suitable application for delicate tissues and has been banned from many hospital pharmacies. Other, more effective chemical debriding agents are now commercially available. Eusol is also known to have damaging systemic effects on debilitated and elderly patients and may contribute to the development of renal failure.

Other novel agents

Rapidly dividing cells depend on a good blood supply to provide nutrients and remove toxic waste materials resulting from metabolism. Direct application of nutritive substances to a wound has never been proven to be beneficial and is never likely to be, as materials such as egg white, traditionally used as topical wound applications, provide excellent culture media for bacteria. Honey is occasionally applied to wounds, not for its nutritive properties, but because its high sugar content renders it strongly hygroscopic, drawing fluid out of the bacterial cells so that they are destroyed. Even more exotic preparations are occasionally tried. Papaya contains the enzyme papain, which can operate as a debriding agent because of its proteolytic action.

Thus, it is apparent that a grain of rationale may underlie the wide range of strange and wonderful substances still occasionally applied to wounds. This does not suggest, however, that novel materials should be encouraged during wound management. Better, more refined applications are commercially available, less messy and usually less unpleasant for the recipient. It is neither logical nor fair to expect the patient to submit to the aesthetically unpleasing home brews regarded favourably by some hospital personnel; and reliance on 'home-made' preparations is unlikely to inspire confidence in the patient or his family.

Simply because something is 'natural' does not imply that it is 'safe'. In the Third World, manure is used to seal the umbilical cord of newborn babies: thousands of infants have died through clostridial infection from spores in the faeces. Often preference for a particular topical agent results because of a spectacular and isolated success in the past.

Some preparations, both 'home-made' and commercially produced, owe their reputation to the 'placebo effect'. In experimenting with the new treatment, special attention has been given to the wound care and overall management of a particular patient, and this, rather than the product, has accounted for the favourable progress made.

Temperature

Wounds require thermal insulation to maintain them at body core temperature. The rate of cell multiplication doubles in wounds maintained at a steady temperature of 37°C compared to the ambient temperature at the skin surface. At lower temperatures, cell division is slowed and may take up to 3 hours to return to its previous level. White cells are especially sensitive to low temperatures and may fail to undergo phagocytosis. Lengthy dressings should not be performed unless essential and should not be employed merely for a daily inspection of the wound.

Preventing contamination, absorption and adherence

To provide optimal protection a dressing must absorb excess exudate (unless aspiration is possible), prevent contamination both of the wound and the surrounding environment and be non-adherent. These properties interact. Exudate must not be allowed to collect in excess quantities or the wound surface may slough, but if the surface of the dressing is allowed to become moist bacteria may gain access from the environment to the wound. Passage in the opposite direction is also possible, so bacteria from a contaminated wound offer a risk of cross-infection to other patients.

Adherence is a major problem, especially in wounds where there is scanty exudate, once healing is under way. Serous exudate dries onto the undersurface of the wound covering and when the dressing is removed the scab and sometimes new tissue are torn away, adding to the patient's discomfort and provoking further inflammation. Of all dressing materials, gauze is the least satisfactory in terms of adherence. Its loose weave is also problematic as bacteria can pass through the mesh. When gauze has been used to cover surgical wounds, fibres have later been isolated from the tissues, where they serve as a focus for infection; and if the dressing is left in place for too long, capillary loops may grow up into it, creating fresh trauma on removal.

Functionally specific wound preparations

In recent years wound management has been revolutionized by modern technology, which has made available a wide range of 'functionally specific' dressing materials, each designed to enhance the management of a particular type of wound. It is no longer possible or desirable to prescribe the same dressing for every wound or every patient. Instead the nursing process must be applied, to:

1. Assess the condition of the wound and the general condition of the patient
2. Decide on a policy of wound care and the physical and psychological nursing care needed to support the patient throughout healing
3. Determine a realistic time span, after which the condition of the wound and patient may be evaluated

4. Implementation
5. Evaluation of the wound and patient. From the re-assessment, the planning cycle is entered again until the wound is fully healed.

The healing of a chronic wound is never easy. The patient and his family may become depressed. He may become apathetic and resist involvement in care planning, especially in the case of a pressure sore, as traditionally this is seen as a hallmark of neglect. He may need encouragement to eat and mobilize, especially if the wound is painful, or he may be reluctant to learn how to apply dressings in preparation for hospital discharge.

Disagreements sometimes occur between members of staff who do not share the same views concerning wound care, especially when the regimen chosen does not provide immediate results. Cost can be a major hurdle, especially in the community, as many preparations are very expensive.

Skill is needed to apply agents and may have to be developed when a particular type of product has not been encountered before. Along with the need to develop skills there is also a need to extend and apply knowledge. For example, the nurse using a streptokinase enzyme preparation (e.g. Varidase) to chemically debride a wound must be aware that all enzymes are proteins. The solution must be prepared and handled gently (proteins are large molecules which denature when roughly handled), stored at a cool temperature and discarded if not used within 48 hours (enzymes are unstable in solution).

Good documentation of care is essential. If the wound is not accurately described and measured (see Ch. 5 for measuring pressure sores), progress may be difficult to detect and it will not be possible to provide feedback to the patient. However, of all the challenging aspects of wound management, the most difficult is perhaps deciding when progress can reasonably be expected to have been made. Chronic wounds do not behave like surgical wounds and cannot be expected to re-epithelialize within 2 or 3 days. Much will depend on the type and location of the wound and the patient's overall condition. It is here that the art and science of nursing meet, the point at which clinical judgement of the individual case complements scientific knowledge. This is an area in which careful documentation of good wound care could help advance nursing knowledge. Individual wards could contribute to the growing research base by collection and storage of meticulously documented care studies, which could be drawn upon to help build protocols for new patients.

Tissue totipotency and cell renewal

Earlier it was pointed out that wound healing occurs through the activity of two types of tissue: replacement of connective tissue by fibroblasts and movement and multiplication of epithelial cells. Not all tissues share this property of regeneration. The ability of a tissue to repair damage sustained through trauma depends on the ability of its cells to undergo mitosis, a phenomenon known as totipotency. Generally, the more highly differentiated (specialized) a tissue has become, the less totipotency is retained by its cells.

Epithelium and the fibroblasts found in connective tissue form a population of labile cells which retain the ability to regenerate throughout the lifetime of the individual. Epithelial cells covering the skin and lining the gastrointestinal system continually replace themselves and are found on external and internal body surfaces where trauma is most likely to be sustained. Cells of many internal organs (e.g. liver, kidneys) are described as stable. They do not normally undergo mitosis, but can do so in response to damage. Some regeneration following trauma is therefore possible. Permanent cells are unable to multiply after the growth phase in early life. Nerves and muscle, both very highly specialized tissues, fall into this category. They cannot regenerate and healing is by granulation with permanent loss of function. This has implications for prognosis in victims of major trauma.

Bone is classified as a connective tissue, as the osteocytes lie in a non-cellular matrix, which in this particular case is reinforced with mineral salts. Regeneration and healing without loss of function are therefore possible after a fracture, following an inflammatory reaction comparable to that operating in soft tissues.

INFECTIONS OF BONES AND JOINTS

Osteomyelitis

Bacteria gain access to bone via the blood from another septic focus elsewhere in the tissues or by direct contamination through trauma. The same pathological processes take place whenever bone becomes infected: necrosis followed by fibrosis. The dead tissue is too bulky for removal by white cells, especially if a thrombus caused by the bacteria has interrupted the blood supply. Repair is inhibited with disrupted osteoblast activity. Irregular remodelling leads to complications:

1. Weakening of the bone with deformity and fracture
2. Formation of a local abscess giving rise to a sinus.

The aim of treatment is to eradicate infection, foreign material and necrotic bone completely; to promote healing and avoid deformity and loss of function. Surgery is accompanied by large doses of antibiotics.

Acute osteomyelitis

Classically, acute osteomyelitis is caused by *Staph. aureus*, but *Brucella* and *Salmonella* (an organism more usually associated with food poisoning) have been isolated from septic bone. This type of infection tends to affect children and young adolescents. Before the era of antibiotics its effects were dramatic and usually rapidly progressive. The organisms gain access to skeletal tissue via the blood, settling in the cancellous tissue of the metaphysis of the long bones, a favourable site because its vascular pattern does not permit ready mobilization of host defences. Figure 8.13 shows how infection and pus formation rapidly involve the shaft of the bone, although spread to the epiphyses is prevented by the cartilaginous plate.

Unless antibiotics are given promptly, the surrounding cortex becomes involved, with ex-

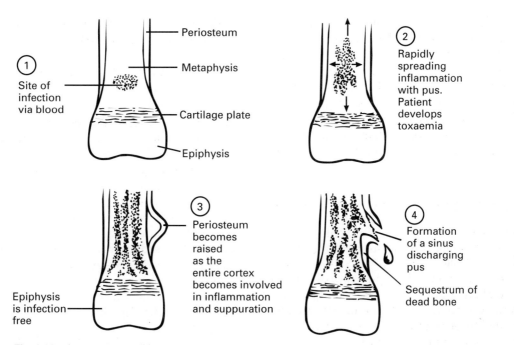

Fig. 8.13 Acute osteomyelitis.

tensive necrosis and severe generalized ill health once bacterial toxins enter the systemic circulation. Accumulating pus raises the periosteum and over time, with lack of treatment, a sinus will evolve. Beneath the periosteum a sequestrum of dead bone remains. This can be removed only by surgical intervention. It imposes the remodelling of newly formed bone, resulting in deformity.

Tuberculous osteomyelitis

The causative organism of this chronic infection is *Mycobacterium tuberculosis*, which enters the body by inhalation, setting up a primary focus of infection in the lung. The bacteria gain access to other tissues, including bones and adjacent joints, via the blood. The skeletal tissues most frequently affected are the spine and actively growing ephiphyses of the long bones. Necrosis and granulation tissue gradually replace affected bones and joints. Abscesses seem particularly likely to develop if there is spinal involvement.

Tuberculous osteomyelitis progresses much more slowly than acute osteomyelitis caused by pyogenic bacteria, because the infection itself is much more chronic, irrespective of the particular tissue concerned. However, preventative health measures have successfully reduced the incidence of tuberculosis in all its forms in the UK today. These include BCG immunization, pasteurization of milk, mass radiography, segregation and antibiotic treatment of infected people with follow-up surveillance of their contacts. Above all, improved living conditions have helped reduce the incidence of this infection, which has always been associated with impoverishment, poor nutrition and overcrowding. Today in the UK the nurse is most likely to encounter pulmonary tuberculosis among members of the vagrant population, usually older people whose poor living conditions and coexisting ill health contribute to reactivation of an old infective focus which developed prior to routine BCG. If tuberculous osteomyelitis is seen, this will almost certainly be in a patient from a Third World country where tuberculosis in children is much more common than in the UK.

Infections of joints

Like osteomyelitis, primary infections of the

joints are rare today, although nosocomial infection can occur.

Infected arthroplasty

Infection remains the most feared complication of total joint replacement operations, although with the incidence now reduced to 1% or less it is much less common than mechanical problems such as loosening. Fears are well founded, for when infection does supervene it is difficult to eradicate because of the resultant chronic inflammation in the presence of foreign materials – metal and polythene implants with their supporting acrylic cement. Several hospital readmissions for revision surgery may be necessary and the final outcome may be an unstable pseudoarthrosis with a shortened limb. A number of risk factors have been associated with an increased risk of sepsis, including rheumatoid arthritis, previous steroid therapy, previous surgery to the joint and a septic focus elsewhere in the body.

Deep infections present in three distinct forms:

1. Acute infection; this manifests up to 3 months after the operation and constitutes approximately 40% of reported cases. However, the incidence is gradually declining, acute infection appearing to be the form most amenable to prophylactic measures presently available.

2. Delayed infection; this occurs between 3 and 24 months after apparently successful surgery. It accounts for about 45% of reported cases of sepsis and its incidence is the most difficult form to reduce, probably because the pathogenic mechanism has yet to be established. It may represent secondary infection or reactivation of quiescent bacteria in the scar tissue around the new joint when the patient's immune response becomes depressed through coincidental ill health.

3. Late blood-borne infection. This accounts for 15% of cases and can occur at any time after arthroplasty, when bacteria gain access to the blood from a septic focus elsewhere in the tissues or following another surgical procedure (e.g. catheterization).

Acute infections present with local inflammatory changes in the wound. The causative organism can usually be cultured from pus. In severe infections, bacteria are also present in the blood. The patient is pyrexial and generally unwell. Delayed sepsis is more difficult to identify. The patient seeks advice with a return of pain, which may be accompanied by loss of movement and sometimes recurrence of deformity. X-rays may suggest the nature of the problem, but scanning with radioactive isotopes may be necessary to confirm it. The isotope is given as an intravenous injection; the labelled particles can be traced with a counter and show up at the site of infection because of the increased local blood supply. The erythrocyte sedimentation rate (ESR) will be raised and fluid aspirated from the infected joint will contain bacteria. An arthrogram performed at the same time will reveal other changes (e.g. loosening of the implant) earlier than they would appear on plain X-ray.

Treatment may vary between centres, although all patients will receive antibiotics. Acute infections may be managed by irrigation of the infected joint for several days with large volumes of saline primed with antibiotics; however, this technique is now seldom used because of the high risk of secondary infection, often with more resistant bacteria. Today the patient is more likely to undergo excisional arthroplasty, removing all implants and all infected soft and bony tissue. Reimplantation using cement loaded with the appropriate antibiotic may be possible, although this does not rule out the need for repeated surgery in future. Gentamicin is widely used because of its broad spectrum effect. Sometimes gentamicin-impregnated beads are packed into the medullary cavity and dead space of the bone for 10–14 days.

Reimplantation following an infected arthroplasty calls for a lengthy and skilled surgical procedure. The outcome cannot be guaranteed, and if there is reason to doubt success, the surgeon may consider it safer to leave the joint as a pseudoarthrosis, especially if the patient is very frail. Later reconversion to arthroplasty may be possible when the general condition has improved and all infection has been eradicated.

A primary infection caused by pyogenic organisms causes painful, acute inflammation with effusion. Complete resolution is possible with prompt antibiotic therapy and rest. Lack of treatment is followed by suppuration, tissue destruction and septicaemia.

Arthritis may complicate gonorrhoea and brucellosis.

Clostridial infections

Clostridia are a group of small bacteria which live freely in the environment, and are able to form highly resistant spores, often carried in the faeces of farm animals. Some species are normal inhabitants of the human gut, although others (e.g. *C. difficile*) can cause severe infective diarrhoea. All members of this group are anaerobic (i.e. they grow without oxygen, most species tolerating oxygen poorly). A number of clostridial infections are relevant in orthopaedics.

Gangrene   Gangrene is a form of tissue necrosis complicated by clostridial infection. Several species are responsible, but most infections are caused by *C. perfringens*. The bacteria multiply in dead tissue, sometimes releasing gas.

Primary (gas) gangrene is a serious complication of wounds under the following conditions:

- Extensive damage to internal tissues following major trauma, e.g. war wounds, road accidents resulting in severe compound fractures (provide source of necrotic tissue)
- Interrupted blood supply (provides source of anaerobic conditions)
- Contamination with soil, water or other foreign matter (provides source of clostridia).

The bacteria rapidly digest muscle because they are able to release powerful proteolytic enzymes. In severe cases, cellulitis proceeds swiftly with the release of gas and there is progression to adjacent, healthy muscular tissue. The patient's life is threatened as toxins enter the systemic circulation, followed by living bacteria causing septicaemia. The diagnosis is obvious on clinical grounds, even before specimens are dispatched to the laboratory.

In the pre-Listerian era, before the need for disinfection became apparent, many operations ended in gas gangrene. Today this dreaded infection is usually acquired outside hospital, but nosocomial infections are not unknown (Lowbury & Lilly 1955). Treatment involves surgical removal of the necrotic tissue and massive doses of penicillin. Exposing the affected site to pure oxygen in a pressure chamber is a very effective adjunct to treatment, owing to clostridial intolerance of aerobic conditions.

Secondary gangrene is the result of mixed bacterial invasion in tissue in which necrosis and putrification are already present. In the form known as 'wet' gangrene the tissue is waterlogged by pre-existing oedema (e.g. occlusion of leg arteries in diabetic patients). 'Dry' gangrene typically occurs in the legs and feet of elderly people suffering from gradual arterial occlusion. Again, diabetics are particularly at risk. Slow putrification occurs, but dry gangrene is possible when the bacterial count is very low.

Tetanus   This severe infection, caused by *C. tetani*, owes its signs and symptoms exclusively to the release of potent toxins by the bacteria; they do not cause tissue destruction. Because this species is strictly anaerobic (entirely intolerant of oxygen), infection depends on deep, penetrating wounds carrying the organisms – which are present in soil contaminated by animal faeces – deep under the skin. Victims of trauma are at obvious risk, but the damage need not be major; puncture with a thorn during gardening has been known to result in tetanus.

Once the bacteria have gained access to the deep tissues they proliferate but remain localized. The muscular spasms typical of the infection commence once toxins are released. Involvement of local nerves results in muscular spasm triggered by minor stimuli. Spread of toxin in the motor nerves causes spasm of the jaws ('lockjaw'), convulsions, opisthotonos and respiratory ventilation spasm. Asphyxia, exhaustion and death are inevitable without treatment.

Patients attending the Accident and Emergency Department must be asked how recently they have received tetanus toxoid, even after minor trauma. The success of this immunization testifies to the importance and value of preventative health measures; tetanus is a rare disease, but *C. tetani* is not an uncommon organism.

HOSPITAL-ACQUIRED INFECTION

So far in this chapter we have discussed a range of infections which may affect the orthopaedic patient; some, like tuberculosis and clostridial infections, are acquired in the community, but many others, notably staphylococcal infections and gram-negative urinary infections, develop mainly after admission. Nosocomial infections are notorious for the manner in which they complicate the course of the original illness and delay recovery, particularly in the patient with an orthopaedic condition. Not surprisingly, the costs of nosocomial infection and its epidemiology have been the subjects of considerable research.

Epidemiology

The most comprehensive study designed to determine the prevalence of infection in hospitals in the UK was conducted in England and Wales in the early 1980s (Meers et al 1981). Details were obtained from 18 163 patients on the acute wards of 43 hospitals with the result that 19.1% were found to be infected. One patient in 10 was estimated to have developed infection in hospital. Respiratory infections were the most frequently recorded, but most of these had been acquired in the community. Urinary tract infections were the most common nosocomial infections (documented in 30.2% of cases), occurring almost exclusively among patients who had an indwelling urethral catheter. Wound infections were the second most frequently encountered class of hospital-acquired infection. Overall, 5% of wounds inspected were judged to have evidence of sepsis. Surgical wounds were categorized according to the scheme shown in Table 8.1. In many cases, infection was present in wounds that, according to the site and operative procedure, should have been clean. Rates of infection recorded in each of the 43 different hospitals were very similar.

The National Prevalence Study provided a 'snapshot' impression of the number of infections present in each institution visited, at the time of the visit only. Possible risk factors such as the close relationship between catheterization and urinary tract infection became apparent but could not be investigated further.

An incidence study sets out to establish the number of new cases affected in a target population over a predetermined span of time and may provide greater information about possible risk factors, providing that an accurate and reliable data-recording system can be maintained.

Cruse and Foord (1980) employed this method of continuous surveillance to monitor the incidence of postoperative wound infection in an 830-bed Canadian hospital over a 10-year period. Daily inspection confirmed that sepsis could develop in wounds categorized as clean (1–2%). More recently, Gastrin and Lovastad (1989), collecting data from 1278 patients undergoing orthopaedic surgery in a Swedish hospital, reported 49 episodes of infection over a period of 1 year. According to wound category, their results were similar to the findings of Cruse and Foord. However, the Swedish authors also analysed their results in terms of specific surgical procedure. Amputation of the lower limb and operations on peripheral nerves most often resulted in infection, and there was a clear relationship between open reduction of fractures and postoperative sepsis.

In the same year Bremmelgaard and colleagues (1988), undertaking continuous computer-assisted surveillance of orthopaedic infections in Denmark over 24 months, found that emergency surgery was most often associated with sepsis. A number of additional risk factors were identified in this study: age, wound contamination, duration of the operation and the date on which surgery was performed.

Like Gastrin and Lovestad, these authors found that infection was most often caused by staphylococci or gram-negative bacilli and that sepsis often became apparent for the first time long after the operation (sometimes 28 days or more), when the patient might already have been discharged. In the Danish study it was calculated that infected patients stayed in hospital for an average of 20.5 days longer than those free of sepsis. In this country it has been estimated that general surgical and orthopaedic patients stay in hospital an average of 12.9 days longer if they develop a wound infection and 5.1 days longer if they develop a urinary infection (Rubenstein et al 1982).

Costs

Nosocomial infection is enormously costly to the National Health Service, not only because of increased bed occupancy, but also through demands of the infected patient for antibiotic therapy, dressing materials, analgesia, laundry and nursing time, especially if isolation precautions are required. Meanwhile, the length of the waiting list for elective admission inevitably increases. A report by the Hospital Infection Working Group (DHSS 1988) estimated that in England and Wales 950 000 bed days are lost as a direct result of nosocomial infection every year, at an annual cost of £111 million. For the patient and his family, nosocomial infection will also have significant costs.

Patients succumbing to hospital-acquired infection experience physical and psychological suffering additional to that already imposed by the original illness or accident, and are likely to face added social and financial problems. Income may be lost through extended hospital stay, and the lasting disability that infection can cause following major orthopaedic surgery could jeopardize future employment prospects altogether. Men as well as women worry about their partner coping alone at home. Child care and other domestic commitments become increasingly difficult as the emergency, short-term help provided by family and friends becomes stretched to the limit. Those who live alone, especially the elderly, may be concerned about leaving the home empty for added weeks or months. Many patients requiring orthopaedic surgery fall into older age groups or will already suffer a degree of incapacitation as a result of long-standing disability. The longer the hospital stay, the more difficult rehabilitation and return to the community will be.

Preventing infection

Figure 8.14 summarizes the many sources of infection which threaten the patient in hospital. All these possible sources are described as exogenous, meaning that they originate either from the environment or from other people. In hospital, there are many opportunities for bacteria living on the skin or in the gastrointestinal tract to be transferred to another, more susceptible site on the same person, such as a wound, where they are able to establish infection. These are called endogenous infections. Many of the precautions taken in the orthopaedic theatre to prevent endogenous infection are costly, but on the ward a great deal depends on inexpensive and relatively simple measures. This view is endorsed by Rahman (1985) who evaluated a new isolation unit. Before the unit was opened, 15 outbreaks of infection had been recorded within the hospital, compared to only one outbreak 5 years afterwards. Success was attributed chiefly to uncomplicated routines and policies, a finding that is in tune with human nature; busy nurses and doctors are more likely to comply with procedures that do not appear to involve endless trouble.

Handwashing

Handwashing is the best example of an inexpensive yet highly effective form of infection control, yet nurses often fail to wash their hands at appropriate times or do so poorly. Hands should be washed:

- Before any aseptic procedure
- Before and after handling patients
- After handling any item that is soiled
- Before handling food
- At once if the hands become visibly soiled.

Adequate technique involves thoroughly lathering all the surfaces, taking care not to neglect the tips of the fingers, webs between fingers, palm and thumb, which are often overlooked. Liquid soap from a dispenser is less likely to become contaminated than a bar of soap, but the mechanical action of the running water is at least

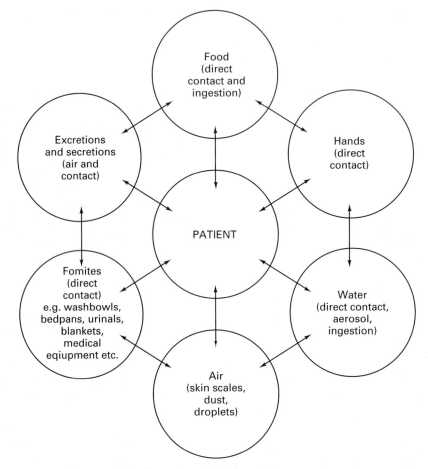

Fig. 8.14 Sources of infection to the patient in hospital.

as important as the detergent in removing micro-organisms. Ideally, rings should be removed before handwashing as bacteria tend to collect beneath them. In some high risk areas an alcohol rub is provided in addition to soap; 70% alcohol is an effective bactericide but again, it must come into contact with the entire surface of the hand and must be allowed to evaporate to be effective. Disposable towels are preferable to avoid recontamination, as are pedal bins.

Hands, like the rest of the skin, are covered by two types of microorganism: a transient flora picked up and shed on skin scales during daily activities, and a permanent flora carried deep in the ducts of the sweat glands. Handwashing can effectively remove the transient population but will never eradicate the permanent flora, so

gloves must be worn when potentially contaminated items are handled and to prolong the effects of hand disinfection when the risk of infection is high (e.g. when catheterizing a patient). Recontamination of the hands is possible if gloves are carelessly removed or if they become punctured.

Decontamination of the hospital environment

Any item within the hospital environment – the structure (e.g. walls and floors), fixtures, fittings and furnishings – can become contaminated with potentially infectious material. When a new hospital is commissioned, care must be taken to ensure that only materials capable of withstanding decontamination procedures are chosen, unless they are intended to be disposable;

the same rule applies whenever refurbishment is necessary.

Decontamination can be achieved at four different levels, each progressively more effective at reducing the threat of infection, but also increasingly expensive, difficult to achieve and more damaging:

1. Cleaning
2. Disinfection
3. Sterilization
4. Incineration.

The method chosen depends on considerations of cost and feasibility. Some very delicate fibre-optic instruments used in theatre can be decontaminated only by chemicals because they cannot withstand autoclaving, although the application of moist heat under pressure is more efficient and less open to performance error. From our earlier discussion it should be apparent that when consideration is given to the prevention of infection, attention must be paid to likely sources of microorganisms, including opportunists and methods of dissemination. Knowledge that all bacteria require moisture and a supply of nutrients is sufficient information for the nurse to deduce that on the ward, clean, dry conditions should prevail. Good ventilation helps disperse airborne bacteria and plenty of sunlight is desirable, as ultraviolet light rays destroy microorganisms. Particular care must be taken in situations where risks of contamination and infection are high. The list below is indicative but not exhaustive:

- Spillages or organic waste material (e.g. blood, pus, vomit, faeces, urine) which have not been cleaned up promptly
- Materials that have been in contact with an infected site (e.g. dressings, 'sharps', excretions and secretions, laboratory specimens)
- The immediate environment of patients who have a particularly virulent infection (e.g. multiresistant staphylococci) or a communicable disease (e.g. tuberculosis)
- All clinical waste
- Any equipment that appears wet or soiled (e.g. baths, mops, medical equipment)

- Raw food (meat, fish) in hospital and ward kitchens.

Cleaning

Although cleaning is not usually part of the nurse's role, she must understand the principles of decontamination by cleaning in order to monitor the performance of domestic staff so that any inadequacies can be reported promptly to their supervisor. The patient to be discharged from hospital with a chronic infection (e.g. HIV) may ask for information about the cleaning of household items. Nurses are responsible for the cleanliness of clinical equipment such as thermometers, and in some high risk areas (theatres, intensive care units), may be required to assist with routine cleaning.

Wherever possible, equipment should be stored clean and dry when not in use. Solutions of disinfectant should not be used for soaking bedpans, urinals etc., because the solution itself rapidly becomes deactivated in the inevitable presence of organic matter. A reservoir of bacteria is rapidly established, providing a source of cross-infection.

Opportunities for cross-infection are reduced if patients have their own thermometers (dry, not standing in solution) and individual creams for skin care, applied with a fresh spatula each time rather than by the nurse's fingers. Individual washbowls, bedpans and urinals are desirable, stored upside-down so that any residual moisture can drain. Flannels, soaps and towels must never be shared. This can be difficult to organize on an orthopaedic unit populated mainly by elderly people with few visitors to replenish these items during a long sojourn in hospital. Visits by hospital volunteers and the mobile shop are to be encouraged.

On orthopaedic units, devices for the relief of pressure are widely used and need careful decontamination because they are in intimate contact with the patient. Sheepskins, foam wedges and pillows should never be washed on the ward, for they dry slowly and the moisture they retain becomes a reservoir of gram-negative bacteria. There is often a reluctance to send this type of equipment to the laundry because ward stocks run low; this leads to hoarding and recirculation, a situation in which all these items can act as fomites.

Cleaning to the required standard in hospital demands equipment, materials and methods not encountered on a domestic scale. Nurses must know the policies and procedures used in their hospital because domestic staff are not always available. Spillages can occur in the middle of the night and must be dealt with by someone at once, using the correct disinfectant (active against bacteria but not destroying the surface) and the correct equipment (the 'dirty' mop reserved for spills, not the 'clean' mop used routinely for the rest of the floor).

Pleasant, clean surroundings are especially important, too, in the orthopaedic unit, where the average stay is longer than in many other parts of the hospital and where the bedfast patient has to perform all activities of living in the same confined area.

Disinfection

Disinfection is destruction of vegetative micro-organisms, but not spores. The aim is to reduce the number of organisms present to a level not likely to result in infection. It can be achieved by heat and by chemical methods. Skill in the use of chemical agents and knowledge of their performance are essential, as a number of pitfalls await the unwary when using chemical disinfectants:

1. Disinfection will not be adequate unless the solution has contact with all contaminated surfaces. Complete immersion of the item is necessary and any lumen must be filled with the fluid. Grease, air pockets etc. prevent contact.

2. A wide range of substances, including residual soaps and the plastic of the bucket holding the solution, neutralize disinfectants and thus reduce their effectiveness.

3. The concentration of the solution is critical. If too dilute, it will be inefficient; if too concentrated it may not perform at the optimal level owing to the presence of additives (e.g. stabilizers) in the increased amount. In hospital, the correct dilution is usually supplied by the pharmacy, but when discharging the patient with HIV or hepatitis B the nurse must be able to advise on the correct dilution of household bleach to apply to blood spillages (1 part bleach, 9 parts water).

4. Most disinfectant solutions are not stable, and because they deteriorate with storage, expiry dates of ward stocks must be checked. The domestic staff must check environmental disinfectants, but the nurse must check the expiry date of wound disinfectants.

5. The speed of action is variable, as are performance and other properties. Some disinfectants act slowly but are suitable for a particular task through some other advantage. Alcohol is suitable as a hand disinfectant because it acts rapidly, but has poor penetration. Hypochlorites act rapidly, and are very cheap and effective at low concentrations, but they are far too corrosive to be applied to the skin. They damage many surfaces and special finishes. Glutaraldehyde is slow in action and expensive, but it is the disinfectant of choice for delicate equipment such as fibreoptic instruments because it does not corrode. It also destroys spores.

6. Disinfectants are not interchangeable as they are not all equally effective against all types of organism. Hypochlorites effectively destroy HIV and hepatitis B. Cetrimide, and to a lesser extent chlorhexidine, destroy gram-positive bacteria more readily than gram-negative ones. Generally, disinfectants which are sufficiently gentle to apply to the skin are not effective as environmental disinfectants. Chlorhexidine, additionally, is too expensive, as it has been specially developed as a non-corrosive, non-toxic, non-allergenic liquid. These properties are costly to achieve.

7. Some parts of the hospital (and the home) are subject to such heavy and rapid recontamination that disinfection is short-lived and must never be relied upon; sinks, drains, etc. fall into this category.

8. Mops and cleaning cloths must be clean if rapid contamination of the fluid which is meant to disinfect is to be avoided. In practice, they often provide reservoirs of infection.

9. In some situations, disinfection is not adequate for a particular patient (e.g. the patient with a very low white cell count will require sterilization rather than disinfection of his crockery, cutlery and bedpans).

The method of heat disinfection most frequently used by nurses on the ward is the bedpan washer. This familiar item of equipment is accompanied by a number of drawbacks, which stem from the need to keep the washing and disinfecting cycles as short as possible. The best machines clean and then maintain moist heat at a temperature of 80°C for at least a minute. In hospitals where macerators have been installed, risks of infection are higher because contaminated aerosols are produced when the door of the machine is slammed shut. Overloading causes the system to become blocked and break down.

Sterilization

Sterilization is defined as the destruction of all microorganisms present, including spores, but this is misleading, as in practice it is not possible to check whether destruction has been absolute despite the use of quality control measures. Sterilization is achieved in hospital by autoclaving suitable items (linen, metal objects) under pressure with steam at 121°C for 15 minutes. The contact of steam with every surface is essential. Delicate items can be chemically sterilized by ethylene oxide gas, 40% formaldehyde gas or 2% glutaraldehyde solution. These substances are noxious and require skilled use. Nurses who work in theatre and outpatient clinics may sometimes be expected to undertake this work. Radiation by ultraviolet and gamma wavelengths is undertaken on a commercial scale for dressings, syringes, needles and the like, but their care becomes the responsibility of the nurse when this equipment reaches the ward or department. Packs must be kept dry and their paper covering undamaged, or their contents can no longer be regarded as sterile. Storage in plastic bags is advisable for items which are seldom used. Storage in a cupboard is better than on open racks, as the

protection from dust and airborne particles is better.

Because sterilization is costly, sterile items should not be used indiscriminately. Sterility is essential under the following circumstances:

1. When equipment will enter part of the body normally free of microorganisms (all surgical instruments, injection needles, catheters, dressings, topical applications)
2. When contamination with bacterial spores in large numbers may occur, or when pathogens are believed to be extremely virulent
3. When a patient is particularly susceptible (e.g. when the white cell count is very low, either through disease such as leukaemia or induced by treatment such as an organ transplant).

Disposal

The disposal of unwanted waste and used materials begins in the ward and theatre, often as the result of a nursing or medical procedure. Unless appropriate action is taken, contamination of the environment or of hospital personnel can occur, as well as a reduction in socially acceptable and aesthetic standards. The DHSS introduced a system of colour-coding for different categories of hospital waste in the mid 1980s (see Table 8.2).

The disposal of 'sharps' deserves special mention because of the potential for accidents to clinical and ancillary staff with associated risks of parenteral infection. The key to safe practice

Table 8.2 Colour-coded bag system for the disposal of hospital waste materials

Colour of bag	Contents	Destination
Red, with alginate-stitched liner	foul/infected linen	laundry
White	soiled linen	laundry
Yellow	clinical waste, including all infectious waste, human tissue	incinerator
Green	waste from offices, non-clinical areas	incinerator

Laboratory specimens likely to be highly infected must be labelled.

should be followed by everyone working in hospital:

- Handling after use should be kept to a minimum. Most accidents occur when needles are resheathed or attempts are made to separate needle and syringe. These practices must be avoided.
- All 'sharps' should be regarded as potentially contaminated and placed in a 'sharps' box as soon as possible after use, by the person who has used them.
- As soon as a 'sharps' container appears full it should be sealed completely and sent for incineration. Attempts should not be made to check that the container is full, as slipping in a finger can result in its puncture.
- If an accident occurs, the victim should report to the occupational health department. Immunoglobulin, protective against hepatitis B, is available, and if necessary tetanus toxoid can be given.

Individuals may be tested for HIV antibody after the appropriate counselling if they wish. Zidovudine can be given prophylactically for HIV, but treatment must be given very soon after the accident. Anyone involved in an accident involving 'sharps' can be reassured that the risks of contracting HIV in this way are very small: only a few cases have been reported world-wide.

The nurse at the ward level is not responsible for the choice of equipment but should have the opportunity to make suggestions which will influence the purchase and availability of suitable items. 'Sharps' containers should be constructed of material thick enough to resist wetting from any fluid released within, and from penetration by a sharp object inside or out. Leakage and puncture are hazards of cheap containers which may present a risk to ancillary staff once the containers have left the ward.

Isolation procedures

Isolation procedures are sometimes essential to contain a source of infection and prevent spread, but should never be undertaken lightly because of the distress they so often generate.

Patients may prefer a single room, but often, especially when confined to bed for a long time, loneliness and boredom supervene. People on a ward together frequently develop a sense of comradeship, particularly if they are suffering from a similar condition, and derive much support from one another. Incarceration in a single room with little in the way of distraction can be depressing and may be detrimental to a disoriented patient. A stigma may be associated with infection, which is made worse by the need for protective clothing. Masks may hamper communication by muffling speech and hiding expression. Rather than isolate the whole patient it may be possible to isolate the site of infection – for example, by covering a wound with an occlusive dressing.

A rational approach is important when nursing patients with diagnosed or suspected infection, taking into consideration:

1. The causative organism if yet identified.
2. The reason for precautions; i.e. is the aim to protect other patients, chiefly the nurse, or the nurse and other patients? If the organism is airborne or spread by contact, everyone in the ward is potentially at risk, although the debilitated patient will probably be much more susceptible than the nurse. If the nurse is handling a contaminated needle, she is concerned primarily with self-protection.

Table 8.3 Spread of infection: faecal–oral route

Conditions requiring enteric precautions	
Examples	*Clostridium difficile* shigella *Salmonella typhi* hepatitis A
Mode of spread	primarily hands of staff but occasionally via equipment, clothing of attendants
Precautions required to prevent transmission	1. single room is preferable, not essential 2. wear gloves and aprons when handling excreta and contaminated articles 3. wash hands after contact with faeces or contaminated articles 4. disinfect, sterilize, or dispose of equipment 5. incinerate waste and treat linen according to local policy for 'infected linen'

Table 8.4 Spread of infection: contact routes

	Conditions requiring wound precautions	Conditions requiring secretion/excretion precautions
Examples	infected discharging wounds pressure sores	urinary tract infections
Mode of spread	primarily hands of staff but can occur from contaminated equipment and articles	
Precautions required to prevent transmission	1. wear gloves and aprons when handling wound, dressings and secretions/excretions 2. wash hands before and after contact with site and immediate environment 3. dispose, disinfect or sterilize equipment 4. incinerate dressings and other contaminated waste	

3. Mode of transmission; this is crucial, as poor understanding can lead to exaggerated and unnecessary precautions. If an infection is spread by contact, a single room is not essential: this is an important point if the only cubicle available would not permit continuous observation of a critically ill or disoriented patient. If an infection is airborne, a single room is essential and the door must be kept shut.

4. Items likely to be contaminated and appropriate methods of decontamination; if the infection is airborne, everything in the patient's room will be potentially contaminated, although those items nearest the source will probably be most heavily contaminated. A patient with hepatitis B is unlikely to contaminate his surroundings providing that he is continent, he is not bleeding, and personal hygiene is of a high standard. Tables 8.3–8.6 illustrate the precautions necessary when preventing infection spread by different routes. A knowledge of the behaviour of pathogenic microorganisms is essential; most nurses are aware that *Salmonella* is spread by the faecal–oral route, but knowledge that it can live freely in the environment, setting up a reservoir of cross-infection from sinks, baths etc., is generally less well appreciated. Among the secrets of successful infection prevention by personnel is the ability to identify gaps in knowledge and know where to find more specialized help – from the hospital infection control policy, the infection control nurse or medical microbiologist.

Effective use of the infection control service

In England and Wales, provision of the hospital infection control service is left to the discretion of

Table 8.5 Spread of infection: parenteral route

Conditions requiring blood precautions	
Examples	hepatitis B, human immune deficiency virus (HIV)
Mode of spread	primarily through inoculation
Precautions required to prevent spread	1. gloves and apron to be worn when handling blood or blood products 2. wash hands after contact with blood 3. cover cuts and abrasions with waterproof dressings 4. adhere strictly to policies for the safe disposal of contaminated needles and sharps 5. dispose of, disinfect, or sterilize equipment and contaminated articles 6. incinerate contaminated waste and deal with contaminated linen according to local policy for 'infected linen'

the individual health district, but all hospitals are required by statute to have an infection control committee and an infection control officer, who is usually its chairman. Infection control nurses are not employed in all hospitals, but when present they play a key role, working with the infection control committee to provide advice about the prevention of infection throughout the hospital and usually also within the community it serves. Work of the committee and its members includes the development of policies to reduce the incidence of infection (e.g. cleaning and disinfection policies, antibiotic policies), disseminating this information to all members of staff and monitoring compliance and effectiveness. Education is therefore a vital activity, often undertaken by the infection control nurse during induction programmes and as part of continuing education for qualified staff.

Table 8.6 Spread of infection: airborne route

	Conditions requiring respiratory precautions	Conditions requiring skin precautions
Examples	chicken pox tuberculosis	*Staphyloccocus aureus* — infected lesions of skin, dry wounds
Mode of spread	air and contact	primarily airborne contamination of hands of staff, fomites, e.g. bedclothes
Precautions required to prevent transmission to contain airborne spread	1. single room (door shut) 2. masks may be required (check on immunity of staff)	1. single room (door shut) 2. masks unnecessary
Precautions required to contain contact spread	3. aprons and gloves worn when in contact with infective skin lesions, when handling secretions (e.g. sputum and contaminated articles) 4. wash hands after contact with infective skin lesions, after handling sputum or contaminated articles 5. dispose, disinfect or sterilize equipment 6. incinerate waste and treat linen according to local policy for 'infected linen'	3. aprons and gloves worn for contact with patient and contaminated articles 4. wash hands before and after contact with patient and environment 5. dispose, disinfect or sterilize equipment 6. incinerate waste and treat linen according to local policy for 'infected linen'

Infection rates are monitored, either throughout the hospital or in high risk areas, of which orthopaedic surgery would be considered a prime example. Outbreaks of infection are investigated by the committee, which advises on methods of control.

Clearly, many hospital departments need to liaise with the infection control team and from time to time representatives will attend committee meetings to discuss problems or make suggestions for improvements in the service. Such representatives could include domestic service managers, CSSD managers, pharmacists, the hospital engineer, and catering and laundry managers. Senior nurses as well as doctors may serve on the infection control committee, helping to establish standards of environmental cleaning and to choose types of equipment necessary to prevent unacceptable levels of infection. Clinical nurses in wards and departments throughout the hospital need to know about the activities of the infection control committee and how to liaise with their nurse representatives. If 'sharps' containers are unsafe, wound preparations available are not of the type required or specific information is needed about the cleaning and decontamination of equipment, the specialist nurse can help provide the answer. Thus, satisfactory infection control measures operate at two levels:

1. At the bedside and during an operation for the benefit of a specific patient
2. Throughout the entire hospital, to provide a pleasant, safe environment to the advantage of everyone.

REFERENCES

Boore J 1978 Prescription for recovery. Royal College of Nursing, London
Bremmelgaard A, Raahave D, Beier-Holdgersen R, Pedersen J V, Anderson S, Søorensen A I 1988 Computer-aided surveillance of surgical infections and identification of risk factors. Journal of Hospital Infection 13: 1–18
Clifford C M 1982 Urinary tract infection. A brief selective review. International Journal of Nursing Studies 19: 213–222
Cruse P J, Foord R 1980 The epidemiology of wound infection. A 10 year prospective study of 62, 939 wounds. Surgical Clinics of North America 60: 27–40
Degl'Innocenti R, De Santis M, Berdondini I, Dei R 1989 Outbreak of *Clostridium difficile* diarrhoea in an orthopaedic unit. Journal of Hospital Infection. 13: 309–314
DHSS 1988, Hospital infection control. Guidance on the control of infection prepared by the joint DHSS/PHLS hospital infection working group. HMSO, London
Duguid J P 1946 The size and duration of air carriage of

respiratory droplets and droplet nuclei. Journal of Hygiene 44: 471–479

Gastrin B, Lovestad A 1989 Postoperative wound infection: relation to different types of operation and wound contamination categories in orthopaedic surgery. Journal of Hospital Infection 13: 387–393

Horan M A 1984 Outbreak of *Shigella sonnei* dysentry on a geriatric assessment ward. Journal of Hospital Infection 5: 210–212

Hughes S P F 1988 The role of antibiotics in preventing infections following total hip replacement. Journal of Hospital Infection II (suppl C): 41–47

Jalovaara P, Puranen J 1989 Air bacterial and particle counts in total hip replacement operations using non-woven and cotton gowns and drapes. Journal of Hospital Infection. 4: 333–338

Lidwell O M, Lowbury E J L, Whyte W, Blowers R, Stanley S J, Lowe D 1983 Bacteria isolated from deep joint sepsis after operation for total hip or knee replacement and the sources of the infections with *Staphylococcus aureus*. Journal of Hospital Infection 1: 19–30

Lowbury E J L, Lilly H A 1955 A selective plate medium for *Clostridium urelchii*. Journal of Pathology & Bacteriology 70: 105

Meers P D, Ayliffe G A J, Emmerson A M, Leigh D A, Mayon-White R L, Mackintosh C A, Strange J L 1981 Report of the National Survey of Infection in Hospitals. Journal of Hospital Infection 2: 23–28

Rahman M 1985 Commissioning a new hospital isolation unit and assessment of its use over the first five years. Journal of Hospital Infection 6: 65–70

Rubenstein E, Green M, Molan M, Ami P, Bernstein L, Rubenstein A 1982 The effects of nosocomial infections on length and costs of hospital stay. Journal of Antimicrobial Chemotherapy 9 (suppl): 93

Taylor L J 1978 An evaluation of hand washing techniques, Parts I and II. Nursing Times 74(2): 54–55; 74(3): 108–109

Sanderson P J 1988 The choice between prophylactic agents for orthopaedic surgery. Journal of Hospital Infection 11: 57–67

Whyte W 1988 The role of clothing and drapes in the operating room. Journal of Hospital Infection 11, Suppl C: 2–17

ANNOTATED FURTHER READING

Ayliffe G A J, Collins B J, Taylor L J, 1990 Hospital-acquired infection: principles and prevention, 2nd edn. John Wright, Bristol. *A useful little book containing essential information, expressed clearly; contains the fundamentals of good infection control practice aimed at a multidisciplinary audience*

Lowbury E J L, Ayliffe G A J, Geddes A M, Williams J D 1990 Control of hospital infection: a practical handbook, 2nd edn. Chapman & Hall, London. *A useful resource book of information; a valuable asset to any ward library*

Mims L A 1987 The pathogenesis of infectious diseases, 3rd edn. Academic Press, New York. *An interesting and detailed account of how microorganisms establish disease in the host; material is presented in considerable depth, but the text is not more technical than necessary*

Playfair J H L 1988 Immunology at a glance, 4th edn.

Blackwell Publications, Oxford. *A more advanced immunology text, presenting information as a series of flow diagrams and notes; a painless way to get to grips with challenging subject matter*

Pratt R J 1991 AIDS: a strategy for nursing care, 3rd edn. Edward Arnold, London. *A useful account of HIV and AIDS. Rather more factual material is presented than nursing care, but a great deal of medical information and guidance for infection control are presented*

Staines N, Brostoff J, James K 1985 Introducing immunology. Gower Medical Publishing, London. *A basic and extremely readable introduction to this complex subject; illustrations are good*

Thomas C G A 1988 Medical microbiology, 6th edn. Balliere Tindall, London. Valuable standard approach to the subject

9

The size of the problem

Peter S. Davis

This chapter aims to provide an overview of the causes, origins, effects, classifications and extent of orthopaedic diseases and conditions. The following chapters will then examine in greater depth specific, common orthopaedic diseases and conditions. The nature of orthopaedic diseases and of orthopaedic nursing often means that the focus of care is predominantly physical. However, it must be remembered that while there is commonality related to the diseases' physical effects and aetiology, social and psychological factors impinge in such a way that each individual will experience ill health differently and thus express illness, in terms of signs and symptoms, in a different way (Boore et al 1987).

The chapter title, 'The size of the problem', with respect to orthopaedic diseases and conditions, implies that it is not merely the number of individuals with orthopaedic conditions that must be considered, although this is enormous, but also the severity and extent of the effects of these conditions on the individual and their cost in terms of resource demands on a health service. The prevalance of orthopaedic diseases and conditions is a national problem and one that society as a whole has yet to address fully. Despite the size and severity of this problem it has not yet been given the priority or attention it deserves. This chapter aims to make clear these issues and how they may be tackled, with particular emphasis on the role of the orthopaedic nurse.

ORIGIN OR CAUSE OF DISEASES AND CONDITIONS

Orthopaedic conditions are classified according to their commonality of effects (signs and symptoms) or to the body tissues affected (bone, soft tissue, joints and nervous system). Concentrating effort and resources predominantly on the more immediate demands of the effects of diseases or ill health at present forms the foundation of our health service. What may be more desirable, and in the long term more cost-effective, is to invest resources in identifying origins and causes to prevent ill health in the first place.

For the health service to be orientated towards prevention and health, a classification derived from cause or origin might be useful. However, it is not always possible to identify the relationship between cause and effect, though knowledge and understanding of this relationship is gradually being acquired and is proving invaluable in the fight against disease and ill health. This chapter will consider the cause or origin of diseases and conditions followed by the effects, although it is often difficult to treat the two concepts separately.

The origin or cause of orthopaedic conditions generally falls into one or more of the following categories:

- environmental factors
- genetic factors
- infection and immunity
- degenerative or neoplastic processes
- trauma.

These causative factors are interdependent; increasingly, links between them are being found and shown to be significant. Orthopaedic conditions due to trauma do not lie within the remit of this text and so will not be considered in any depth.

Environmental factors

Environmental factors that may be the cause or origin of a disease either exist within the individual (internal) or emanate from outside (external).

Internal

As the link between cause and effect is tenuous, it is often difficult to identify conclusively the internal factors that may lead to disease or ill health. However, a clear example of an internal factor is that of hormonal status. As oestrogen protects against bone loss, postmenopausal women are at a significantly greater risk of problems such as vertebral collapse and bone fracture due to osteoporosis than premenopausal women. This risk increases with age as the amount of bone loss increases due to reduced oestrogen levels.

Crawford Adams (1986) suggests that in female babies one type of congenital dislocation of the hip may be due to the ligament-relaxing hormone relaxin. This is secreted by the fetal uterus in response to oestrogens and progesterone reaching the fetal circulation, and leads to the joint instability associated with the condition, which may explain its higher incidence in girls.

External

External causes include those that are physical, sociocultural and politicoeconomic. Health and safety hazards in the workplace, home and outside environment lead to substantial numbers of occupational diseases and injuries each year. Injuries in the form of accidents are significant. There were 13 041 accidental deaths in Great Britain in 1987 (Central Statistical Office 1989). These include those due to accidents on the road, rail or other forms of transport (42% were road accidents) and those occurring at work or at home (38% were home or residential accidents). Importantly, between 1966 and 1986 the number of fatal home accidents in England and Wales was reduced from 7500 to 4500 and is now amongst the lowest in Europe.

The number of fatalities does not directly affect the role of the orthopaedic nurse. However, with the increasingly important role of the nurse as a health promoter, every opportunity should be taken to educate individuals in safety and the preventative aspects of health. Similarly, the orthopaedic nurse's role may not be that of caring for individuals immediately following injury, but the secondary and tertiary needs of these individuals ensure that most orthopaedic nurses will nurse people with traumatic injuries at some stage after the initial injury.

The majority of non-fatal home accidents involve falls. In 1987 in England and Wales, 60% of accidents amongst women between the ages of 65–74 years involved falls; this figure increases to 76% for those aged 75 years or over. The figures for men in the same age groups were 40% and 68%, respectively (Central Statistical Office 1989). In total, there were 107 253 home accidents.

During 1987, 69 000 people were killed or seriously injured in road accidents in Great Britain. The rate per thousand of those aged 15–19 years was three times that for the rest of the population, with the rate for users of two-wheeled vehicles 6.5 times that for the rest of the population. The importance of identifying the cause of road accidents can be clearly seen from road traffic accident statistics: the number of breath tests administered following accidents rose from 37 000 in 1977 to 65 000 in 1987; positive results from the tests fell from approximately 32% to 17%, respectively.

In 1987–88, injuries as a result of work activity numbered more than 188 000 in the UK (Central Statistical Office 1989). A third of the 150 000 reports of injuries requiring 3 days or less off work were sprains and strains, of which half affected the back. In nursing, three-quarters of a million working days are lost per year due to back pain, one in six being due to patient-handling incidents (Stubbs et al 1983). The prevalence of back pain in the nursing profession is second only to its prevalence in heavy industry. In a study carried out by Moffett and colleagues (1990), 64% of student nurses reported low back pain at some stage during a 20-month period,

Genetic factors

Congenital deformities or malformations of an orthopaedic nature are attributable to faulty development of the fetus and are present at birth, though they may not be recognized until later.

The incidence varies among different races. In the UK about 1–2% of infants are born with significant developmental abnormalities affecting the skeletomotor system (Crawford-Adams 1986). Examples of these deformities or anomalies are osteogenesis imperfecta, spina bifida and congenital dislocation of the hip. (For a more extensive list with further detail see Crawford-Adams 1986.)

Congenital deformities (i.e. those existing at the time of birth) may be caused by genetic or environmental factors or a combination of the two. Environmental factors may be internal or external, as previously discussed, and may be dietetic, hormonal, chemical, physical or infective in nature.

Genetic causes may be:

- Single genes of large effect, e.g. achondroplasia
- Chromosomal aberrations, e.g. Down's syndrome.

In addition, there may be multifactorial causation; for example, in the case of spina bifida and congenital dislocation of the hip.

A genetic defect is not always inherited from an affected parent or parents: it may occur from a fresh mutation in the gamete.

Genetic predisposition and environmental triggers

An important factor in the causation of disease and cancers is thought to be the link between a genetic predisposition and an environmental trigger; that is, the individual is not destined to develop a disease or cancer, but if he encounters a trigger then the risk of developing the disease or tumour increases. Examples of orthopaedic conditions to which a predisposition may exist include certain types of osteoarthritis, ankylosing spondylitis, gouty arthritis, idiopathic scoliosis, osteochrondritis dissecans, Dupuytren's contracture and many of the rheumatoid diseases (Crawford-Adams 1986).

The existence of a link between genetic predisposition and environmental trigger has been demonstrated in rheumatoid diseases such as systemic lupus erythematosus and rheumatoid arthritis. The mechanisms by which a particular part of the gene complex, known as an allele, gives rise to the disease state is poorly understood for most of these conditions (Davey 1989). For example, it is not known why some people who have an 'increased risk' allele for a particular disorder remain well, while others become ill. Nor is it conclusively known what triggers the onset of the condition, although environmental factors are important. It can be shown, however, from statistical association, that in comparison to individuals with some other allele, individuals with HLA allele DR4 have a 5.8 times greater risk of developing rheumatoid arthritis (Davey 1989), while those with HLA B27 have an 87.4 times increased risk of developing ankylosing spondylitis and a 37.0 times increased risk of developing Reiter's disease (arthritis of the lower spine).

An example of a potential environmental trigger associated with rheumatoid arthritis is that of diet. Brigg (1989) highlights the current revival of interest in the possibility that the disease might be caused by a sensitivity to certain foods in the diet. Interestingly, some therapeutic success has also been achieved using dietary manipulation with diagnosed sufferers.

Congenital disorders

As yet there is little that can be done to prevent the effects of inherited disorders and deformities, although the more that can be discovered about their origins or causes the closer we come to their prevention. However, the ethical dilemmas that surround possible interventions, such as genetic engineering, prenatal screening and termination of pregnancy, are presenting our society with difficult choices and much conflict of interest.

Although some genetically inherited disorders, such as congenital dislocation of the hip, can be treated successfully either conservatively or through surgery, this is far from always the case, and relatively little can be achieved with the majority of congenital deformities and disorders. Increasingly, more is being understood about

these deformities and disorders which would help health care professionals when advising parents prior to conception or early in pregnancy. It is now possible in some cases to detect whether a woman is a carrier for a particular condition or to diagnose prenatally the existence of an inherited deformity in a fetus. This ability to determine carriers and to diagnose deformities prenatally raises religious and ethical dilemmas for health care professionals and for the parents affected: nurses, in particular, are implicated in these issues through their involvement in the process of screening parents, the fetus and the newly born infant, and also through key roles in genetic counselling and the termination of pregnancies. It is estimated that 11–13% of severe childhood disability, both mental and physical, could be prevented if antenatal and neonatal screening tests and treatments were effectively implemented (King's Fund 1988).

As a result of antenatal investigative screening such as amniocentesis or chorionic villus sampling, parents can now be informed if there is a fetal deformity or abnormality. However, before these investigations are carried out, parents should be informed of the procedure, the information it provides, potential risks and possible outcomes; some parents would not consider a termination of pregnancy, and therefore to put the mother and fetus at risk if no action is to be taken from the results of the investigation would be undesirable. (Chorionic villus sampling is a technique that entails the taking of a small sample of fetal tissue for genetic and chromosomal analysis at 8–11 weeks of pregnancy.)

The acquisition of greater diagnostic and treatment capabilities is enabling genetic counsellors and knowledgeable, skilled health carers to help potential parents make decisions about the risks of genetic disorders. For example, parents with an only child who has osteogenesis imperfecta may wish to know the risk of having subsequent children with the same condition; or a newly diagnosed rheumatoid arthritic mother of two young children would perhaps want to discuss the chances of her two children, and any subsequent children, developing the disease.

Nurses are able to provide a continuity of

contact in caring for individuals and families affected by diseases of genetic origin. They are able to assume a general health education role to overcome the considerable lack of knowledge and the fear that surround physical handicaps and diseases.

Infection

Infection of bone and infections generally have been discussed in Chapter 8. The perspective used was predominantly one of prevention, which assumed that by understanding the causes of infection and systematically organizing nursing care, nurses and doctors can minimize the risks to patients and others. However, in spite of the preventative measures now available, acute haematogenous osteomyelitis still remains one of the important diseases of childhood, although tuberculous and syphilitic infections of bone are diminishing as the causative diseases are being attacked through primary and secondary prevention.

Immunity

The immune response is a major line of defence when the body is threatened by infection, and is initiated during the inflammatory response. It involves lymphocytes which are found in the blood and lymphoid tissues. The response can be divided into two broad categories:

- Humoral immunity
- Cell-mediated immunity.

Humoral immunity is developed when the body produces antibodies which are transported in body fluids such as the blood and lymph, for example the antibodies produced by the auto-immune response in rheumatoid arthritis. Antibodies are members of a group of proteins known collectively as immunoglobulins, and are produced in response to antigens, which are invading or foreign cell proteins.

Cell-mediated immunity is developed when cells are produced consisting of one variety of lymphocyte which is capable of destroying the invading or foreign cell by direct action rather than through the action of antibodies.

Immunity may be acquired through active stimulation of the immune system of an individual (for example, BCG (Bacille Calmette-Guérin) vaccination consists of weakened bacteria which protect the individual against tuberculosis), while neutralized preparations of microbial toxins – toxoids – protect against tetanus.

Immune response to infection

Viruses Antiviral antibodies restrict the spread of viruses predominantly within tissue fluids and particularly from infected cells. They are not significantly effective in the control of viral infections. Cell-mediated immunity controls viral infections by the production of immune system cells which act against the modified antigens of infected cells. Viruses continue to be a significant health problem as so many of them undergo variations which are slight enough to prevent the production of new antibodies but are different enough not to react with existing antibodies; thus, no immunity to the new viruses exists within the individual.

Bacteria Antibacterial antibodies enhance phagocytosis of the invading cells; they also neutralize the toxins produced by bacteria. Cell-mediated immune responses are of importance when they act against infecting bacterial cells that continue to grow within a cell, for example tuberculosis.

Cancer Membrane antigens of tumour cells, which are not present on normal cells, may be recognized as foreign (see Ch. 14). There is at present some debate as to the relative importance of immune and non-immune protection against cancer.

Diseases and HLA antigens

Human leukocyte antibody (HLA) antigens are used in tissue typing for transplantation surgery to match donor with recipient: the closer the match the less chance of rejection due to immune responses. The HLA antigens are similar to antigens on other tissue cells of the individual and are used as they are relatively straightforward to obtain and to analyse through a blood sample. These antigens are membrane markers on cells, providing the basis of the body's recognition of self and non-self. They are derived from a large number of genes known as the major histocompatibility complex (MHC) and are inherited in the normal way.

Increased understanding of immune responses may be of benefit in the future when person-to-person bone transplantation is developed. It has already been applied in bone marrow transplantation procedures.

Autoimmunity

The discovery of a link between genetics and disease has extended our existing knowledge of the causation of diseases. There is a well-documented link between anklosing spondylitis and the HLA-B27 antigen (Elves 1986). In the UK the HLA-B27 antigen is found on the tissue cells of only 5–10% of the general population, whereas 90% of individuals with ankylosing spondylitis are found to have tissue type HLA-B27. These types of links are increasingly being discovered in similar autoimmune orthopaedic diseases.

In autoimmune diseases, the individual produces antibodies which act against him, and this may have catastrophic effects. As yet there is no one factor or cause for this phenomenon which can be identified. Probably, each disease manifests itself in a multifactorial way, which includes immunological variations, genetic and hormonal changes, and viral infections. But, as discussed above, there is an undoubted connection between the development of autoimmune diseases and an inherited tendency or predisposition (Holme 1987).

Many autoimmune diseases are orthopaedic, for example, systemic lupus erythematosus and rheumatoid arthritis. In rheumatoid arthritis, antibodies react against the IgG immunoglobulins to produce complexes which, when deposited in the joints and other affected tissues, initiate inflammatory processes causing damage. (See Chs 11 and 12 for more details of these diseases and conditions.)

Degenerative processes

With increased age there is a gradual loss of muscular strength and stamina due to muscle cell atrophy. The accompanying loss of elastic fibres and collagen in muscle tissue, tendons and joint ligaments leads to reduced flexibility and increased stiffness. In bone, naturally occurring osteoporotic changes weaken the skeleton. These natural degenerative changes, related to age, have associated effects on the mobility of the individual which do not become obvious to health care services until further problems, such as a fracture, occur. Many of these individuals need community care and their numbers are growing: by 2001 there will be 9.0 million people aged 65 years and over (HMSO 1989). Growth in the size of this population will be greatest amongst the very elderly, with nearly a doubling of those aged over 85 years between 1986 and 2001. Other projections suggest that there will be just under 900 000 severely disabled adults in the UK aged 65 years and over by 2001 (HMSO 1989). These demographic changes are having a greater effect on orthopaedic services than any other part of the health service as degenerative diseases affect the musculoskeletal system more than any other system.

Osteoporosis

Osteoporosis is not a disease associated with abnormal bone composition: it is generally believed that the chemical composition of osteoporotic bone is no different from normal bone – there is just less of it (Nordin 1983).

Primary osteoporosis has two phases:

1. Senile osteoporosis, which is a protracted slow phase that occurs in both sexes and is commensurate with age
2. Postmenopausal osteoporosis, a transient accelerated phase which occurs in women after the menopause, bone loss being in excess of that expected with age.

Owing to the growing elderly population, the Office of Health Economics (1990) predicts that as the number of elderly people increases the number of hip fractures due to osteoporosis will also increase. In 1985 in England there were 43 230 fractures of the hip with an average hospital stay of 29.8 days. This represents one in 10 orthopaedic beds at any one time at a cost of £122.5 million per year.

Osteoporotic fractures in the elderly represent a major health care and social problem and are largely preventable. As bone loss is inevitable with advancing age, what must be identified and prevented is excessive bone loss. Identifiable risk factors are given in Table 9.1. An understanding of these factors will enable nurses, in their health promotion role, to educate individuals and encourage and support lifestyle changes to minimize the risk of fractures and deformities. Areas in which changes can be made include diet, exercise and hormone replacement therapy.

Screening procedures to identify at-risk individuals are being developed to aid primary and secondary prevention. At present there is no entirely satisfactory method of identification. However, bone mineral content can be measured accurately with dual-photon absorptiometry and quantitative computerized tomography, but these techniques are expensive and time-consuming. Cheaper methods are becoming available and it may be possible in the near future to provide cheap, quick mass screening techniques that would be very cost-effective for the health service.

Degenerative joint disease

Degenerative joint disease, or osteoarthritis, is the commonest type of arthritis and affects most people, to some degree, over the age of 75 years (Graves 1988). (See Ch. 10 for the in-depth nursing care of individuals with osteoarthritis.) The prevalent negative perception of old age, that functional capacity decreases with age largely owing to diseases such as osteoarthritis, is to be discouraged in the health care professions. Studies (King's Fund 1988) have shown that up to three-quarters of elderly people aged over 65 years see themselves as healthy for their age, and there is now clear evidence that self-perception of health among the elderly is an accurate positive indicator of future mortality. However, it is also clear from these and other studies (Office of Health Economics 1982) that joint disease, of which degenerative joint disease is by far the largest proportion, has a significantly inhibiting effect, nationally, on the ability of the elderly to carry out activities of living owing to impaired physical mobility (see Table 9.2).

Table 9.1   Risk factors associated with osteoporosis

Risk factor	Effects
Age and gender	by the age of 70 years bone mass has declined by 30% or more in women, less in men
Hormonal	oestrogens tend to protect bone against the resorbing actions of pararthyroid hormone. Decline of oestrogen at the menopause is associated with a rise in bone resorption
Parity	the increased oestrogen in pregnancy and/or the use of oral contraceptives may be protective of bone mass
Body build	obese postmenopausal women are less likely to experience fractures than slim women, as obesity increases the amount of biologically available oestrogen. Also, greater body weight places more stress on bones stimulating new bone formation
Genetic	black people have a higher skeletal mass than Whites and therefore sustain fewer fractures. Recent studies have also shown a family history of osteoporosis
Physical activity	the effect of gravity and the tension of contracting muscles help to maintain a positive balance between bone formation and resorption. Reduced amounts of physical exercise due to lifestyle or prolonged bed rest, etc. have the reverse effect
Dietary	reduced calcium absorption due to age and/or inadequate intake as a result of poor diet exacerbate osteoporotic effects. Sufficient vitamin D is also important. Recently, flouride has been shown to be an effective stimulator of sustained bone deposition
Alcohol	alcohol has a negative effect on bone mass
Cigarette smoking	there is an association between smoking and risk of fracture due to several reasons including the fact that smoking decreases oestrogen concentrations
Medications	steroid therapy decreases bone formation and increases resorption
Falling	the increased risk of falling due to age increases the risk of fracture

Table 9.2 Mobility and health at age 65 years and over

General Household Survey (1980)		Scottish Clackmannan Study (1976)	
Indicator	%	Indicator	%
General health, good/fair	76	General health, good for age	61
Unable to go out alone	12		
Unable to wash all over alone	9		
Unable to shop	14		
Unable to cook	7		
		Trouble with joints	17
		Trouble with back	9

Crawford Adams (1986) emphasizes that age alone is not the cause of osteoarthritis. Although it is caused by wear and tear, there is also nearly always a triggering or causative factor(s) that accelerates the degenerative process. These factors may be:

- congenital abnormal development
- irregularity of joint surfaces from a previous fracture
- internal derangements, such as a loose body or torn meniscus
- previous disease leaving a damaged joint, for example rheumatoid arthritis or haemophilia
- malalignment of a joint, e.g. due to trauma
- obesity.

It is important to recognize that these factors do not condemn the individual to osteoarthritis or relate directly to its severity. For instance, obesity has not been shown directly to cause osteoarthritis; however, if the individual has a predisposition, then the disease is more likely to develop in the overweight and also to progress more quickly.

Degenerative joint disease clearly has an effect on a large proportion of the population. Fortunately for many sufferers, since the 1940s surgical developments in the form of joint replacements have transformed their care, relieving them of chronic pain and disability. Of all the joint replacement operations, those for the hips have been the most outstandingly successful. In 1978 15 300 total hip replacements for osteoarthritis were performed in National Health Service (NHS) hospitals in England and Wales at a cost of £18 million (Office of Health Economics 1982). Since then, in Wales, these operations

have increased by 50% and knee replacement operations have more than trebled (HMSO 1989).

As yet, supply or throughput has not met the demand for joint replacement surgery. This situation is not improved by the confusion that exists over the actual sizes of waiting lists and the vast differences in throughput for this surgery between one health authority and another.

Yates (1982) was amongst the first to look at the number of hospital beds and orthopaedic waiting lists; he made some staggering revelations about the size and maintenance of waiting lists and the apparent lack of efficient use of operating sessions in some health authorities. Solutions to problems such as inadequate bed numbers, inaccurate or misrepresented waiting lists and invalid or unreliable statistical analyses and predictions have yet to be provided. The drastically reduced length of time of a hospital admission, increasing community care provision post-discharge and the market economy approach adopted by the NHS and the Community Care Act further complicate the debate surrounding these issues.

Neoplastic processes

Neoplasia, the proliferation of cell masses without normal control to form tumours which do not have any useful function, may occur in any body cells that have the potential to divide. The process may be triggered or caused by one or several of the factors already discussed, i.e. environment, heredity, immunity and infection, and trauma.

There are several theories about the initiation and process of carcinogenesis. There is, however, overwhelming evidence that cancer is a genetic disease, as it is the genetic material that is or becomes abnormal (McKenna 1987). This does not necessarily mean that it is hereditary, as the majority of tumours arise from abnormalities of the genetic material after conception; therefore, these cells are not passed on to future generations.

Environmental factors, in the form of carcinogens, are difficult to link conclusively with the causation of specific cancers. However, cigarette smoke and lung cancer, and ultraviolet light and skin cancer are two examples where a definite link has been established. Viruses that cause cancer or trigger the neoplastic processes – oncoviruses – are at present being investigated; for example, viral infections obtained during sexual intercourse and their link with cancer of the cervix.

The efficiency and state of the immune system of the individual are of importance in the development of cancer. Individuals with a relatively poor immune system, or who are immunosuppressed, have been shown to be more prone to develop cancers. Increasing evidence is also becoming available that demonstrates a link between the general well-being, and in particular the psychological state, of an individual and cancer. It is suggested that a negative attitude to life, and specifically the fear of developing cancer, predisposes an individual to developing the disease. Many complementary therapies aim at nurturing a positive mental attitude within the cancer sufferer in order to slow, halt or even cure the disease. The approach depends on the mind–body link of holism referred to in Chapter 1. While the mechanisms of this approach and its success are not fully understood as yet, there are increasing numbers of successful cases.

Classification of tumours

Bone tumours may be either benign or malignant; the latter may also be either primary or secondary (see Ch. 14 for further details). Although malignant bone tumours are more commonly secondary, significant numbers of primary bone tumours still occur. Through surgery and

chemotherapy, cure or increased survival times are being achieved. Statistics on the diagnosis and treatment of malignant bone tumours demonstrate the relationship between mortality ratios and the availability of specific regional health service provision (see Table 9.3). It is apparent that North East Thames, which has a regional and national bone tumour service, has a far lower mortality ratio than its neighbouring region, North West Thames. Early detection, rapid treatment and the ready availability of local specialized health care professionals seem to have produced a 50% decrease in the mortality rate within North East Thames compared to the standardized mortality ratios for England and Wales generally. The West Midlands, which also has a regional and national centre and works closely with that of North East Thames, shows a significantly lower mortality ratio as well (Office of Population Censuses and Surveys 1985).

THE NURSE'S ROLE IN THE PREVENTION OF ILL-HEALTH

To return to the theme of this chapter, the size of the problem is vast; orthopaedic conditions make great demands on health care provision

Table 9.3 Standardized mortality ratios of bone and cartilage cancer by sex (adapted from Office of Population Censuses and Surveys 1985 Mortality Statistics for England and Wales, HMSO)

Regional health authority	Mortality ratios	
	Male	Female
England and Wales	100	100
Northern	96	109
Yorkshire	82	172
Trent	77	83
East Anglian	80	106
North West Thames	144	112
North East Thames	44	67
South East Thames	89	87
South West Thames	131	120
Wessex	121	56
Oxford	137	75
South Western	119	87
West Midlands	51	76
Mersey	125	52
North Western	141	72

as well as adversely affecting the quality of individuals' lives. The remaining chapters in this book describe orthopaedic nursing within a curative framework. But as this chapter emphasizes, prevention is becoming an increasingly important aspect of care and the nurse's role in this should not be undervalued.

Prevention of ill-health may be primary, secondary or tertiary (Ewles & Simnett 1985):

1. Primary prevention is directed at healthy people, and aims to prevent ill-health arising in the first place.

2. Secondary prevention stops ill-health from moving to a chronic or irreversible stage and restores the person to his former state of health.

3. Tertiary prevention helps patients and relatives to make the most of their potential for healthy living in situations of established ill-health problems.

The role of the orthopaedic nurse in primary prevention may be, for example, to encourage an individual to participate in physical activity throughout his life. The increased strength, suppleness and stamina acquired would prevent many of the falls which occur as a result of the ageing process. Lindsay (1985) reports how physical activity may help to slow down the osteoporotic process which accompanies ageing. The King's Fund (1988) proposes four general objectives related to physical activity:

1. To encourage participation in appropriate, regular physical activity in all age groups and sectors of the community

2. To provide cheap, accessible sport and recreation facilities for all members of the community

3. To increase public and professional understanding of the importance of physical activity in the maintenance of health

4. To create a social climate in which regular physical activity is seen as a normal part of work and leisure.

These objectives would require support in the form of financial backing for bodies such as the Sports Council and tax relief for employers to encourage the building of better sports and recreational facilities at work.

Secondary prevention is often achieved through screening programmes. The nurse's role in this may be, for example, to carry out the simple test for idiopathic scoliosis now undertaken in many schools during regular medical examinations.

The nurse's role in tertiary prevention could be to identify the need for and to support an obese patient in a weight reduction programme. This is often beneficial to those with osteoarthritis of the lower weight bearing limbs both before and after surgery.

Perhaps the size of the problem should be perceived as directly related not to the range of orthopaedic diseases and conditions, but to the orthopaedic nurse's ability to respond in an open-minded and knowledgeable way.

REFERENCES

Boore J R P, Champion R, Ferguson M C 1987 Nursing the physically ill adult. Churchill Livingstone, Edinburgh

Brigg D 1989 Dietary manipulation in arthritis. Nursing Standard 3(47): 25–26

Central Statistical Office 1989 Social trends 19, HMSO, London

Crawford Adams J C 1986 Outline of orthopaedics, 10th edn. Churchill Livingstone, Edinburgh

Davey B 1989 Immunology. Open University Press, Milton Keynes

Elves M W 1986 Principles of genetics. In: Powell M (ed) Orthopaedic nursing & rehabilitation, 9th edn. Churchill Livingstone, Edinburgh

Ewles L, Simnett I 1985 Promoting health. John Wiley, Chichester

General Household Survey (1990) Office of Population Census & Surveys 1985. HMSO, London

Graves M 1988 Physiologic changes. In Hogstel M O (ed) Nursing care of the older adult. John Wiley & Sons, New York

Her Majesty's Stationary Office 1989 Caring for people. HMSO, London

Holme D J 1987 Infection and immunity. In: Boore J R P et al (eds) Nursing the physically ill adult. Churchill Livingstone, Edinburgh

King Edward's Hospital Fund for London 1988 The nation's health. King's Fund, London

Lindsay R 1985 Prevention of osteoporosis. In: Muir Gray J A (ed) Prevention of disease in the elderly. Churchill Livingstone, Edinburgh

McKenna P G 1987 Degenerative and neoplastic processes. In: Boore J R P et al (eds) Nursing the physically ill adult. Churchill Livingstone, Edinburgh

Moffett J A, Hughes G I, Griffiths P 1990 A longitudinal study of low back pain in student nurses. Unpublished paper

Nordin B E C 1983 In : Office of Health Economics 1990. Osteoporosis & risk of fracture. Office of Health Economics, London

Office of Health Economics 1982 Hip replacement & the NHS. Office of Health Economics, London

Office of Health Economics 1990 Osteoporosis and risk of fracture. Office of Health Economics, London

Office of Population Census & Surveys 1985 General household survey. HMSO, London

Scottish Clackmannan Study (1976) Office of Population Census & Surveys 1985. HMSO, London

Stubbs D A et al 1983 Back pain in the nursing profession. Ergonomics 26(8): 755–765

Yates J 1982 Hospital beds. William Heinemann, London

10

Osteoarthritis

*Elizabeth O'Brien   Lorraine Rundell
Nicholas Hext*

INTRODUCTION

This chapter discusses the demography and morbidity of osteoarthritis. To demonstrate the effects of the disease on an individual, a care study is presented and this is used to make explicit the general principles of nursing care that apply. It is to be hoped that these general principles will be transferable to the care of other individuals who suffer from this disease.

PRESENTATION OF SYMPTOMS AND DIAGNOSIS

Pain is the most prominent feature of osteoarthritis (Dobree 1988) and is usually the reason why medical advice is first sought. The sufferer classically complains of a gradual increase in pain in the affected joints over some months, or even years. Initially, pain is present only when the affected joints (e.g. hip, knee, shoulder) are active, but as the disease progresses the pain persists even at rest, until ultimately sleep may be disturbed.

With the progression of the disease, movements become more restricted (Adams 1990), mobility is impaired and there are significant changes in gait (Table 10.1), to accommodate these movement restrictions.

The diagnosis of osteoarthritis is made from the patient's presenting history, which takes into account age, past history and presenting symptoms. The diagnosis can be confirmed on clinical examination of the affected joints (Table 10.2) and radiographic examination (Table 10.3).

Table 10.1 Alterations in gait due to osteoarthritis (from Banwell & Gall 1988)

Joint affected	Differences in gait
Hip	Trendelenburg gait pattern
	antalgic hip gait – leaning body to affected side on weight bearing
	hip flexion contracture and resultant increase of lumbar lordosis – Thomas' sign
	apparent leg shortening on affected side
	shortened step on affected side
Knee	genu varus deformity – bow legs
Ankle	decreased plantar- and dorsiflexion
Forefoot	shortening stride length of opposite lower extremity due to metatarsophalangeal degeneration causing rigidity of the great toe

Table 10.2 Clinical examination of joints affected by osteoarthritis

Examine for:
Pain
Reduced range of motion
Fixed flexion deformity in hip joint
Crepitus
Signs of bony enlargement – osteophyte formation
Excess synovial fluid
Local warmth over joint
Heberden's nodes – osteophytic lumps on distal interphalangeal joints
Bouchard's nodes – osteophytic lumps on proximal interphalangeal joints

Table 10.3 Radiographic changes in osteoarthritis

Narrowing of joint space
Subchondral sclerosis
Spurring at joint margins
Subluxation
Juxta-articular or subchondral cysts

PATHOPHYSIOLOGY

Osteoarthritis is a disease of one or more synovial joints, characterized by degeneration of the cartilage and changes in the underlying bone. It is also referred to as arthrosis, osteoarthrosis and degenerative joint disease. Osteoarthritis begins with an increase in synovial fluid within the articular cartilage. Further chemical changes within the cartilage follow, preceding alterations in the chondroblasts. Bone at the joint margin hypertrophies to form osteophytes. These spread into the original articular cartilage, causing

thinning or complete destruction and thus a reduction in joint space. As the cartilage thins, underlying bone is exposed and in response there may be some cyst formation and osteosclerosis of subchondral bone. Although there is no primary change to the capsular or synovial membrane, continuing mechanical change may eventually distort the normal joint anatomy, leading to malalignment (see Figs 10.1 and 10.2).

In Britain osteoarthritis affects nearly 10% of the population; 17% of those who consult their GPs over rheumatic complaints are found to have osteoarthritis (Leitch 1987). Croft (1990) noted that between 1955 and 1981, the number of such referrals more than doubled and showed a marked female predominance.

As 'ageing is the primary cause of osteoarthritis' (Brusseau 1988), it follows that the incidence of osteoarthritis will increase with a growing elderly population.

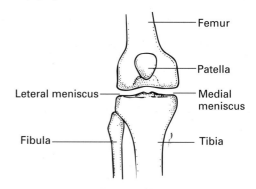

Figure 10.1 The normal knee joint, anterior-posterior view. (Adapted from McRae 1990.)

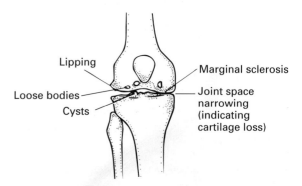

Figure 10.2 An osteoarthritic knee joint, anterior-posterior view. (Adapted from McRae 1990.)

WHICH JOINTS DOES OSTEOARTHRITIS AFFECT AND WHAT ARE THE CAUSES?

Osteoarthritis, unlike rheumatoid arthritis, is not an inflammatory disease and does not affect all body systems or cause systemic symptoms. Most commonly, it affects the weight-bearing joints (see Table 10.4), but there are marked differences between the causes of primary and secondary osteoarthritis (see Table 10.5).

A CARE STUDY

After the diagnosis of osteoarthritis has been made, the choice of treatment is dependent upon the severity of the disease; often reassurance and education about the disease are sufficient to provide the mild sufferer with the peace of mind

Table 10.4 Joints commonly and less commonly affected by osteoarthritis

Joints commonly affected	Joints less commonly affected
Distal interphalangeal	wrists
First carpometacarpal	hips
First metatarsophalangeal	lateral metatarsophalangeal
Knees	shoulder

Table 10.5 Primary and secondary osteoarthritis

Primary	Secondary
Idiopathic	previous trauma or disease such as: joint infections inflammatory arthritis avascular necrosis intra-articular fracture joint dysplasias congenital hip dislocation Perthes' disease acromegaly scoliosis Paget's disease rheumatoid arthritis gout history of surgery to affected area differing leg lengths (Bird 1990, Hornsby 1985)
Mostly females in UK due to hormone imbalance	affects males and females equally
Rare below 50 years of age	rising incidence with age (Croft 1990)
Affects many joints	affects isolated joints

to continue life, knowing that the pain is not due to a life-threatening illness.

If treatment is required, then whatever form it takes, the sufferer will still have to make adaptations to his lifestyle in order to ensure that his quality of life remains at an acceptable level; at present, with the increasing demands for surgery and rising waiting lists, it may be several years before a surgical option is made available to him.

To illustrate the many difficulties encountered by the sufferer of osteoarthritis and how they can be overcome, a care study of a 64-year-old grandmother, for this purpose named Janet, has been interspersed throughout this chapter with more general comments on the treatment of osteoarthritis.

Janet was diagnosed as suffering from osteoarthritis of both knees 14 years ago, and has lived with the resulting pain and disability since that time. She was admitted to hospital to undergo left total knee replacement surgery. Janet is married with two adult daughters and three grandchildren and lives with her husband in a three-bedroomed bungalow, with one flight of stairs leading to the loft. Until the age of 50 years her only previous medical history of note concerned a uterine prolapse repair following her second pregnancy.

Janet began to experience menopausal symptoms from the age of 49 years, which when coupled with concurrent family problems resulted in a nervous breakdown, for which she received inpatient electroconvulsive therapy (ECT) and made a full recovery. Shortly after this, at the age of 50 years she began to notice pain in her knees, particularly when kneeling.

With the worsening pain, kneeling became impossible, and after examination by her general practitioner osteoarthritis was diagnosed. Initial referral was to an athletic clinic where the effusions in her knees were aspirated. However, the pain continued to increase and the aspirations were soon discontinued.

In desperation, Janet turned to complementary therapies and found the most effective pain relief was massage. For the past 12.5 years, she has 'lived' for her weekly therapy sessions and also a week's holiday a year to a naturopathy clinic where she has tried several complementary therapies.

Hormonal changes during the menopause have been identified as a causative factor of cartilaginous changes leading to primary osteoarthritis (Dobree 1988).

The impact of osteoarthritis on Janet's life and its treatment may be suitably expressed within the framework of the Activities of Living model of nursing (Roper et al 1980). (See Ch. 5 for a full description of this model.)

Communicating

Communicating her fears and anxieties about the forthcoming surgery posed no difficulties for Janet.

Not every sufferer of osteoarthritis is able to communicate his feelings, nor adequately describe his pain and its effect. Providing sufficient information and an explanation of the proposed treatment and surgery by all health care workers involved with the osteoarthritic patient is vital. As osteoarthritis is not directly life-threatening, complete and direct sharing of information should occur. The sufferer may benefit from involvement with self-help groups such as those organized by the Arthritis and Rheumatism Council (ARC).

Breathing

Under normal circumstances, the breathing of an individual with osteoarthritis is not compromised. However, chest infections can result if mobility is severely restricted, and breathing cannot therefore be disregarded, especially in the case of the very elderly sufferer or those with other underlying medical conditions.

Eating and drinking

As Janet was overweight when osteoarthritis was diagnosed, she was advised to reduce her weight and lost approximately 10 kg by eating her usual diet but in smaller quantities.

Ideally, patients with osteoarthritis should keep as close to their normal ideal body weight as possible, as 'during walking, the knee bears a weight two or three times the total body weight' (Quintet 1986).

A sensible weight-loss programme should be undertaken if appropriate, but it is important that the nurse, or other health care professionals, assess the sufferer and his circumstances with care before suggesting that he needs to lose weight. Tact must always be employed and accompanying factors, such as those listed below, taken into account:

1. The amount of exercise undertaken inevitably decreases as mobilizing becomes more painful, and the sufferer often resorts to 'comfort eating' out of boredom.
2. For elderly sufferers living alone, shopping and cooking can prove so laborious that their main source of sustenance is likely to be sugary or fatty snacks and convenience foods.

Eliminating

Since undergoing the repair of a uterine prolapse at the age of 30 years, Janet has suffered from frequency and urgency of micturition. This has posed few problems until the progression of her osteoarthritis led to a reduced ability to hurry and an increased difficulty in rising from chairs. To compensate Janet began to wear pant liners in order to minimize the dribbling incontinence that she invariably suffered before reaching the lavatory. Because Janet lived in a bungalow, her inability to climb stairs posed no problems to her elimination needs.

Urgency and frequency of micturition become more common as a person ages; in females, this is due to lax pelvic floor muscles and in the male due to benign prostatic enlargement. Normally the urge to pass urine is felt at 50% bladder capacity but in the elderly this can be as much as 90%, which means that the time available for an elderly person to reach the lavatory before voiding is much reduced (Garret 1983). As osteoarthritis is commonly associated with increasing age, incontinence can be a result of the physical limitation of reaching the bathroom in time rather than any urological dysfunction.

This difficulty can be overcome with the use of household adaptations and aids, or in extreme cases, a suitably located commode. (See also Ch. 5 for examples of aids.)

Constipation is a well-known consequence of reduced mobility, especially when strong analgesia is taken. Alterations to diet may need to be considered in order to counteract constipation before the sufferer requires ever-increasing quantities of aperient in order to defaecate regularly.

Personal cleansing and dressing

In order to facilitate bathing, Janet had handles fitted to her bath and she purchased a non-slip mat. These enabled her, with some difficulty, to get in and out of the bath, but she preferred to use the shower, as this was more straightforward.

Janet could dress independently, although she had difficulty in reaching her feet and relied upon her husband to help her put on footwear.

In general, the limitation of mobility that osteoarthritis causes greatly affects the sufferer's ability to wash and dress independently; this is especially so in those with osteoarthritis of the hip or spine who find bending almost impossible. Baths can no longer be climbed into; the pain caused by twisting may make backs difficult to wash; and feet may remain inflexibly out of reach, despite a range of innovative postures that the sufferer may attempt. It is very important for the sufferer to maintain his independence and self-esteem by continuing to carry out these intimate tasks if at all possible. There are many bathing aids available to assist him with personal hygiene, although many sufferers find their own ways of adapting. For this reason, a talk with a fellow osteoarthritic, or literature written by other sufferers, could prove useful for those having difficulties in washing or dressing.

Controlling body temperature

Janet had no difficulties in controlling body temperature as she lived in a comfortable, centrally heated bungalow with her husband for companionship.

However, there is a significant risk of hypothermia for the frail, inactive, elderly sufferer living alone. Adequate social support from within the community should be ensured for these people and the availability of government grants for home improvements or help with heating bills should be investigated. The sufferer may also be encouraged to perform exercises that can assist the maintenance of core temperature.

Mobilizing

Pain was the principal limiting factor to Janet's mobility. She described the pain experienced in her knees as 'toothache' within the joints. She experienced it constantly but, typically, it was less severe whilst she was resting. Several alternative therapies had been tried in addition to massage, such as hot wax and heat treatments, hydrotherapy and acupuncture. All except acupuncture proved effective, to some degree, in reducing the pain. Janet tried Royal Jelly and Oil of Evening Primrose. She found Royal Jelly ineffective but felt that the Oil of Evening Primrose improved her feeling of general well-being, and thus made her more tolerant of the pain and disability. Ice packs also helped, and Janet kept two bags of frozen peas on hand especially for this purpose. Initially, non-steroidal anti-inflammatory drugs were prescribed for pain relief, but these proved to be ineffective for Janet.

The use of an analgesic such as Aspirin or Paracetamol is often of benefit to the 'mild' sufferer. (Aspirin has more anti-inflammatory properties than Paracetamol.) Although Duckworth (1984) states that, 'Anti-inflammatory analgesics are of little help in osteoarthritis', this is principally because the nature of the disease is not due to an inflammatory reaction. However, other surgeons (Dandy 1989, Crawford Adams 1990), believe that non-steroidal anti-inflammatory drugs (NSAIDs) provide effective relief of pain caused by inflammatory reactions secondary to the disease process. In regular doses, they exhibit both analgesic and anti-inflammatory properties, making them an appropriate form of treatment. They must, however, be used with caution, as the side-effects can be many and varied (gastric irritation is the most common). A total of 60% of all patients will respond to the use of any NSAID (British National Formulary 1990), but the remaining 40% may respond to only one or two, if any. A response to a NSAID should be seen within 48 hours of its initiation, but if deemed appropriate, the drug should be taken for a period of up to 3 weeks before full efficacy can be properly assessed.

The application of an ice pack or heat pad locally to the affected joint may also be of some temporary comfort to the sufferer. By dulling sensation and reducing swelling the ice will allow very temporary relief, whilst the heat pad will provide a feeling of comfort.

For 12 years Janet had walked the mile to her local shop with minimal discomfort but, gradually, walking became increasingly difficult and hurrying impossible. Ascending and descending stairs were similarly problematic, and for the past 5 years Janet had managed by crawling up and down the stairs on her hands and knees, a practice that was less acceptable in public places.

One year from diagnosis, Janet's knees had deteriorated to 70° of flexion in the right knee and 80° in the left. Movement medially and laterally against resistance was very poor.

The physiotherapy and massage that Janet received on a weekly basis began with light massage and progressed to the application of friction and stress on the affected joint. The simple exercises that the therapist prescribed were carried out with great enthusiasm and determination by Janet. Janet's husband bought her an exercise bicycle and rowing machine, which both provide excellent exercises for sufferers of osteoarthritis if they can be tolerated. Janet found these exercises very beneficial until about 2 years ago, when further deterioration became apparent and she could no longer tolerate her normal pattern of mobilizing.

Most sufferers of osteoarthritis find their mobility decreases with the progression of the disease. Pain and stiffness are the usual limiting factors. For the sufferer whose mobility becomes severely affected, and whose ability to perform even simple functional tasks is reduced, referral to an occupational therapist may be useful. A home assessment can be made during which the occupational therapist assesses the sufferer's environment and gives advice on possible adaptations and alterations which could help him to either maintain or regain his independence. Major improvements may be performed with the financial support of the social services, but the sufferer can make many small and inexpensive adaptations to his own environment to make it more manageable. Table 10.6 indicates how different aids can assist the sufferer of osteoarthritis.

The community or hospital-based physiotherapist can provide the sufferer with programmes of active and passive exercises which may be performed at home. In addition, a course of hydrotherapy may be prescribed. The warm water and easing of joint load provide an environment within which the sufferer may exercise more freely, improving both muscle tone and range of movement in the affected joint.

Osteoarthritis is in many cases associated with years of obesity. At the very least, the overweight osteoarthritic will be increasing the load placed upon his already impaired joints, leading to greater discomfort and a more rapid progression of the disease. The cessation or modification of activities stressful to the diseased joint (sports, active hobbies) may also help to ease discomfort. The physiotherapist can again be of use by assessing the stance and mobility of the sufferer, and providing walking aids or advice on improving posture.

Carers, whether in hospital or a community setting, must make every effort to ensure some form of exercise is continued for as long as can be tolerated, so as to avoid the many complications associated with reduced mobility.

Working and playing

Janet's sedentary job as a part-time audio-typist allowed her to stay in employment until she was 62 years old, as a colleague drove her to and from work.

Her hobbies included knitting and cooking for the Women's Royal Voluntary Service (WRVS) one afternoon a week, which she was able to maintain without difficulty. She was also a keen gardener, but found that she required increasingly longer rest periods and that her inability to kneel hampered her gardening.

Statistics published in the USA (Kramer et al

Table 10.6 Aids and adaptations

Osteoarthritis of the trapeziometacarpal or interphalangeal joints makes gripping or fine movements difficult to perform	• clothes can be adapted to include Velcro or zippers which are easier to manage than buttons • extension levers fitted to taps provide more leverage when they are switched on and off • bottle openers with large, easily held handles are available to open jars and bottles • large-handled cutlery is available
Osteoarthritis of the lumbar spine and hips can limit bending; involvement of the cervical spine prevents the sufferer from looking upwards	• handle extensions can be fitted to house dusters and cleaners • a 'helping hand' can be used for reaching too high or too low • long-handled shoe horns and bath sponges limit the need to bend and twist • a stocking aid allows the sufferer to wear socks or tights even when the feet cannot be reached
Osteoarthritis of the hips, knees and lumbar spine makes it difficult to get up from low seating	• a high straight-backed chair with arms is essential to enable the sufferer to get up independently. When this becomes more difficult, sprung chairs can help users to a standing position • raised toilet seats are available to fit over a normal household toilet and can also come attached to rails; they effectively provide seat arms around the toilet from which to rise
When bathing becomes difficult	• a non-slip mat and the fitting of handles or rails increase safety and reduce the risk of falling when getting into and out of the bath • a simple board and bath seat set will allow the sufferer to continue bathing activities when he can no longer lift legs over the bath edge
Generalized slower mobility	• installation of a cordless telephone prevents the need to hurry from one room to another to answer the the telephone • remote control television and other electronically controlled entertainments (e.g. hi-fi music centres) mean that the sufferer does not have to rise so frequently • an entryphone for those living in flats not only increases personal safety but can obviate the need for a trip downstairs to answer the door

1983) show that 60 million days of work were lost in a year as a result of osteoarthritis. Those employed in more physical work suffer a higher chance of enforced early retirement or longer periods of sick leave due to the disease. Alternative jobs are not always available, and the possibility of changing professions beyond the age of 50 years may be impossible for many people when there are high unemployment and few retraining facilities. Their financial security may become compromised and they may suffer from severe loss of self-esteem.

It is vital that a social worker or employment counsellor with an understanding of the difficulties faced by the sufferer is available to discuss the benefits and social support on offer. For many, leaving full-time employment is an opportunity to take up new interests and spend more time on hobbies. Keeping active increases morale and ensures that some exercise is taken.

Some hobbies, however, such as sporting or do-it-yourself activities, cannot always be continued in comfort. Decreasing mobility diminishes interest in active pursuits and the sufferer feels forced to spend more time indoors. Morale drops with the onset of boredom, and when coupled with constant pain, it is perhaps not surprising that a number of sufferers become depressed. Support of family and friends is vital in this situation. The sufferer must be encouraged to feel of value and to take up different interests.

Expressing sexuality

Janet was very fortunate in having an understanding husband who remained supporting and loving throughout her illness. Nevertheless, there were occasions when their relationship was placed under great strain; when her pain was at its worst she became very frustrated and irritable. Fortunately, the physical relationship she shared with her husband was largely unaffected. They continued to share a double bed, and both benefited from the comfort of being physically close to one another.

Janet had always taken great pride in her appearance. She continued to dress in elegant clothes and wear make-up, even though she did not always feel like doing so. She tended to choose clothes to hide her 'misshapen' knees and bowed legs. Fortunately, Janet was able to adapt without a severe change of body image.

Many sufferers cannot adapt to a new body image as clothes which previously suited them no longer fall correctly, or they look unattractive. Certain styles become difficult to wear, and shopping for clothes becomes a tiring activity. Putting on make-up, shaving or visiting the hairdresser become activities that can easily be missed, resulting in a poor body image and loss of self-esteem.

The Arthritis and Rheumatism Council (ARC) found that: 'two out of three people with arthritis of the hip joint experienced some difficulty with their sex lives which they felt was entirely due to their arthritis' (ARC 1989). It is unfortunate that difficulties which make the sufferer less agile and cause discomfort with conventional sexual positions, force many couples to stop having intercourse altogether. For some couples, this may be a natural progression of their relationship into later life, but for others it may be an unnatural loss of intimacy, adding to the stress placed upon the relationship. Frequently, sufferers are too embarrassed to discuss these problems with their doctor or a Relate counsellor. Most solutions offered involve the use of alternative positions (SPOD 1990), but this must be approached in a sensitive and tactful manner, as traditional attitudes and limited sex education have led to the view that the 'missionary position' is the only normal combination and that other positions are somehow unnatural. Providing advice on alternative sexual techniques requires the nurse not only to provide information but also to give reassurance that an alternative practice is equally as acceptable.

The degree to which physical relationships are affected depends which joint(s) are osteoarthritic:

- Osteoarthritis of the hands and feet may appear to be the least troublesome disability, but the loss of fine movements in the hand can make undressing difficult and foreplay clumsy.
- Osteoarthritis of the knee or hip makes kneeling difficult, and the active role in the missionary position can become very uncomfortable. The passive role is therefore advised, although it is not always tolerated in practice, especially by men.
- Osteoarthritis of the hip can prevent abduction and thus render intercourse almost impossible for females.

A useful resource is SPOD (Association to aid the Sexual and Personal Relationships of People with a Disability), who have produced frank and easy-to-understand information leaflets on positions and relationships (SPOD 1990).

Sleeping

On an average night, Janet wakes up approximately three times due to her osteoarthritis. This does not significantly tire her.

Many sufferers find constant sleepless nights very exhausting. Stronger or alternative analgesia may be required or a mild form of night sedation when appropriate. It must be ensured, however, that these methods are closely monitored and that they are used only as a short-term remedy. If a sedative is taken over an extended period it could prove ineffective, as tolerance to it will develop. The sufferer may wish to try alternative, herbal remedies or may compensate for loss of sleep by taking a rest during the day.

Dying

Life expectancy is seldom reduced by a diagnosis of osteoarthritis. The Office for Population Census and Survey (OPCS 1990) for the years 1987/1988/1989 show that only 0.17% of the total number of deaths is due to osteoarthritis (0.07% of male and 0.27% of female deaths). From almost 577 000 deaths in 1989, less than 1000 were due to osteoarthritis or associated conditions. The figures serve to emphasize that osteoarthritis is not a life-threatening disease, but one that requires the sufferer to adapt when necessary to its impositions.

TOTAL JOINT REPLACEMENT

The great advances made in joint replacement surgery over the past few decades have provided benefits which can transform the lives of those suffering from osteoarthritis. The recipient of a synthetic joint can with reasonable certainty expect lower pain levels, greater mobility, increased range of joint movement and, often most importantly, a lowered dependence on friends and relatives. The implications for the patient who has for many years been debilitated by an osteoarthritic joint(s) are myriad, reaching into many facets of daily life.

The most common surgical procedure in advanced osteoarthritis of the hip joint is the replacement of both the acetabular and femoral components. As the prosthetic joint should ideally provide many years of untroubled service, a low friction surface contact is essential. This is usually obtained by the use of a dense polyethylene cup and a metal/metal alloy femoral component. The individual parts are secured by the compound methyl methacrylate, which has properties similar to human bone.

Research into improved design of prostheses and fixatives more closely resembling bone are constantly yielding results, providing the orthopaedic surgeon with a greater range of options to offer the individual patient. One of the most recently developed prostheses is the model which does not require the methyl methacrylate fixative. Greater preparation of the bony contact areas is required; the prosthesis is then tightly forced into the femoral shaft. The theoretical advantage of using this type of prosthesis is that it enables younger patients to undergo total joint replacement because, with this type of prosthesis, more cortical bone is preserved

where cement would normally be placed, thus increasing the options for later revisions.

The period of bedrest following a cementless total joint replacement is extended to approximately 4–5 days rather than the standard 2, and the patient is instructed to walk non-weight-bearing using crutches for a further period of at least 6 weeks. This enables the prosthesis to become firmly incorporated into the femoral stem. All other care is as for a standard joint replacement. Figures 10.3 to 10.6 illustrate different types of joint prostheses.

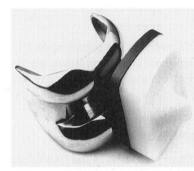

Figure 10.3   Insall Burstein total knee prosthesis.

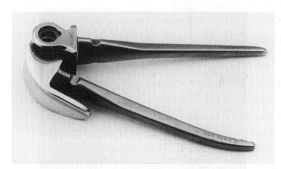

Figure 10.4   Stanmore total knee prosthesis.

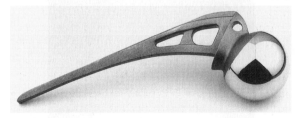

Figure 10.5   Austin Moore hip prosthesis (femoral component).

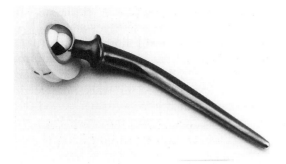

Figure 10.6   Stanmore total hip prosthesis.

Preparation of the patient undergoing total joint replacement of the lower limb

Figures 10.7 and 10.8 are preoperative X-rays taken of Janet's left knee. They show clearly the presence of osteoarthritis, with a reduction in the joint space and a worn articular cartilage, particularly on the lateral side.

Psychological preparation

A thorough explanation of the procedure should be given by a member of the surgical team. Expe-

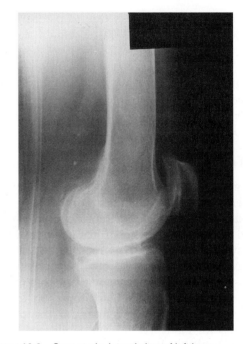

Figure 10.8   Care study, lateral view of left knee.

rience has shown, however, that this task often falls to the nursing staff. The nurse should explain all likely procedures and outcomes frankly without alarming the patient unnecessarily. Factors such as equipment likely to be used, pain control and positioning should all be discussed.

This early preoperative period is an ideal time to include friends, relatives or partners who may become involved in providing care and support following the patient's discharge from hospital.

Physical preparation

Preoperative preparation is based on the following guidelines:

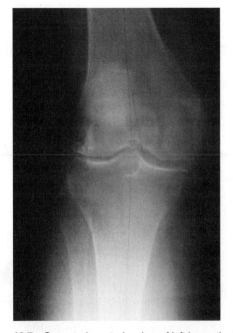

Figure 10.7   Care study, anterior view of left knee, the joint space is reduced, particularly laterally.

- A ward specimen of urine is obtained and tested using a reagent stick. If any signs of a urinary tract infection are present, a sterile specimen should be sent to the laboratory for microscopy and culture. This will indicate the presence of any such infection, which may be treated as deemed appropriate by the surgical team.
- The prescription of preoperative and postoperative antibiotic cover depends upon the

individual surgeon's preference. All patients have some form of antibiotic cover, as the infection of a prosthetic joint is a serious complication, often leading to many months or even years of expensive treatment with little chance of complete success in eradicating the infection. Infection occurs in approximately 1 : 100 replacement operations (Hughes 1988).

- Preoperative skin preparation should be confined to bathing and the use of fresh linen/clothing. Some studies, however, advocate the use of a 4% chlorhexidine gluconate solution for use when the patient showers prior to elective surgery (Van Diemen 1985). Shaving of the operative site is best performed in the sterile conditions of the theatre, immediately before surgery. The skin is aseptically cleansed, before and after shaving with a sterile safety razor. An occlusive clear film dressing is then applied to the area to minimize the risk of infection from adjacent skin bacteria.

- The physiotherapist will assess the patient before surgery to determine the range of movement within the joint to be operated upon and to determine the patient's respiratory capabilities in order to identify any actual or potential problems. The physiotherapist will also go through the exercises to be carried out postoperatively, practising each one with the patient. A typical programme consists of:
  — Deep breathing and coughing exercises to prevent the development of postoperative chest infection
  — Dorsi- and plantarflexion exercises to deter the formation of a deep vein thrombosis
  — Exercises to strengthen the quadriceps muscles, preventing flexion deformity of the knee.

- It is advisable for patients to attempt to open their bowels prior to surgery – especially in cases where an uncemented prosthesis will be used or a prolonged period of bedrest is indicated; this will preserve their peace of mind in the postoperative phase, by reducing the threat of having to defaecate whilst on bedrest. The nurse may be required to assist this process by the provision of prescribed aperients or suppositories.

- It is advisable to administer any intramuscular medication in the preoperative and postoperative phases to the unaffected side to further reduce the risk of infecting the prosthetic material.

Postoperative care of the patient undergoing total hip replacement

Janet was taken to theatre and had an Insall Burstein total knee replacement. As in Figures 10.7 and 10.8 (preoperative), the X-rays in Figures 10.9 and 10.10 are of the left knee in the anterior and lateral views, taken after surgery.

Maintaining a safe environment: observations

On her return to the ward area, Janet's observations of blood pressure, pulse and respiration were comparable to their preoperative recordings and their frequency soon reduced accordingly. The neurovascular status of the left foot was satisfactory and was similar to that of the right.

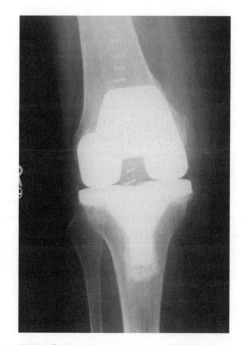

Figure 10.9 Care study, anterior view of left knee following the insertion of an Insall Burstein total knee prosthesis.

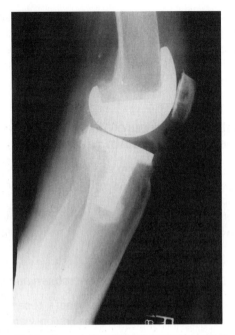

Figure 10.10 Care study, lateral view of left knee following the insertion of an Insall Burstein total knee prosthesis.

If possible, the ward bed should be in the theatre recovery area with a fresh change of linen and a bed cradle so that the postoperative patient can be transferred directly to the bed, minimizing patient discomfort and risk.

Observations of pulse, blood pressure and respiratory rate are initially made and recorded each half hour; this rate of observation is reduced as their stability and resemblance to the preoperative baseline occur. The neurovascular status of the affected limb is ascertained by checking its degree of colour, warmth, sensation and movement and the presence of foot pulses. These parameters are then compared to those of the unaffected limb; any abnormality is noted and reported to the surgical staff immediately. Marking the location of the foot pulse, usually the dorsalis pedis artery, with a cross or other such mark will ensure all staff observe the same area.

Wound care

One vacuum drainage bottle was used in Janet's wound. This was removed 48 hours after surgery, when a little more than 400 ml of bloody fluid had been collected. Wound closure was carried out with stainless steel clips, which were removed 11 days later without incident. Janet's wound dressing consisted of wool and crêpe bandaging, which did not become soiled as there was minimal oozing from the wound itself. The bandaging was removed 48 hours after surgery, and a clean, sterile dressing applied.

If a vacuum drainage system is in situ, this must be checked regularly for drainage, patency and maintenance of the vacuum. The collection vessel should be changed only when full or when the vacuum is lost; the amount of drainage should be recorded on the patient's fluid balance chart. Unless heavy drainage continues, drains should be removed approximately 24 hours after surgery (Willett et al 1988). The use of a closed drainage system in the postoperative joint replacement patient remains a topic of some controversy among surgeons (Willett et al 1988, Cobb 1990).

The type of initial wound dressing applied in theatre varies from a large airstrip dressing to one of wool and gauze. Whatever dressing is used it should be regularly assessed for oozing and may be reinforced if necessary with a pressure dressing. The layers of dressing first applied should be left in place for at least 48 hours unless this is contraindicated.

The sutures or clips used in wound closure are removed 10 to 12 days after hip replacement operations and 10 to 14 days after knee operations, providing that there are no contraindications.

Pressure risk areas

Pressure area care was carried out with relative ease. Janet was able to lie comfortably on her right side when supported by pillows, and assisted the nurses by using the overhead trapeze to support some of her body weight when her position was changed. No breakdown of pressure risk areas occurred.

The patient should be on a firm bed with its lower end raised to assist venous return and to decrease the amount of swelling in the knee. This increases comfort, and lessens the risk of sacral pressure sore development as the shear forces are reduced (see Ch. 5).

The artificial knee recipient may be nursed on his side at any postoperative stage, although the level of comfort obtained in this position will vary greatly. At least two nurses must assist the patient to turn: one to support the affected limb and one to place pillows between the legs and in the back for support. When the patient is lying flat in bed, a pillow should not be placed beneath his knee as this may promote the development of a flexion deformity.

Positioning

Positioning of the hip replacement patient entails the additional risk of prosthetic dislocation. To prevent dislocation of the prosthesis, abduction of the affected limb must always be maintained in the postoperative period. This can be achieved with the use of a triangular abduction wedge, pillows or other similar equipment. The bed should be fitted with an overhead trapeze (monkey pole) to enable the patient to assist with pressure area relief and to use bedpans.

The patient should be nursed initially in the supine position; he should never flex the hip joints to an angle of 90° or more (45° if the hip was replaced from a posterior angle) to reduce the risk of dislocation.

Unless the surgeon instructs otherwise, the patient may be turned onto his unaffected side in the immediate postoperative period. A minimum of two nurses are required for this: one to support the affected limb and one to turn the patient onto his unaffected side. Once the patient is in place, the affected limb is positioned safely and pillows are put on both sides of the body to maintain comfort and stability. At least one to two pillows are placed between the legs to maintain adequate abduction and to ease discomfort caused by the weight of the upper leg.

While the patient is being turned, pressure risk areas may be checked and compared with their preoperative condition. Any deterioration in the condition of a pressure area must be dealt with as a matter of urgency.

Some orthopaedic centres still advocate lifting patients who require pressure area care, rather than turning them onto one side, to further re-duce the risk of hip dislocation. This is not, however, recommended as it puts the patient and nurse at risk of injury (Love 1986).

Pain relief

Janet experienced relatively little pain during the initial postoperative 48 hours. What pain she did have was controlled to her satisfaction by intramuscular opiates and later oral Omnopon and Aspirin (the analgesic of choice, as Janet had no previous history of gastric problems). Later, analgesia was restricted to the occasional dose of Paracetamol at Janet's own request.

It is important for the patient to obtain effective pain relief following surgery so that he can begin an early programme of both limb and deep breathing exercises in relative comfort. Intramuscular analgesia (opiates / anti-inflammatories) should be administered throughout the initial postoperative period. Antispasmodics are often effective in counteracting muscular spasm, which can be a source of severe postoperative discomfort.

Breathing

Janet's respiratory status was never a cause for concern in the postoperative phase. She performed the deep breathing exercises that she had learnt preoperatively from the physiotherapist, at regular intervals whilst on bed rest.

On returning from the recovery area, the patient may receive oxygen therapy until he is fully awake, depending upon both the individual patient and the anaesthetist. As soon as possible, the patient should begin a programme of deep breathing exercises for a short period each waking hour. The nurse in constant attendance is in an ideal position to encourage and assist with these exercises.

Eating and drinking

Janet was able to take sips of water within a few hours of returning to the ward. She expressed no feelings of nausea and was soon taking free fluids. An intravenous infusion was maintained during the first postoperative night but was removed the following morning. Although Janet's appetite was reduced for several days, she was able to take a full, normal diet quickly.

Eliminating

Micturition was not a problem for Janet as she managed to pass 300 ml of urine within a few hours of returning from theatre. A 'slipper' bedpan was used with relative ease as Janet was able to lift herself onto the pan using the overhead trapeze.

Defaecation did not occur until the third postoperative day, when Janet managed to reach the toilet without help from the nursing staff.

The act of eliminating potentially entails much discomfort and embarrassment for the joint replacement patient in the period prior to ambulation. Bedpans in particular press on and around the wound area when sat on. By being sensitive to the patient's needs, the nurse may do much to make this activity more bearable.

Several factors may influence the patient's ability to micturate. These include anaesthesia, pain and discomfort, the patient's position, prostatic hypertrophy and excessive anxiety. The use of a slipper bedpan is preferable to the conventional deeper type, as it is easier to position and less uncomfortable: the patient may either be rolled or lifted onto it. If he is rolled, the maintenance of leg abduction is paramount in the hip replacement patient.

An inability to micturate often will result in urinary catheterization being necessary, although in some cases the surgeon will authorize the use of a commode which is placed adjacent to the bed. This will enable the patient to sit in relative comfort in an effort to micturate.

With an early ambulation programme, the patient should not develop constipation, although poor nutritional status, low fluid intake and the effects of strong analgesia may combine to cause it. The nurse can give dietary advice and, if necessary, involve the dietitian to prevent constipation occurring, but if it becomes a problem, the use of an oral aperient should be considered before suppositories or enemas.

Personal cleansing

During the initial postoperative period, Janet had to meet her hygiene needs with a daily bed bath; she needed help only in washing her back and feet. On these occasions an entire change of linen was given to promote a feeling of freshness which was greatly appreciated by Janet.

Once mobile, Janet was able to use the bathroom, and sat by the sink to wash. Full bathing commenced 4 days after surgery; a hoist was used to lower Janet into the bath. Prior to discharge, Janet was able to use the bathing boards to enter and exit the bath. These occasions were greatly appreciated by Janet, who had always maintained high standards of hygiene. The soothing effect of the warm water also enabled Janet to commence flexion exercises on the left knee in greater comfort.

Throughout the initial postoperative period, prior to ambulation, the patient will require assistance in meeting his daily hygiene needs: a bed bath, given daily or more frequently, is the only possible way.

Although confined to bed, the patient should be allowed and encouraged to maintain maximum independence within the limits of safety. The provision of frequent changes of water and placing toiletries, towels, flannels and the nurse call bell within easy reach of the patient will enable him to wash in privacy.

The time spent by the nurse in assisting the patient to meet his hygiene needs is an ideal opportunity for the nurse to educate the patient in aspects such as wound care, positioning and mobility. During this period the nurse will also be able to evaluate the patient's skin for signs of fungal infection, rashes and pressure area breakdown.

Once mobile, the patient may wash in the bathroom, providing that a safe environment is maintained. When given clearance by the surgeon, the patient can be assisted to take a shower or bath.

Before discharge, the occupational therapist may assess the patient for bathing/dressing and provide him with advice and devices such as bathing boards, a raised toilet seat, a helping hand or a stocking fitter. Figure 10.11 illustrates

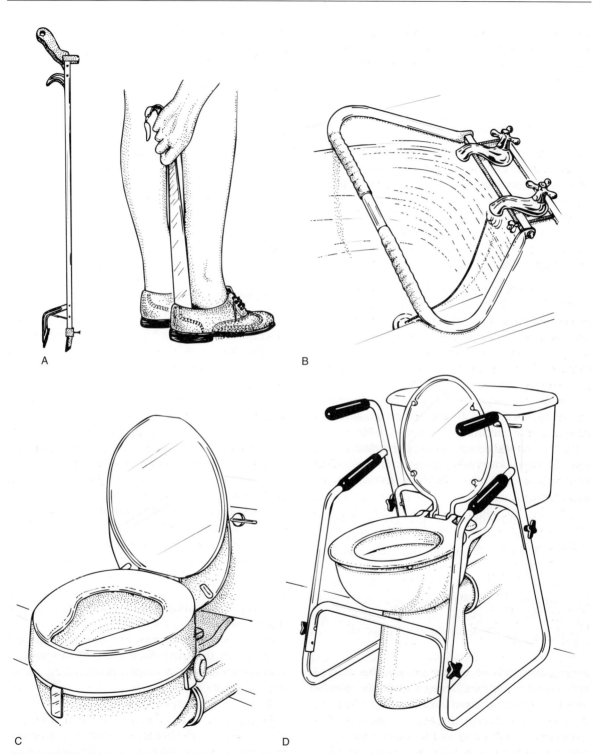

A

B

C

D

Figure 10.11 Aids to independence in the home: A. Easy reacher and shoe horn; B. Bath support rail; C. Raised toilet seat and lid; D. Bathroom system frame. (From Independence in the home (catalogue), The Boots Company, with permission.)

some of the aids commonly available to people in hospital or the community, which may be purchased from the occupational therapist or at some major high street stores.

Controlling body temperature

On her return to the ward, Janet's temperature was 35.2°C per axilla. A space blanket was placed next to her body and supplemented with extra bedlinen. Within 2 hours, the axillary temperature had risen above 36°C and the space blanket was removed.

Mobilizing

Janet began to use the continuous passive motion (CPM) machine 24 hours after surgery, initially with a modest degree of flexion (10° to 40°), but as she found this easier to tolerate, greater angles were introduced, until 90° of flexion was achieved. The machine was used for a total of 6 hours daily in divided periods of 1 to 2 hours. In addition to these exercises, the physiotherapist encouraged regular active flexion exercises on the edge of the bed. By the 9th postoperative day, Janet was able to actively flex the knee to 90°.

Janet performed both dorsi- and plantarflexion exercises at regular intervals in the postoperative period. The bed was also tilted initially to prevent venous congestion.

Deep vein thrombosis is the greatest single threat to postoperative recovery (Walker et al 1985) and is a major complication of lower limb surgery. There are, however, several ways in which the threat can be reduced; see Chapter 5. In addition, simply elevating the lower end of the bed by an angle of only 10° will increase blood flow in the lower limbs by as much as 30%.

Janet started walking on the 3rd day after surgery, with the aid of crutches. These were easily accepted and Janet had progressed to sticks by the time of her discharge 9 days later. By then, Janet could also safely and effectively negotiate stairs, which was a source of great pleasure, although not needed in her bungalow.

Before the patient starts walking again a check X-ray is taken to ensure that the new prosthesis is correctly located and positioned. The surgeon decides when postoperative mobilization should commence: this is usually after 1–3 days for the patient without complications. Mobilization is initiated by the physiotherapist or nurse, who decides which walking aid is the most appropriate. Usually, the patient is taught to stand and begins to walk gently with a walking frame, proceeding to crutches and finally to a stick (or sticks) by the time of discharge. Each progression is monitored carefully by the nursing or physiotherapy staff before the use of less supportive equipment is allowed.

Exercises for knee replacement surgery

Following knee replacement surgery, a CPM machine may be used to assist the patient by putting his knee through a series of pre-set flexion/extension movements with no active effort on his part. Exercises to build up the quadriceps muscles are also encouraged: the patient attempts to straight leg raise and to force the knee down on to a flat, firm surface. An active flexion of 90° is aimed for prior to discharge; if necessary the physiotherapist can arrange treatment on an outpatient basis. Unless the patient continues to exercise following discharge, the knee joint may soon stiffen and require further treatment, possibly a return to theatre for manipulation under a general anaesthetic.

Exercises for hip replacement surgery

To prevent accidental adduction and possible dislocation of the new hip joint, the patient is taught to leave the bed on the affected side and to enter on the unaffected side. In this way, a state of abduction is always maintained in the affected joint.

The physiotherapist or nurse should discuss with the patient whether he is able to continue this at home as the home setting may not permit such movements; for example, the bed may be placed against a wall or the patient may have slept on one side of a double bed for many years and refuse to change. In such instances, members of the multidisciplinary team should suggest other ways of maintaining safety, which may be initiated in the hospital.

The nurse or physiotherapist should ensure that the patient fully understands which activities he can undertake on discharge from hospital. The advice that the nurse should give to the patient before he is discharged is included later in this chapter.

Sleeping

Janet was frequently disturbed during her first postoperative night. Although the nursing staff tried to co-ordinate events to allow for longer periods of rest, this was not always possible. Turning, observations, drug administration, use of bedpans and other activities allowed little time for quality sleep. During subsequent nights, however, there was little disturbance, and Janet soon returned to a regular sleeping pattern. The use of a mild analgesic and assistance with position changes facilitated this.

Sleep can be disturbed in the period following joint replacement due to discomfort, nursing procedures, infusions, noise from fellow patients and many other factors. The nurse may help the patient to obtain a good night's rest by putting him in a comfortable position, providing the appropriate prescribed medication and generally considering the effects of ward noise levels and light. A mild sedative is often effective, particularly for the first-time user.

Communicating

Janet was discharged home 11 days following surgery. As Janet's husband was able to provide support, the multidisciplinary team had few arrangements to make for her care. She was given an outpatient appointment for 6 weeks after surgery, a letter for her general practitioner, outlining all treatment received, and a week's supply of an oral analgesic, although she seldom required these.

The physiotherapist felt that there was no need to arrange outpatient treatment, but reinforced the need for regular exercise. The occupational therapist provided Janet with a long-handled shoe horn and a stocking aid, and Janet's husband purchased a bathing seat from the local branch of a high street chemist, and also provided transport.

The confident, self-caring patient who is sent home with inadequate preparation may soon encounter unexpected difficulties. The nurse should carry out a thorough assessment of a patient's social situation upon his admission to hospital, to identify any areas liable to cause problems at a later date and to alert other members of the multidisciplinary team to his needs.

The nurse should try to determine the following when assessing the patient:

1. Suitability of accommodation; the nurse should identify areas such as the presence of lifts or stairs, toilet and bathing facilities, proximity to shops, size of residence and number of inhabitants, and type of accommodation.

2. Home support; the presence of family or friends should be looked into, and any areas where support may be lacking identified. Once such lack of support has been discussed, the nurse may, with the patient's knowledge and consent, involve relevant services and voluntary organizations such as home help and local authority housing departments.

Working and playing

Janet intended to resume her work with the Women's Royal Voluntary Service after a period of rest of 3–4 months. She felt that this period would allow her to concentrate on recovery without having commitments which would become unenjoyable chores if she embarked on them prematurely. She did, however, intend to begin a little light gardening. She realized that movement would have to be restricted to bending or sitting, but the personal satisfaction it gave her made it worthwhile.

The resumption of working or spare time activities will depend on how much additional strain is put on the new joint prosthesis during the activity. Those activities that are very physical may place an unnecessary degree of stress upon the joint and may have to be curtailed or modified. The nurse should discuss with the patient what activities he can undertake before discharge and suggest alternatives if necessary.

Sexuality

Janet soon began to use make-up again and took great care in making herself look presentable. Even whilst on bedrest she was able to use her hair-styling wand to enhance her appearance and improve her self-image. When mobile, Janet also dressed during the day, wearing loose-fitting cotton dresses (the ward temperature was always high) and flat shoes.

The question of resuming sexual relations did not arise, although Janet did confide that initially her husband was going to sleep in the spare bedroom, to allow her to exercise during the night if she awoke.

Many patients want to raise the question of when it is safe to resume sexual relations following surgery but find it too embarrassing to do so. The nurse should provide the opportunity or even initiate such a discussion, allowing the patient to decide how much information is required. The advice usually given to patients following total hip replacement surgery is that it is safe to resume sexual intercourse in the passive role at approximately 6 weeks. Patients following knee replacement surgery may resume sexual relations at any time but they may find that the passive role is the most comfortable. For the patient who finds taking the passive role in love-making undesirable or not acceptable, the safety factor must be stressed at all times.

Longer-term complications of joint replacement surgery

Longer-term complications of joint replacement surgery include the following:

- A fractured femoral component
- Pain resulting from infection
- A loose femoral component; in total hip

arthroplasty this is now the most common complication of that procedure (Ling 1981).

Stem fracture of the femoral, tibial or humeral prosthetic component is usually related to metal fatigue. As Charnley (1975) reported: 'Stem fractures did not present a serious problem until the 1970s even though joint replacement has been performed in Britain since the early 1960s'.

Sudden onset of pain is the usual feature of prosthetic stem fracture, although in some cases the fracture may be asymptomatic for some time. Diagnosis is made following radiographic examination, and treatment is revision of the affected component.

If the prosthetic component becomes loose, the treatment of choice is a revision arthroplasty, providing that there is adequate bone stock, as every revision of the arthroplasty will require fresh reaming into the active bone. After such operations the patient is instructed to continue to use crutches for 4–6 weeks, to allow adequate time for healing to occur.

Rehabilitation of the post-joint replacement patient

On discharge from hospital, patients are offered advice on how best to protect their new joints. The provision of printed information sheets is the most effective way of ensuring that patients receive advice essential to their progress; these should be given in conjunction with advice from the physiotherapist and the occupational therapist.

The patient should be most careful during the first 3 months following surgery when muscle and tissue surrounding the joint are healing and consequently less stable:

- The patient is advised to use crutches or sticks when mobilizing.
- A stair rail, if available, should be used for ascending and descending stairs: the patient should be taught to lead with the good leg when climbing and with the healing one when descending.
- When picking up objects from the floor, the patient is advised to hold onto a firm surface with the healing limb extended posteriorly to

avoid putting excessive, unnecessary strain on the less stable hip.

- Walking is excellent exercise and can be increased gradually.
- Use of an upright chair with arms is advisable; low chairs and sofas should be avoided.
- Bathing aids, as supplied or suggested by the occupational therapist, are useful. Feet can be washed with long-handled sponges and dried with a handle with a towel attached.
- Driving can usually be commenced after 4–6 weeks, provided that insurance cover is available.
- Dancing: ballroom dancing is safe, but the patient must avoid sudden twisting which puts extra strain on the new joint.
- If the ankles swell, they should be elevated when resting.
- The patient may find that he tires more easily because of the nature of this surgery.
- Body weight should be kept as close to the patient's ideal weight as possible, as it is a major cause of stress on the new lower limb prosthesis.
- Any infection, even as seemingly minor as a septic finger or chest infection, must be reported to the patient's general practitioner and appropriate treatment given, as the foreign body of the prosthesis will act as a focus for sepsis.

A success rate of 100% following joint replacement surgery cannot be guaranteed, but results show that 95% of patients are free from pain and in time regain three-quarters of the range of movement of a normal, undiseased joint (Arthritis Research Council 1989).

OTHER OPERATIONS FOR TREATING OSTEOARTHRITIC HIPS/ KNEES

Osteotomy

An osteotomy is the surgical division of a bone and may be used by surgeons in a variety of circumstances. In the older osteoarthritic patient, however, osteotomy is usually performed to redistribute the load placed upon an already diseased joint in the hope of easing discomfort, and in the young patient, to postpone the need for joint replacement surgery.

Arthrodesis

An arthrodesis is the surgical fusion of a joint into a position that enables the patient to retain maximum function. The patient sacrifices all movement within the athrodesed joint but is free of pain. It is performed on patients who have severely disabling pain from advanced disease, and may be carried out on one or more joints.

CONCLUSION

The orthopaedic nurse has a significant role to play in the care of the individual with osteoarthritis. This may extend from the early stages of the disease process, when the patient is seeking information and wants to understand what is happening to him, to the period when nursing care is required during the various forms of therapy. Whatever the nature of the care required it will be long term, and the nurse delivering it will need to be knowledgeable and skilled.

REFERENCES

Adams J C, Hamblen D L 1990 Outline of orthopaedics, 11th edn. Churchill Livingstone, Edinburgh, p 117
Arthritis & Rheumatism Council 1989 Sexual aspects and parenthood. ARC, London
Banwell G F, Gall V 1988 Physical therapy management of arthritis. Churchill Livingstone, Edinburgh
Bird H 1990 Osteoarthritis 1. Practice Nurse 13(1): 24–26
Brusseau B 1988 Overcoming rheumatism and arthritis naturally. Century Hutchinson, London
Charnley J 1975 Fracture of femoral prostheses in total hip replacement. Clinical Orthopaedics and Related Research 111: 105
Cobb J P 1990 Why use drains? Journal of Bone & Joint Surgery 72B
Croft P 1990 Review of the UK data on rheumatic disease. 3. Osteoarthritis. British Journal of Rheumatology 29(5): 391–395
Dandy D J 1989 Essential orthopaedics & trauma. Churchill Livingstone, Edinburgh, p 72
Dickens W, Lewith G T 1989 A single, blind, controlled and

randomized clinical trial to evaluate the effect of acupuncture in the treatment of trapezio-metacarpal osteoarthritis (study). Complementary Medical Research 3(2): 5–8

Dobree C 1988 Arthritis: your questions answered. Ebury Press, London

Duckworth T 1984 Lecture notes on orthopaedics and fractures, 2nd ed. Blackwell Scientific, Oxford, ch 39, p 255

Garret J 1983 Health needs of the elderly, the essentials of nursing. Macmillan, London

Hornsby V 1985 Osteoarthritis of the hip joint. Nursing 44: 1318–1320

Hughes S P F 1988 The role of antibiotics in preventing infection following total hip replacement. Journal of Hospital Infection 11 (suppl C): 41–47

Kramer J S, Yelling E H, Epstein W V 1983 Social and economic impacts of four musculoskeletal conditions. Arthritis & Rheumatism 26: 901

Leitch M 1987 Living with arthritis. Collins, London, p 8–9

Ling R S M 1981 Loosening experiences at Exeter. Orthopaedic Transactions 5: 351

Love C 1986 Do you lift or roll? Nursing Times 82(29): 44–46

McRae R 1990 Clinical orthopaedic examination, 3rd edn. Churchill Lingstone, Edinburgh, p 202

Offices for Population Censuses & Surveys. 1990 Mortality & morbidity figures. HMSO, London

Quintet R 1986 Therapies to keep the osteoarthritic patient mobile. Geriatric Medicine 16(11): 23–26

Roper N, Logan W, Tierney A 1980 The elements of nursing. Churchill Livingstone, Edinburgh

SPOD 1990 Physical handicap and sexual intercourse: positions. Resource & Information Leaflet No 2. SPOD, London

Van Diemen A H 1985 Prevention of postoperative infection using chlorhexidine soap. Ziekenhuis Hygiene & Infektiepreventie 4: 123–127

Walker I D, Davidson J F 1985 Fibrinolysis. In: Thompson J R (ed) Blood coagulation and homeostasis. A practical guide, 3rd edn. Churchill Livingstone, Edinburgh

Weinberger M, Tierney W, Booker P, Hiner S 1990 Social support, stress and functional status in patients with osteoarthritis. Social Science and Medicine 3(4): 503–508

Willett K M et al 1988 The effect of suction drains after total hip replacement. Journal of Bone & Joint Surgery 70b(4): 604–610

FURTHER READING

Adams J C (1990) Outline of orthopaedics, 11th edn. Churchill Livingstone, Edinburgh

Dandy D J (1989) Essential orthopaedics and trauma. Churchill Livingstone, Edinburgh

Farrell J (1986) Illustrated guide to orthopaedic nursing, 3rd edn. Lippincott, London

Footner A (1987) Orthopaedic nursing. Bailliere Tindall, London

Powell M (1986) Orthopaedic nursing and rehabilitation, 9th edn. Churchill Livingstone, Edinburgh

Which 1989 Living with arthritis. Which way to health June: 24–27

11

Rheumatoid arthritis

Amanda Matthew
Carol A. Humphreys

INTRODUCTION TO RHEUMATOID ARTHRITIS

This chapter describes our present understanding of rheumatoid arthritis. It describes the available information reflecting our significant but incomplete knowledge of the disease. To demonstrate the enormity of the effect the disease process has on sufferers, two case studies are presented and these are related to the relevant nursing care.

HISTORICAL PERSPECTIVE

Rheumatic diseases have been recognized since the 5th century BC under the general term of arthritis. Gout, for example, is now known to be one of the commonest rheumatic diseases and was referred to by Hippocrates as 'the most violent, tenacious and painful of joint affections' (Copeman & Scott 1978). Unlike osteoarthrosis, which was observed in the skeletons of the ape man, rheumatoid arthritis (RA) was not clearly described before the 19th century. Although rheumatoid arthritis is unique to man, there is a rheumatic disease seen in primates which bears some resemblance to it (Boyle & Buchanan 1971).

Around the middle of the 19th century, Sir Archibald Garrod first applied the term rheumatoid arthritis to an 'inflammatory affection of joints' (Copeman & Scott 1978).

DIAGNOSIS AND ONSET

The disease is diagnosed when the rheumatoid

Table 11.1 Criteria for diagnosis of rheumatoid arthritis: the disease is diagnosed when at least four of these are present

Morning stiffness
Arthritis of three or more joint areas
Arthritis of hand joints
Symmetrical arthritis
Rheumatoid nodules
Serum rheumatoid factor
Radiological changes

patient fulfils at least four of the criteria shown in Table 11.1. Criteria 1 to 4 must have been present for at least 6 weeks.

The most common sites of involvement are the synovial joints of the hands, wrists, feet, knees and neck. Other synovial joints that may be involved are those of the lumbar spine, anterior chest wall, shoulder, elbow, hip and occasionally the temporomandibular joint. Periarticular manifestations of the disease may be present in muscles, tendons, tendon sheaths and bursae.

In 80% of all patients with rheumatoid arthritis there is widespread predominantly peripheral symmetrical polyarthritis; monoarticular onset occurs in about 20% of all cases, usually in the knee or wrist (Edmonds & Hughes 1985). The patient complains of pain and stiffness with functional impairment or weakness and soft tissue swelling in the affected joints. Early morning joint stiffness is a particular feature. This is related to an accumulation of local oedema in the joint capsule and associated structures. In the inflamed joint the increase of fluid causes further swelling of tissues that are already stretched.

The effects of the disease may vary in severity from chronic disability to relatively minor clinical manifestations. A general feeling of ill health may precede the arthritis for several months.

Acute, irregular attacks of pain and swelling usually affecting only one or two joints for 2–3 days are known as a 'palindromic onset'. Some of these patients will develop rheumatoid arthritis, while others will develop systemic lupus erythematosus (SLE) or another inflammatory joint disease.

Rheumatoid arthritis runs a prolonged fluctuating course with remissions and exacerbations; the latter may be induced by pregnancy (Edmonds & Hughes 1985), with a flare of activity in the puerperium (Wood 1978, Dieppe et al 1985). Use of the contraceptive pill may have a possible protective effect which may postpone or modify the onset of RA (Silman & Vandenbroucke 1989). These associations suggest that hormonal factors may be influential.

EPIDEMIOLOGY

Rheumatoid arthritis is a common disease which appears to have a world-wide distribution. It is a chronic, systemic, articular inflammatory disease of the synovial membrane affecting approximately 1.5 million people in the UK (Hickling & Golding 1984). The overall prevalence rate for RA in the adult population is 1%. In the UK, one in four patients visit their general practitioner with an 'arthritic' problem (Wright & Haslock 1984).

There is a marked sex difference in the incidence of RA; the disease is three times more common in women than in men (Kraag 1989). The prevalence of RA increases with age in both sexes, with the difference ratio remaining relatively constant. It is more prevalent among people between the ages of 20 and 60 years with a peak incidence in women of between 40 and 60 years. Recent research from the USA and the UK shows that there may be a decline in the incidence of RA, particularly in females.

ENVIRONMENTAL FACTORS

There appears to be no direct cause and effect relationship between the incidence of RA and a person's occupation. A link between social status and rheumatic disease remains unproven. The relationship between diet and rheumatoid disease remains uncertain, but it receives considerable attention. Where there is a tendency towards obesity, this may exacerbate a chronic arthritis of the joints.

Ambient temperature and pain threshold

A certain mythology exists in people's minds about the effect of climatic changes on disease progression. There is often considered to be a greater frequency of the disease in cold, wet climatic conditions. Patients will talk about an increase in joint stiffness and associated pain in damp weather. Warmth and sunshine are regarded as having the opposite effect.

However, in a study carried out by Boyle and colleagues in 1967 in which a comparison was made between tribes of American Indians inhabiting two different climatic regions, there was found to be no statistically significant difference in the prevalence of rheumatoid arthritis.

Patients also frequently associate rheumatism with the weather; they may find the information sheet *Rheumatism and the Weather* published by the Arthritis and Rheumatism Council useful (ARC 1988).

GENETIC ASPECTS

Wood (1978) suggests that the principal clues likely to emerge from family studies are environmental rather than inherited. However, where there is a family history of the disease, individuals have an increased frequency of the human leukocyte antigen (HLA) HLA-DR4 and are considered genetically predisposed to rheumatoid disease (Holland & Jayson 1981).

AETIOLOGY

The cause of rheumatoid arthritis is still unknown. Many factors have been examined in an attempt to unravel the mystery of this disease: infective, metabolic, allergy-related, immunological, etc. It is a complex disease with many theories about polyarthritic changes occurring in conjunction with bacterial infections such as gonorrhoea and pneumococcal pneumonia, and viral illnesses. Investigations were made into the immunological aspects of rheumatoid arthritis with the discovery of the rheumatoid factor by Waaler in 1940 and by Rose and co-workers in 1948.

A connection between the aetiology and the prognosis of rheumatoid arthritis, and emotional and psychological factors, is suggested by the observation that emotional stress and anxiety precipitate deterioration (Elliot 1979, Dieppe et al 1985). Rheumatoid arthritis creates major life stresses for patients and families who encounter the disease. The stress often associated with the disease may be due to any one of the following factors: its uncertain pathogenesis, unpredictable course, and the potential for physical disability.

Despite intensive research, the causative agent is still unknown; however, there are three hypotheses that might be significant:

1. Immunological
2. Genetic
3. Infective.

Immunological

Some people argue that rheumatoid arthritis is caused by an autoimmune response. Complex immunological processes may play a central role in antigen/antibody production activating the immune response and causing polymorphonuclear leukocytes to migrate into the joint. The polymorphs then phagocytose immune complexes, resulting in inflammation and subsequent synovitis.

An alteration in the body's own proteins may occur, with the formation of antibodies. Rheumatoid blood contains substances which act as antibodies to gamma globulin; these substances are known as rheumatoid factors (RF). Rheumatoid factors consist of immunoglobulins (IgM and IgG) which behave as autoantibodies reacting with a patient's own gamma globulin. RFs may be detected both in the serum and in the synovium of most patients with rheumatoid arthritis.

Patients with rheumatoid arthritis may be termed 'seropositive' or 'seronegative' to the presence of RF in the serum. Olsen (1989) states that early studies indicate a less severe course for seronegative than for seropositive disease.

Infective

Intra-articular infective agents seem a likely cause of RA, stimulating immunological changes in the synovium and joint fluid. Various viruses have been isolated but, as yet, no organism has been identified. It is possible that infection with a microorganism can initiate RF production in genetically susceptible individuals. The production of RF is thought to be self-perpetuating, i.e. it does not depend on the continued presence of the initiating infection. The agents currently being considered are the Epstein-Barr Virus (EBV), mycobacteria and retroviruses.

PATHOLOGY

The pathological changes which occur in rheumatoid arthritis are centred on the synovial joints. Articular synovial tissue is the target, with altered pathology affecting non-articular tissues, i.e. the synovial membranes of tendon sheaths and bursae. Figure 11.1 illustrates a typical synovial joint.

The pathological changes proceed in three stages (Fig. 11.2):

- Stage 1   Cellular
- Stage 2   Inflammatory
- Stage 3   Destructive.

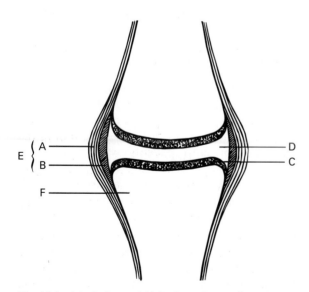

Fig. 11.1 A typical synovial joint (from Gunn 1992, with permission): A. Fibrous capsule; B. Synovial membrane; C. Articular hyaline cartilage; D. Joint cavity filled with synovial fluid; E. Joint capsule; F. Articulating bone.

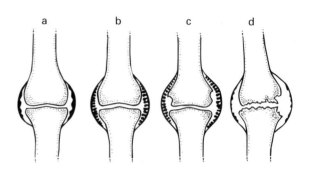

Fig. 11.2 Three stages of rheumatoid arthritis: A. The normal joint; B. Stage 1, cellular phase; C. Stage 2, inflammatory phase; D. Stage 3, destructive phase.

Cellular phase

In the early stages of the disease the synovial membrane is initially affected. The joints are warm, swollen and tender and movement is limited. These features are a result of inflammation of the synovium, oedema, hypertrophy and joint effusions.

The lymphocytes and plasma cells aggregate to form lymphoid follicles, synthesizing and secreting rheumatoid factors which react with immunoglobulins to form immune complexes.

Inflammatory phase

Activation of the complement system results in the accumulation of large numbers of granulocytes in the synovial fluid. During the inflammatory process the granulocytes are destroyed, releasing lysozomal enzymes.

Destructive phase

Primary destruction occurs in the avascular hyaline articular cartilage. Local damage leads to irreversible tissue injury with little possibility of hyaline cartilage regeneration. Vascular granulation tissue known as 'pannus' produces destructive proteases and collagenases which erode demineralized cartilage and bone. The pannus forms a marginal erosive process, working inwards until all cartilage is destroyed. Opposing articular cartilage becomes linked by fibrous tissue, forming collagenous adhesions.

Persistent synovitis and large effusions along with osteoporotic changes cause abnormal stress on the joint. Instability of the joint occurs through destruction of the articular cartilage, joint capsule and ligaments, resulting in instability with subluxation and gross deformity characteristic of rheumatoid arthritis.

CLINICAL FEATURES

'Rheumatoid disease' is a more suitable term to use when describing rheumatoid arthritis, since there are so many systemic features as well as extra-articular features to consider.

The pattern of emergence is one of generalized joint stiffness affecting first the metacarpophalangeal (MCP) joints of the hands. Joint stiffness is most noticeable after periods of inactivity, occurring early in the mornings and lasting between 30 minutes and several hours. This is accompanied by signs of synovitis:

- warmth of affected joints
- pain
- tenderness
- swelling of joints
- oedema of the hands and feet
- atrophy of nearby muscles
- muscle wasting becomes obvious.

The presence of stiff painful joints affects the patient's ability to function normally. Performing simple activities of daily living becomes difficult, with loss of hand power and grip being prominent. The onset of rheumatoid arthritis may be accompanied by symptoms of malaise, fatigue, anorexia, weight loss, fever and myalgia.

Symmetrical joint involvement is usual with the disease progressing to the feet, elbows, shoulders, knees and ankles. Asymmetrical involvement may be an early presentation, especially when the large joints are targeted.

Specific articular features

The classical distribution of joint involvement is shown in Figure 11.3. Some of the characteristic features in rheumatoid arthritic joints are described below.

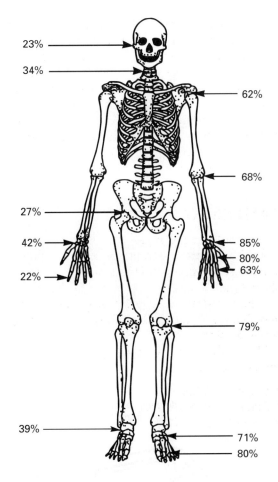

Fig. 11.3 The classical distribution of joint involvement in rheumatoid arthritis. (From Dieppe et al 1985, with permission.)

Hands

Early in the disease there is muscle wasting with swelling of the MCP joints and spindling of the proximal interphalangeal (PIP) joints. Tenosynovitis leads to impaired function with loss of grip and 'triggering' of the finger (Fig. 11.4).

Palmar subluxation of the MCP joints results in swan-neck (Fig. 11.5) and boutonnière or button-hole (Fig. 11.6) deformities of the fingers. Other characteristics associated with rheumatoid arthritis include ulnar (Fig. 11.7) or radial deviation of the hand and Z-deformity of the thumb (Fig. 11.8). Deviation is due partly to synovitis of the MCP joints and rupture of the 4th and 5th extensor tendons (Fig. 11.9).

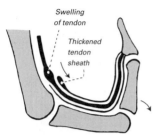

Fig. 11.4 Trigger finger deformity. (From Adams 1990, with permission.)

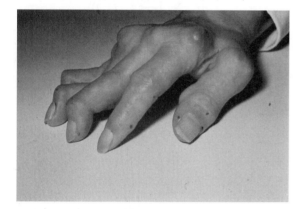

Fig. 11.5 Swan neck deformity of middle, ring and little fingers. (From Dr R Jubb, with permission.)

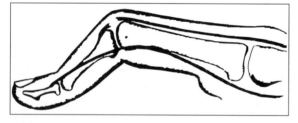

Fig. 11.6 Boutonnière deformity. (From Kane 1981, with permission.)

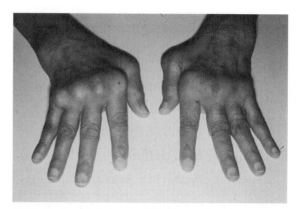

Fig. 11.7 Ulnar deviation. (From Dr R Jubb, with permission.)

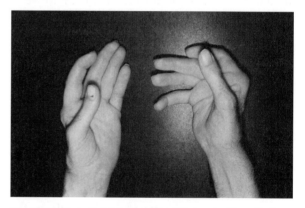

Fig. 11.8 Early Z-deformity of the left thumb. (From Dr R Jubb, with permission.)

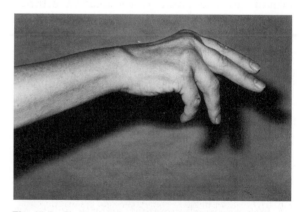

Fig. 11.9 Rupture of the extensor tendons 4th and 5th fingers. (From Dr R Jubb, with permission.)

These deformities, although debilitating, still allow modified movement to which the patient can adapt.

The fingers of a rheumatoid arthritic often appear shortened and floppy. This shortening and 'telescoping' is typical in severe cases of the disease (Fig. 11.10).

Wrists

Initially, soft tissue swelling and synovial hyper-

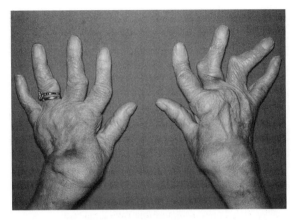

Fig. 11.10 Shortening and telescoping of the fingers. (From Dr R Jubb, with permission.)

trophy are present with ulnar nerve entrapment, causing wasting of the dorsal interossei. A common occurrence is prominence of the ulnar styloid due to inflammation and subluxation in the radio-ulnar joint, with the ulnar head being pulled upwards by the dorsal carpal ligaments, producing a 'dinner-fork' deformity. Instability from joint subluxation and rupture of tendons results in severe loss of grip. Carpal tunnel syndrome with compression of the median nerve may occur, with extensive pain which is severe at night.

Feet

Pain and tenderness from synovitis of the metatarsophalangeal (MTP) joints occur early. Synovitis and oedema around the metatarsal heads

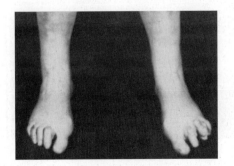

Fig. 11.11 Synovitis and oedema around the metatarsal heads push the toes apart, allowing 'daylight' to be seen between them. (From Powell 1986, with permission.)

push the toes apart, allowing 'daylight' to be seen between them (Fig. 11.11).

Destruction of the MTP joints leads to subluxation of the metatarsal heads, where unprotected bone must bear the patient's full weight. The toes become clawed with painful callosities, and pressure sores develop under the 2nd and 3rd metatarsal heads and over the proximal interphalangeal (PIP) joints in particular (Fig. 11.12). Comfortable shoes are very difficult to find, and ill-fitting footwear increases the problems associated with pressure lesions.

Hallux valgus deformity often occurs with a prominent bunion (bursa), and the toes can be seen to override one another. The foot appears flattened due to collapse of the longitudinal arch.

Ankle

The ankle joint has very little synovial tissue and therefore is not greatly affected by rheumatoid arthritis. Pain is common due to tendinitis of the posterior and peroneal tendons.

The subtalar joint is more involved, being responsible for inversion of the ankle. Valgus deformity is usually due to joint changes of the talonavicular joint.

Knees

Fixed flexion deformities may occur early as a result of synovitis and joint effusions (Fig. 11.13), and there is evidence of quadriceps muscle wasting. The knee becomes unstable due to laxity of the lateral and medial ligaments and instability of the anterior and posterior cruciate ligaments. The patella may become mobile.

High intra-articular pressure may give rise to the rupture of bursae at the back of the knee, with leakage of synovial fluid into the calf producing severe pain, swelling and tenderness. This acute rupture of a Baker's cyst (Fig. 11.14) may be confused with a deep vein thrombosis, as the patient presents with a positive Homans' sign. An arthrogram will clarify the diagnosis.

Cervical spine

Cervical spine involvement is a frequent cause

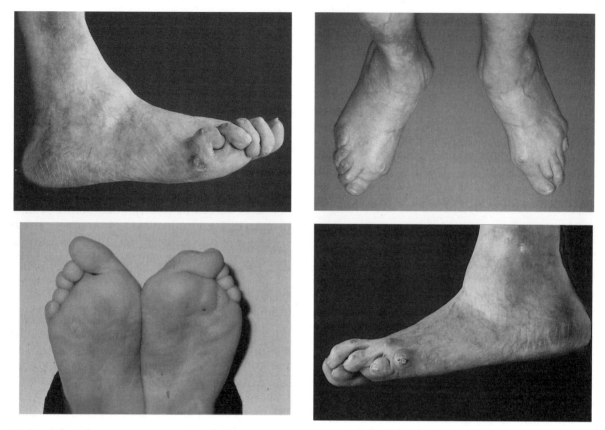

Fig. 11.12   Callosities over the metatarsal heads; such sites are prone to the development of pressure sores. (From Mr J L Plewes, with permission.)

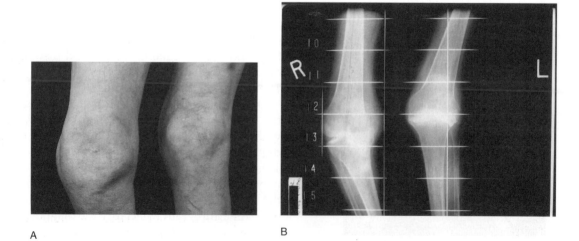

A

B

Fig. 11.13   A. Valgus and varus deformity of the knees – 'windswept' knees. There is also evidence of muscle wasting on the left. B. X-ray appearance of this deformity. (From Mr J L Plewes, with permission.)

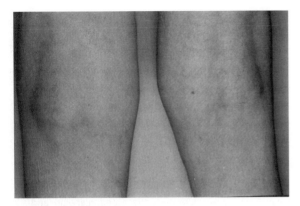

Fig. 11.14 Baker's cyst. (From Dr R Jubb, with permission.)

of pain and associated disability and may lead to upper limb paraesthesia or, if severe, quadriplegia. Changes are seen primarily at the atlantoaxial joint, with further multiple subluxations occurring between C2 and C6 (Fig. 11.15).

Rheumatoid changes affect the synovial-lined bursae surrounding the odontoid peg at the atlantoaxial joint. Normally the odontoid peg is held in place against the anterior arch of the atlas by the transverse ligament of the atlas. Synovitis

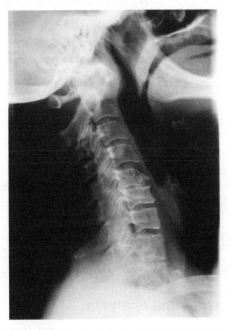

Fig. 11.15 Rheumatoid changes of the cervical spine. (From Mr J L Plewes, with permission.)

results in changes to the odontoid peg including erosion, a reduction in size, and weakness and laxity of the transverse ligament. These changes lead to instability of the head on the neck, particularly during flexion.

Cervical involvement may cause pressure on the vertebrobasilar artery resulting in transient vertigo, ocular disturbances and hemiparesis. Vertical subluxation, in which the odontoid peg is pushed up into the foramen magnum, may also be seen on X-ray.

The patient with rheumatoid arthritis of the neck is most at risk when requiring a general anaesthetic. The anaesthetist would probably advise that the patient should wear a cervical collar for support during surgery.

Shoulder joint

This joint has the widest range of movement. An affected shoulder joint considerably limits the patient's functional ability and independence. The primary site of inflammation is the glenohumeral joint, with involvement of the acromioclavicular joint. External rotation, internal rotation, abduction and elevation are all affected, making it difficult for the patient to carry out activities of living such as combing hair or dressing. As the disease progresses the shoulder may become fixed, with the majority of movement coming from the scapula.

Elbow

Pain, stiffness and joint deformity will limit movement at the elbow. There is early loss of extension and reduced flexion resulting in fixed flexion deformity. Bursitis may be present. Extra-articular features such as rheumatoid nodules are common around the extensor aspect of the elbow (Fig. 11.16).

Hip

The hip joint is not frequently affected. In patients with evidence of hip disease there is limitation of movement with referred pain to the knee. Synovitis causes pain on weight-bearing.

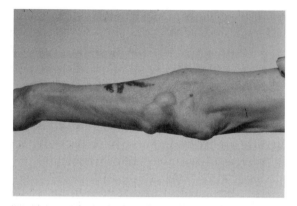

Fig. 11.16 Rheumatoid nodules at the elbow joint. (From Dr R Jubb, with permission.)

Extra-articular features

Rheumatoid arthritis predominantly affects articular joints. Periarticular features occur outside the joint and involve soft tissue structures (Table 11.2). Non-articular systemic features are common (Table 11.3). Of rheumatoid arthritic patients, 75% present with two or more extra-articular features which are generally associated with seropositivity. The presence of extra-articular features may be indicative of the severity of the disease and an adverse prognosis.

There are many extra-articular features associated with rheumatoid arthritis, but the presence of nodules is very characteristic and therefore requires further explanation.

Nodules Nodules are a major extra-articular feature of rheumatoid arthritis. They are commonly subcutaneous, though they may be intradermal, subperiosteal or found in a number of organs including the heart and lung. They are seen over pressure points, and are commonly found at the elbow (Fig. 11.16). They may also occur along tendons, favouring the Achilles tendon.

In the heart they may lead to mitral valve disease. Nodules may occur in the lung, and on chest X-ray can be confused with neoplasms. A needle biopsy of the nodule will confirm the diagnosis. The presence of nodules tends to signify an adverse prognosis.

INVESTIGATIONS

Investigations into rheumatoid arthritis are

Table 11.2 Periarticular features of rheumatoid arthritis

Features	Clinical manifestations
Nodules	20–30% of cases usually below the elbow, but may develop anywhere, e.g. pleural nodules 3–20 mm in diameter usually firm, non-tender and mobile, often multiple generally in seropositive patients, but may be seen in seronegative patients as a result of treatment signify an adverse prognosis
Tenosynovitis	involving hands and wrists affects extensor tendon sheath, and flexor tendons causes: pain, tenderness, local swelling, trigger finger and flexion deformity
Bursitis	causes swelling and discomfort usually over the olecranon
Synovial cysts	predominantly posterior to the knee (Baker's cyst) raised intraarticular pressure. Synovial fluid leaks from cyst into calf muscles producing: swelling, severe pain, tenderness and a positive Homans' sign (closely resembling a deep-vein thrombosis)
Muscle wasting	muscle weakness and wasting are very common, caused by reflex inhibition of muscles controlling an inflamed joint inflammatory myositis and steroid myopathy may occur
Ligament laxity	leads to hypermobility and joint deformity, e.g. ulnar deviation, atlantoaxial subluxation

mainly clinical, and include blood tests and X-rays. Haematology results support the diagnosis, but may have limited value. Some of the commonest haematological investigations are listed in Table 11.4. The most useful diagnostic test is radiological examination of the affected joints.

Haematological investigations

These are listed in Table 11.4.

Synovial fluid analysis

Analysis of synovial fluid is useful if only to exclude other conditions such as infection and the presence of crystals. Synovial fluid in RA is

Table 11.3 Non-articular manifestations of rheumatoid arthritis

System	Clinical manifestations
General	malaise, possible fever, tiredness, myalgia, anaemia, anorexia and depression
Vasculitis	nail-fold lesions and splinter haemorrhages large vessel arteritis chronic leg ulcers and peripheral neuropathy Raynaud's phenomenon
Haemopoietic	anaemia lymphadenopathy thrombocytosis Felty's syndrome
Cardiac	pericarditis pericardial effusion nodules
Respiratory	pleurisy pleural effusion nodules Caplan's syndrome fibrosing alveolitis
Neuromuscular	muscle wasting entrapment neuropathy peripheral neuropathy
Eye	keratoconjunctivitis episcleritis scleritis scleromalacia performans drug-induced cataracts and retinopathy nodule formation Sjogren's syndrome

light yellow in colour, watery and opaque due to a high white cell count.

A synovial biopsy may be obtained for histological examination. The findings are synonymous with changes in other forms of inflammatory disease and are not specific to RA.

Radiology

Plain X-rays (Fig. 11.17) are essential in the diagnosis and assessment of disease progression in bone and joint diseases.

In the early stages of RA the X-ray findings reflect inflammation due to synovitis: soft tissue swelling, and periarticular osteoporosis – particularly of the PIP, MCP and MTP joints. Erosions appear in the bone, initially at the junction of the synovium with the articular cartilage. These gradually increase in size to form defects in the bone. Narrowing of joint spaces occurs as a result of continued destruction of cartilage.

In later stages of the disease juxta-articular osteoporosis and soft tissue swelling are less pronounced, but erosions develop a firm outline. Further bone destruction is evident. Joint subluxation and deformity become apparent and ankylosis of the carpus may be seen.

In addition to plain films, special techniques may be used to provide greater anatomical detail, such as computed tomography, scintigraphy, magnetic resonance imaging, ultrasound and arthrography.

DRUG THERAPY

A wide selection of drugs is available for the treatment of RA. They will not provide a complete cure but may offer some relief of symptoms. Many patients will use drug therapy in conjunction with some of the other approaches outlined in this chapter.

Drugs used in the treatment of RA can be classified as follows:

1. Analgesics
2. Non-steroidal anti-inflammatory drugs (NSAIDs)
3. Disease-modifying antirheumatic drugs (DMARDs)
4. Corticosteroids
5. Immunosuppressive drugs.

Analgesics

In general, analgesics are used in conjunction with NSAIDs. Patients, especially the elderly, should be aware of the commonest side-effect of analgesics, i.e. constipation, particularly in the case of codeine and dihydrocodeine.

Non-steroidal anti-inflammatory drugs (NSAIDs)

NSAIDs are the drugs used initially in the treatment of RA (first-line-drugs), providing analgesia while controlling inflammation (Fig. 11.18).

Table 11.4 Haematological investigations in rheumatoid arthritis

Rheumatoid factor Test: Latex fixation tests Sheep cell agglutination test (SCAT) (Rose Waaler test)	rheumatoid factors react against the Fc portion of altered gamma globulin seropositive/seronegative refers to the presence or absence of IgM antiglobulin in the serum high titres of RF correlate with disease activity the presence of increased levels from the other major immunoglobulin classes: IgG, IgA, IgM RFs indicate chronic disease activity and a poor prognosis
Antinuclear antibodies Test: Antinuclear antibody test (ANA)	often a positive low titre in rheumatoid arthritis greater significance in Sjogren's syndrome and systemic lupus erythematosis
Anaemia Test: Haemoglobin (Hb)	associated with most chronic diseases drug-induced (related to gastrointestinal bleeding) serum iron is low, and there may be a poor response to oral iron serum ferritin may be normal or high bone marrow stores may be normal or increased
Sedimentation rate Test: Erythrocyte sedimentation rate (ESR) (Plasma viscosity)	generally raised reflecting disease activity elevation may be disproportionate to disease activity, suggesting concurrent illness
Reactive proteins Test: C-reactive proteins (CRP) Serum amyloid-A protein (SAA)	C-reactive proteins are associated more with SLE and Sjogren's syndrome serum amyloid-A develops into secondary amyloidosis levels may be high in RA and Still's disease
Complement levels Test: C1q binding Total haemolytic complement (CH50)	circulating levels of the complement component C1q may be elevated, remaining stable over a period of time as the levels of C1q are relative to disease progression, serum C1q levels can be used as a useful predictor detected by the haemolysis of red blood cells components of complement are also acute phase reactants and raised levels are found in RA significant test in SLE
Hyaluronic acid Test: Serum hyaluronic acid	increased levels of serum hyaluronic acid may be a useful disease marker for synovitis

They do not halt the disease process, and destruction of cartilage and bone continues. There is a wide range of drugs available in this category but their use is accompanied by several side-effects.

The most toxic effect is damage to the gastric mucosa, leading to ulceration, bleeding and perforation. Gastric ulcers are produced predominantly by a local effect, although NSAIDs may exacerbate acute peptic ulcers. It is likely that patients with RA have an increased susceptibility to drug-induced mucosal damage. Age may also be a factor, as well as alcohol, smoking, stress or combinations of other drugs. Gastric irritation may be overcome by giving enteric-coated tablets or using rectal preparations, for example, indomethacin suppositories. Nearly all NSAIDs have the propensity to impair renal function. Although it is possible to overcome some side-effects with more drugs, it is essential that the patient understands the nature of his drug therapy. The importance of positive nurse–patient interaction cannot be over emphasized.

Some drug regimens are so complex in the number and timing of dosages that good compliance is difficult to achieve. Non-compliance may lead to exacerbation of the disease process; thus, it is far better for the patient if the regimen is kept simple.

Disease-modifying antirheumatic drugs (DMARDs)

Patients with RA who do not respond to NSAIDs within a few months should be treated aggressively with DMARDs (second-line drugs). These drugs have:

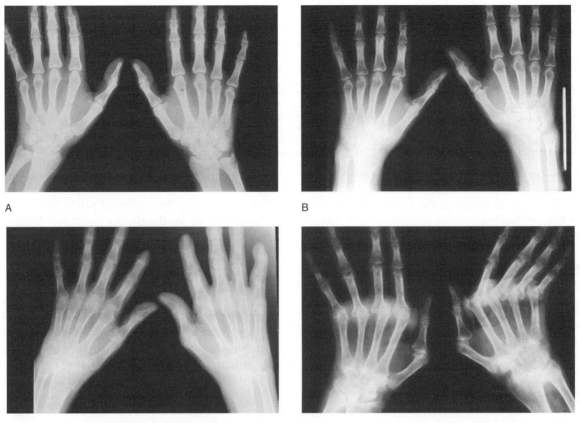

Fig. 11.17 X-rays of hands showing disease progression (from Dr R Jubb, with permission): A. Initial presentation; B. 5 years later; C. 10 years later; D. Advanced rheumatoid arthritis.

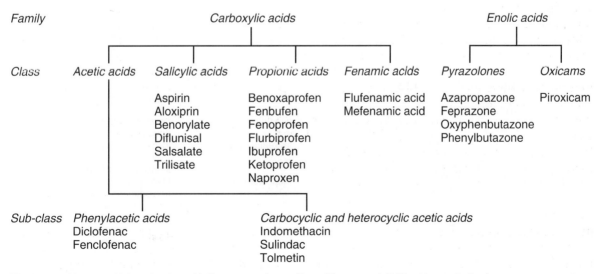

Family			Carboxylic acids				Enolic acids	

Class	Acetic acids	Salicylic acids	Propionic acids	Fenamic acids	Pyrazolones	Oxicams
		Aspirin	Benoxaprofen	Flufenamic acid	Azapropazone	Piroxicam
		Aloxiprin	Fenbufen	Mefenamic acid	Feprazone	
		Benorylate	Fenoprofen		Oxyphenbutazone	
		Diflunisal	Flurbiprofen		Phenylbutazone	
		Salsalate	Ibuprofen			
		Trilisate	Ketoprofen			
			Naproxen			

Sub-class	Phenylacetic acids	Carbocyclic and heterocyclic acetic acids
	Diclofenac	Indomethacin
	Fenclofenac	Sulindac
		Tolmetin

Fig. 11.18 Non-steroidal analgesic anti-inflammatory drugs. (From Dieppe et al 1985, with permission.)

Table 11.5 Disease-modifying antirheumatic drugs (DMARDs)

Agent	Delay in efficacy	Side-effects
Gold injection	4–6 months	pruritic skin rash, stomatitis, proteinuria, haematological effects
Oral gold (Auranofin)	4–6 months	diarrhoea, nausea, rash, proteinuria, haematological effects (frequency of adverse reactions are less compared to gold injections)
Methotrexate	3–4 months	nausea, stomatitis, alopecia or leukopaenia, gastrointestinal intolerance
Hydroxychloroquine	4–6 months	macular degeneration; less frequently: rash, nausea, myopathy (opthalmic effects are reversible)
Sulphasalazine (EC)		nausea, headache, rash haematological effects, hepatic effects
D-penicillamine	12 months	rash, loss of taste, stomatitis, proteinuria, haematological effects
Cyclosporin		impaired liver and renal function, gastrointestinal disturbances, gum hyperplasia

- The ability to suppress the rheumatoid disease process
- Slow onset of action, requiring 3–12 months of therapy
- Frequent mild reactions
- Rare severe reactions.

DMARDs may cause serious toxicity (Table 11.5) more commonly than do NSAIDs; nevertheless, the majority of patients who can tolerate these agents will benefit from them.

Corticosteroids

Corticosteroids are likely to offer greater relief than any other group of drugs due to their anti-inflammatory and immunosuppressive properties. However, steroids have far-reaching systemic side-effects (Table 11.6) and should be used in small doses with caution. The use of corticosteroids should be limited to patients suffering from progressive disease or to the elderly.

Immunosuppressive drugs

These drugs are reserved for those patients who have failed to respond to DMARDs. Immunosuppressive drugs have minimal, non-specific anti-inflammatory actions. These agents should be used in those patients for whom the potential benefits outweigh the potential toxicity.

Intra-articular therapy

Local injection therapy may help to restore comfort and mobility to joints and other synovial structures. It may be employed safely as a means of treatment or for diagnostic purposes. Various agents are used.

PROGNOSIS

The prognosis for the individual with RA is often quite positive. Out of 100 people with RA, 30 will recover completely within a few years, 60 will continue to have joint pain, swelling and exacerbations of their disease leaving them with mild disability, and five will go on to develop

Table 11.6 Side-effects of corticosteroids

System affected	Side-effects
Cardiovascular system	congestive cardiac failure hypertension
Central nervous system	alteration in mood psychosis benign intracranial hypertension
Endocrine/metabolic	Cushingoid features: moon face, truncal obesity, buffalo hump, hirsuitism hyperglycaemia adrenal insufficiency impotence, altered menstrual cycle
Gastrointestinal	peptic ulceration pancreatitis
Immunological	increased susceptibility to infection immune suppression
Musculoskeletal	myopathy osteoporosis avascular necrosis
Ocular	glaucoma posterior subcapsular cataracts
Skin	thin friable skin bruising striae, impaired wound healing

Table 11.7 Classification of rheumatoid arthritis (from Rideout 1992)

Stage	Clinical manifestations	Functional manifestations
Early	no evidence of joint destruction	no loss of functional capacity
Moderate	evidence of some destruction of cartilage and probably of subchondral bone; no deformity but full range of motion may be limited; adjacent muscle atrophy present	able to carry out usual activities despite some discomfort and limited joint mobility
Severe	cartilage and bone destruction quite evident; muscle atrophy and joint deformities such as hyperextension, flexion contracture, ulnar deviation and subluxation present	functional capacity impaired with occupational and self-care activities quite limited
Terminal	criteria of severe stage plus fibrous or bony ankylosis present	confined to a wheelchair or bed; not able to carry out self-care; dependent

severe disease and extensive disability. Table 11.7 offers a classification of RA.

PSYCHOLOGICAL ASPECTS

The image that most people have of arthritis is of crippled bodies in wheelchairs, totally dependent on others.

A period of grieving usually follows the diagnosis, and periods of denial, avoidance, fear, anxiety, anger, despondency, withdrawal and depression are all coping strategies that the patient uses.

The difficulty is that often there is no positive proof of diagnosis, as the rheumatoid factor can be negative; and physicians cannot reliably predict a prognosis, so patients are often left feeling very uncertain about what future they can expect.

As time passes and their body changes shape, they have to come to terms with a change in their body image. What ideas they had about themselves – for example, a handsome young athlete or pretty young woman – have changed to future images of crippled worthless human beings.

From this it can be deduced that patients suffering from rheumatoid arthritis need a great deal of psychological care and understanding, and that all health professionals involved in their care need to be aware of the psychological changes patients experience to be able to fulfil their particular role in the patient's overall care.

The patient and his family should be educated about the disease process, the prevention of deformity, and the maintenance of health and well-being; they should also be made aware of the occasions when medical help must be sought.

Patient counselling on all aspects of the disease will help to avoid misunderstandings and uncertainty. Close relatives should be involved in these discussions so that they can understand the implications of the disease and have an opportunity to discuss their own fears and anxieties.

SOCIOLOGICAL ASPECTS

The physical environment of the rheumatoid arthritis patient is an important factor in the management of his disease. As RA is a life-long process, it is essential that the optimum environmental conditions are achieved to promote the patient's health and well-being. Ultimately the nurse is striving to maintain a good quality of life for the sufferer, his family and friends.

Modifications will almost certainly be required in the home, and gadgets may be needed for the patient to continue with the routine acts of daily living. These aids provide a visual sign that the patient has some form of disability. Many patients find it embarrassing to use such gadgets in front of their friends and relatives. To overcome this stigma and accept these modifications, the patient and his family require time and counselling.

Patients may occasionally find it necessary to change roles within the family. The husband of a female sufferer may take on additional domestic chores, whilst the wife of a male sufferer may find that she needs to go back to work full-time to enable her husband to work part-time. Obviously, these changes can cause emotional, social and psychological trauma to the patient and his family. It is important that nurses recognize this and equip themselves with the necessary knowledge and expertise to help their patients cope with these radical changes in lifestyle.

NURSING MANAGEMENT

The rheumatology health care team traditionally is comprised of a consultant rheumatologist, other medical staff, nurses, physiotherapists, occupational therapists and social workers. The degree of provision for the rheumatoid sufferer varies throughout the country. The major goal for the health care team is to facilitate a holistic approach towards each patient.

The nurse's aim in the management of rheumatoid arthritis is to facilitate the aims of the patient and his family. This will require programmes of care to be adapted symptomatically according to individual needs. The prime aim for the patient is to return to an independent, 'normal' lifestyle as quickly and uneventfully as possible. In the newly diagnosed patient, programmes may focus on the psychological aspect of care rather than the physical aspects. Patients will require counselling to reassure them and their families about their disease.

The manner in which the newly diagnosed patient is nursed can have a considerable effect on the way in which he comes to terms with the disease process later on. It is seen as a 'blueprint of care' for the rest of the patient's life; it is therefore essential that physical, social, psychological and emotional support is given from the outset.

The aims of care for the rheumatoid arthritic patient in hospital are:

1. To reduce pain and stiffness
2. To prevent deformity
3. To maintain the patient's self-esteem.

Pain management

The use of a pain chart (see Ch. 7) is an invaluable tool for measuring the degree of pain experienced and assessing any improvement or deterioration in the level of pain.

Pain and stiffness are the commonest complaints of the rheumatoid arthritis patient. These symptoms prevent him from functioning normally. Analgesia is perhaps the first method the team would consider to reduce pain. Complementary therapies may also be used.

Other measures that may be employed initially, or in combination with analgesia, are described below.

Rest

It is important for the patient to have enough rest, but a good night's sleep is often not enough. The patient is advised to sleep for an hour during the afternoon, to prevent him from becoming fatigued by the end of the day. This may be easy for the housewife who can schedule daily chores to allow for an afternoon nap, but for the working man or woman it may be very difficult.

He may have to negotiate with his employer for a longer midday break, or perhaps take a couple of shorter breaks during the day to allow him to rest. It is important to work out a regimen that suits the individual and then negotiate for this with the employer. Some patients will find a sympathetic ear; other employers may not be so considerate.

Resting splints can be made to support the hands, feet, knees and wrists in the optimum position. Patients should be encouraged to use these resting splints whenever possible to support their joints.

Many patients derive benefit from listening to relaxation tapes when trying to rest. Alternatively, classes are available where patients may learn about other relaxation techniques which can be used at work or in the home.

Application of heat and cold

The benefits of heat or cold on a joint can be established only through individual trial and error. Some patients find that the application of heat to a painful joint is soothing; others may find ice packs have a greater effect. Whichever method is used, the utmost care should be taken to prevent injury to the patient. To avoid an unwanted reaction, a patch test may be carried out prior to the initial application.

Dry heat may be applied by using a hot water bottle wrapped in a towel, or an electric heat pad. Wet heat using a hydropack can be safely applied. The hydropack is preheated and then wrapped in towels before being applied to the skin. Warm wax is an alternative method. The wax is heated to body temperature and the patient immerses his hands or feet in the wax, allowing it to accumulate over the skin. This may be left on for approximately an hour before being peeled off and reheated for use later.

Ice packs consist of crushed ice in a damp cloth bag. To prevent ice burns, arachis oil or a similar preparation should be applied to the skin first. At home an excellent substitute for crushed ice is a packet of frozen peas wrapped in a damp cloth. The ice packs can be left in place for up to 15 minutes.

Warm baths and hydrotherapy

Early morning stiffness may persist for several hours, causing severe problems for the patient. For many, a warm bath first thing in the morning is of considerable benefit. Ideally the temperature of the water should be 97°F, and the whole body should be immersed in the water. The water supports the patient's stiff limbs and the heat soothes his painful joints, enabling him to move more freely. After 15 to 20 minutes the patient should experience a noticeable improvement in his symptoms.

Most rheumatology departments have ready access to baths, such as the Parker bath (Fig. 11.19). Without these warm water baths, patients almost certainly would not be able to carry out their physiotherapy routine. It is for this reason that hydrotherapy can be an important part of treatment, and rheumatology units find that their hydrotherapy pools are indispensable.

Prevention of deformity

One of the aims in the management of RA is the prevention of joint deformity through patient

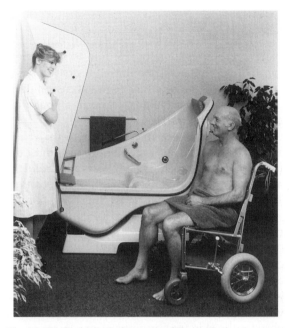

Fig. 11.19 Parker bath (courtesy of Parker Bath Developments Ltd).

education and the use of splints. Deformity will reduce joint function.

Patient education forms a vital part of the patient's care. In the prevention of deformity, patients must be able to recognize the signs and symptoms that indicate a deterioration in their joints.

The occupational therapist (OT) is a key figure in educating the patient in all aspects of joint protection. She assesses the functional status of the patient before making recommendations about adapting behaviour to protect the joints. For example, when polishing a table, the patient is advised to use circular movements towards the body, instead of using circular movements away from the body which increases the risk of ulnar deviation.

Before being discharged from hospital, the patient may be invited to arrange a home visit with the OT so that she can assess the home environment and offer advice on possible modifications or ways to overcome potential difficulties. The OT may advise the patient about his work environment by suggesting possible adaptations or the use of aids that may enhance mobility, efficiency and independence.

Use of splints

The nurse and physiotherapist introduce the patient to splints by allowing him to wear them for short periods of time initially, gradually increasing the duration as he grows accustomed to their use. It is particularly important that they are worn during resting periods.

Resting splints are made for the legs, wrists and hands (Fig. 11.20). Lower limb splints are full-length (they include the foot), and hold the ankle and knee joint in the optimum position. This principle applies to wrist and hand splints, which must also support the joints in the optimum functional position.

Splints are made of plaster of Paris, or more commonly now of a light-weight material such as 'Fractomed', which can be remoulded as the joint changes shape. The nurse should take care when applying and removing the splints, to observe the skin for any signs of pressure.

Positioning

The patient is encouraged to sit upright in bed, well supported by pillows (Fig. 11.21). The natural curves of the spine are supported and spinal deformities are prevented. If the patient is not wearing his splints, the legs should be stretched out with the knees straight and the feet should be resting with the ankle joint at 90° of flexion.

To maintain the position of the feet, a foot board or a rolled-up pillow can be secured to the sides of the bed by a drawsheet (donkey). The patient is strongly discouraged from putting a pillow under the knees as this can lead to flexion deformities.

When the patient is sitting, the chair should be high enough for him to be able to get out of it easily, so reducing the strain on his joints. The chair should encourage a good posture, providing support for the patient's spine while enabling him to place his feet firmly on the floor.

Maintaining self-esteem

Self-esteem is as important for those with physical disability as it is for healthy individuals. Self-esteem embraces the concepts of ego or ego strength, inner self, identity, self-image, personality, self-concept, self-worth, self-respect and self-satisfaction. Self-acceptance, which is fundamental to high self-esteem, may be challenged when previous aspirations, roles and relation-

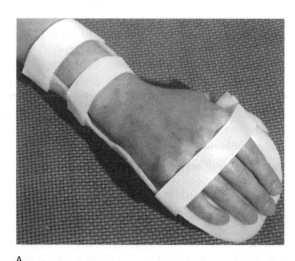

A   B

Fig. 11.20 Wrist and hand splints support the joints in the optimum functional position: A. Resting splint; B. Working splint. (From Turner et al 1992, with permission.)

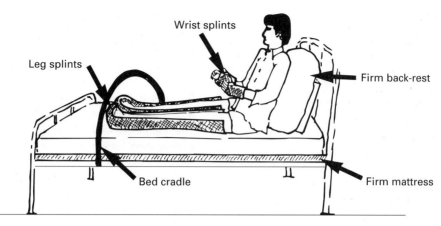

Fig. 11.21 Correct body posture while on bedrest. (From Dieppe et al 1985, with permission.)

ships have to be changed because of illness (Pigg-Smith et al 1985).

According to Maslow's hierarchy of needs (Fig. 11.22), many basic needs have to be met before a person is able to satisfy his esteem needs. This can be quite a chore for the healthy individual, but it is far more difficult for those suffering from a chronic disabling disease such as RA.

With the onset of RA the patient's roles in sexual, family, social and work relationships change. In particular, a hospital admission can take away from the patient control of his own destiny: he is no longer able to handle his own affairs. This increased dependency drastically affects the patient's self-esteem.

Following the initial diagnosis, patients often engage in activities that can cause further damage to their joints. In this way, the patient is trying to appear unaffected by his disease. It is a basic human need for an individual to feel in control of his life and destiny. The patient who continually makes excuses for missing a clinic appointment, or for not performing his exercise programme, may be using denial as a coping strategy.

Conversely, some patients need to satisfy their desire for knowledge of their disease, repeatedly directing the same questions to different members of the health care team. By acting in this way they test the validity of the information they have been given while striving to find the ultimate answer to their problem themselves.

When patients display these types of coping mechanisms it is important that the nurse recognizes this behaviour. She may then show the patient that she is available to listen to his fears and anxieties about the disease and how it will affect his daily activities. The nurse and patient should work towards identifying the positive aspects of the patient's life and relationships, and

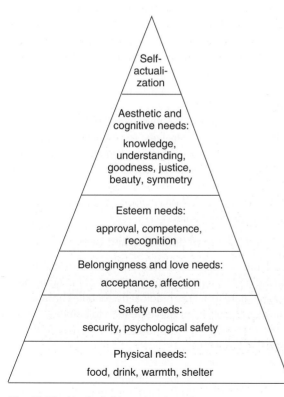

Fig. 11.22 Maslow's hierarchy of needs.

steer away from the negative ones with which the patient may be more concerned.

Changes in body image may also affect the patient's self-esteem (see Ch. 9). At first these may not be physical signs of disease progression; the fact that the patient is experiencing pain, stiffness and fatigue can alter his perception of his body image. Once physical changes occur, the patient will see a visual alteration of his body image. These changes will have a psychological effect on the patient and those people around him.

Sexual relationships may be difficult due to pain, stiffness and fatigue. It may be necessary for the patient to adopt unorthodox positions for sexual intercourse (see Ch. 10). The partner may be afraid of physical contact when touching or caressing the patient for fear of hurting him. If these problems do arise then the patient and his partner should be encouraged to talk to each other about their feelings and the ways in which they might overcome their difficulties.

Using Orem's self-care model with a newly diagnosed rheumatoid arthritis patient

Orem's self-care model is based on how the patient performs self-care. It centres around patient achievement or non-achievement and not on nursing intervention.

There are five assessment stages of the model (Aggleton & Chalmers 1985a):

1. Demand for self-care:
   - sufficient intake of air, water and nutrition
   - satisfactory elimination
   - activity balanced with rest
   - time spent alone balanced with time spent with others
   - prevention of danger to self
   - being 'normal'
2. Ability to carry out the above
3. What are the deficits in self-care and why
4. Does the present state allow the patient to engage safely in self-care
5. Assess potential for self-care in the future.

Orem's self-care model may be implemented using the nursing process of assessment, planning, implementation and evaluation.

Care study 1

Steve is a 40-year-old man who has been admitted with a 'flare' of rheumatoid arthritis in his right knee. The diagnosis of rheumatoid arthritis was made 6 months ago. Steve is married with two young sons aged 10 and 12 years, and works as a shop floor supervisor for a large car manufacturer.

Assessment

Demand for self-care:

1. Intake of water, nutrition and air: Steve was able to satisfy these needs independently.
2. Elimination: Steve expressed no problems with bowel or bladder function.
3. Activity balanced with rest: Steve's main problem was the 'flare' of arthritis in his right knee and the resultant immobility.
4. Time spent alone balanced with time spent with others: At present Steve was having time off work because of the exacerbation of his disease. This was causing him some stress as he feared losing his job due to prolonged sickness.
5. Prevention of danger to self: No problems were identified.
6. Being 'normal': Steve was expressing anger about his disease. He was abrupt when questioned about the things with which he needed help and persistently asked when he would be able to go home and get back to work. His wife was present on admission and also appeared anxious about her husband's present state of health.

Identification of deficits in self-care:

1. Immobility: This is due to physical deficit. Steve will be able to assist in the treatment of his right knee, but the 'flare' requires medical treatment. There was a knowledge deficit, as Steve needed to be taught about the treatment of a 'flare' and the importance of rest (see Table 11.8).
2. Socioeconomic factors: Steve was very concerned about the amount of time he was away from work. He felt insecure because of the possibility that

Table 11.8 Goal-setting and care planning (see care study 1 in text)

Goal	Plan of Care
1. For Steve to have the necessary knowledge and confidence to deal with a 'flare' in his arthritis	Educate Steve about the nature of a 'flare' and the usual form of treatment. Assist in maintaining Steve's joints in the optimum position with good posture and the use of resting splints. Teach skills in joint protection. Assist in maintaining usual standards of hygiene until able to do so independently. Teach the necessary skills to prevent complications of bed rest.
2. For Steve to feel able to cope with the internal conflict that he feels about being away from work	Educate Steve about all aspects of his disease, in particular the expected course of his disease. Teach the necessary skills that will help him to remain at work; • resting during meal breaks to conserve energy • use of working splints when writing or carrying out administrative duties • daily exercise regimen to help strengthen muscles, so protecting joints • ensure that the occupational health department is aware of his disease, and his needs whilst at work.
3. Steve and his wife should have all the information they require so that they are able to cope with the long-term implications of RA	Educate Steve and his wife about all aspects of RA, concentrating on a positive approach. Teach adaptation skills to enable as much independence as possible. Offer counselling so that Steve and his wife are given the opportunity to discuss their fears and apprehensions, and learn how to cope with their new situation.

he might have to leave his job due to his sickness record. This conflicted with the behaviour that he saw as being socially and culturally acceptable, for example, as the 'bread winner' in the family. In view of these issues Steve needed the knowledge and skills to be able to adapt to his situation.

3. Psychological factors: Steve expressed anger about his current admission to hospital. This indicated that Steve was lacking in the motivation he required to enable him to deal with his disease and to take responsibility for it. Steve received the necessary education to enable him to develop his knowledge and skills and therefore cope with his disease effectively.

Implementation

The primary aim in implementing this care plan was for Steve to achieve self-care. The emphasis was mainly on the involvement of Steve's wife and family. The nursing staff discussed all aspects of Steve's education and retraining with his wife so that the couple continued their close involvement with each other while at home.

Evaluation

Evaluation of the care plan is through the observation of Steve's progress in the performance of the stated self-care activities. The evaluation should centre around Steve's achievement or non-achievement and not around the nursing intervention.

Using Roper's activities of living model with a terminal rheumatoid arthritis patient

Roper's model is based on the twelve activities of living:

1. Maintaining a safe environment
2. Communicating
3. Breathing
4. Eating and drinking
5. Eliminating
6. Dressing and cleansing
7. Mobilizing
8. Controlling body temperature
9. Working and playing

10. Sexuality
11. Sleeping
12. Dying.

Roper's model is implemented using the nursing process which comprises assessment, planning, implementation and evaluation (Aggleton & Chalmers 1985b).

After assessing the patient's ability to perform the twelve activities of living the nurse decides whether:

1. There is no problem (N), i.e. the patient is independent in that activity
2. There is a potential problem (P), i.e. the patient is able to perform the activity with the use of aids, but might change
3. There is an actual problem (A), in that the patient is unable to perform the specific activity.

The assessment is intended to be ongoing so that any changes can be identified as soon as they occur.

Care study 2

Joan is a 62-year-old woman who has had rheumatoid arthritis for 20 years. During the last 5 years her disease has been progressive, leaving her with increasing disability, joint destruction and deformity. She was admitted to hospital with loss of normal function of both arms due to subluxation of the cervical vertebrae and compression of the spinal cord.

Joan is married with two daughters, who are both married with families of their own. Joan's husband is retired and is very much involved with his wife's care at home.

Assessment

Maintaining a safe environment (N) Although increasing loss of function prevented Joan from maintaining her own environment, she recognized potentially dangerous situations and summoned help.

Communicating (N) Joan had no problems; she was able to hear and speak well.

Breathing (P) Joan had orthopnea. She felt claustrophobic when lying down, so she slept in the semi-recumbent position using four pillows.

Eating and drinking (A) Joan was unable to feed herself. Her appetite was poor.

Eliminating (P) Joan was prone to constipation. She had no problem with micturition.

Dressing and cleansing (A) Joan was unable to do either due to loss of function in her arms.

Mobilizing (A) Joan suffered from early morning stiffness for 3–4 hours. However, she was mobile using a pulpit frame and could walk 10 yards. A valgus deformity of both knees, and a fixed flexion deformity of her right knee prevented greater mobilization.

Controlling body temperature (N) Temperature on admission was within normal limits. Joan usually wore two layers of clothes because she felt the cold.

Working and playing (N) Joan was retired. She enjoyed watching the television and listening to the radio.

Sexuality (A) Joan was acutely aware of the change in her body image. She was distressed by the recent advancement of her disabilities and her increasing dependence on her husband.

Sleeping (N) Joan slept well without night sedation.

Dying (P) Although this was not discussed on admission, later conversation revealed Joan's fears that her life was coming to an end. She did express the desire for her life to end if she was going to remain dependent on her husband and family.

The assessment is summarized in Table 11.9; two potential problems were identified:

1. Breathing
2. Eliminating.

Joan should be reassessed on a daily basis so that these problems can be monitored.

Care plan

1. Inability to eat and drink independently:
Full assessment of functional ability to be carried out by the occupational therapist. Assistance should be given at mealtimes when the patient is eating and drinking.
● Sit beside the patient on the same level
● Cut food into bite-size pieces before offering to patient
● Wait for patient to finish her mouthful before offering more food or drink

Table 11.9 Identification of problems and goals (see care study 2 in text)

Problem	Goal
1. Joan is unable to feed herself or drink independently	Joan should have adequate diet and fluids to satisfy her needs
2. Joan is unable to maintain her own hygiene needs or dress independently	Joan will be helped to wash and dress to her satisfaction
3. Joan has reduced mobility	Maximum mobility should be achieved
4. Joan is concerned about the changes in her body image and increasing dependence on her husband. Joan wants her life to end if she is to remain dependent	To help Joan feel happier with her body image and to provide support and guidance for her and her husband in coping with her increased dependence

- Offer a drink regularly in between meals, and position drinks close to patient so that she is able to drink from a straw independently
- Encourage family participation.

2. Inability to maintain hygiene needs and dress unaided:
- Maintain patient's privacy at all times
- Assist with a wash at the bedside, or use the bath/ shower
- Observe skin for any lesions or signs of pressure
- Dry skin well after washing
- Assist patient to dress in clothes in which she feels comfortable
- Care for mouth and teeth by offering to brush teeth after meals and prior to bedtime
- Brush/comb hair as necessary
- Ensure anal and vulval areas are clean and dry after elimination and offer handwashing facilities.

3. Reduced mobility:
- Physiotherapist to assess present mobility status and potential
- Assist with mobility as needed
- Ensure Joan has a high chair to sit in, allowing an easier exit from the chair
- Educate Joan about the need to change her position regularly, giving assistance where necessary
- Observe pressure areas for any signs of pressure
- Assist with exercise programme in the absence of the physiotherapist.

4. Psychological needs due to increased dependence on others and change in body image:
- Give Joan the opportunity to discuss her fears and apprehension by asking open questions
- Use non-verbal communication by:
  — sitting by the patient on the same level
  — leaning towards the patient
  — maintaining eye contact
- Use opportune moments to talk in privacy, for example while attending to hygiene
- Listen to Joan attentively
- Provide Joan with all the information she needs to enable her to cope with her increasing dependence; for example, agencies that may provide support such as home help and district nurse
- Involve the occupational therapist in teaching adaptation techniques for the various gadgets and aids that may benefit Joan and her family
- Involve Joan's husband and family in all aspects of care and decision-making
- Use positive reinforcement rather than concentrating on the negative aspects of Joan's ability
- Refer Joan and her husband to support groups in their area such as 'Arthritis Care'.

Implementation

All members of the multidisciplinary team are involved in the implementation of the care plan. Each person has a specific role to play and is responsible for different aspects of care. Joan is dependent on those people around her for maintaining her activities of daily living. Her husband, who is her main carer at home, is also involved with her care in hospital. He participates in the planning of his wife's care so that continuity can be maintained between the hospital and home. This is an obvious advantage for Joan, in that she has someone she loves and trusts who is involved in her care. In addition, her husband benefits by having gained confidence in his own actions at the hospital to continue caring for his wife at home.

Evaluation

The process of evaluation is carried out on a day-to-day basis. All aspects of care are evaluated for their effectiveness, and care plans are adjusted accordingly. Any new problems can be identified, goals set and care plans revised.

Exacerbation of rheumatoid arthritis – a 'flare-up'

The rheumatoid arthritis patient will have periods of exacerbations of joint inflammation which are known as 'flare-ups'. One or more joints become red, hot, swollen and very painful. The patient is nearly always admitted to hospital for rest and further treatment.

Rest

Rest can vary according to the joints affected. If the joints of the upper limbs are affected, then it may not be necessary to have complete bedrest, but only to rest the affected joint. The patient will feel unwell and generally tired and should be encouraged to rest during the day as much as possible.

When weight-bearing joints such as the knees are involved, then it is necessary to have complete bedrest. Complete bedrest is very difficult for many patients to accept. It takes away their independence, making them dependent on the nurse for assistance. The nurse should be aware of the need to educate her patient about resting the joints completely during a 'flare-up'. He should be allowed to go to the toilet and bathroom areas in a wheelchair. This limitation of activity may be quite alarming to many patients until they understand the principles of bedrest.

The patient should be encouraged to sit upright in bed supported by pillows to maintain the joints in the optimum position. The knees should be straight and the ankles at 90° of flexion. Resting splints should be worn whilst the patient is in bed.

Bedrest is maintained for 7–10 days or until the cessation of symptoms. During a 'flare-up', patients may find an early morning bath effective in helping to reduce stiffness and relieve joint pain.

Care should be taken to prevent the complications of bedrest. Patients should be told why they must change their position, to avoid pressure sore development; they should also perform deep breathing and leg exercises. The physiotherapist is very involved in the patient's care at this stage. In addition to routine exercises, she will teach isometric exercises to minimize muscle atrophy.

In patients with upper limb involvement, the nurse will need to assist with activities of living.

Remobilization

Remobilization after a period of complete rest should be a gradual process. Initially the patient should walk only short distances, for example to the bathroom and back, resting on his bed for a while afterwards.

The physiotherapist will advise on mobility, suggesting any aids, such as the walking frame or walking stick, that may be of use. The patient may then be ready to progress to a more vigorous exercise programme that will build up the muscles around the joint.

When the patient has reached this stage he should be encouraged to dress. This has a dual purpose. First, it provides an opportunity to carry out a dressing assessment, and second, it enables the patient to readjust to his normal lifestyle. By dressing, the individual is able to discard his 'sick role'. Patients are encouraged to do more for themselves until they reach their usual level of independence.

Rehabilitation

Rehabilitation occurs simultaneously with remobilization. The occupational therapist is the key health care professional in the rehabilitation of the patient. The emphasis is on the restoration of normal function, adjustment and retraining.

The patient is no longer a passive recipient of care, but is encouraged to take responsibility, with the help of staff, for his rehabilitation, to achieve a maximum level of functioning. The relationship between patient and the health care professional is therefore one of mutual participation (Morgan 1986).

The OT assesses the patient's level of function and then suggests ways in which he could adapt to perform tasks in order to save energy. She may also offer advice about the numerous gadgets and adaptations available for use during normal daily activities.

Going home

Discharge home can cause as much anxiety for the patient as his initial admission to hospital. Many patients worry about coping back in their home environment. They may express concern about daily activities such as looking after the children, continuing with family relationships or returning to work.

Care of the individual with RA involves members of the community services as well as those based within the hospital setting. In order to continue with adequate care at home this service should be utilized.

The community health care team is comprised of the patient's general practitioner, health visitor, district nurse, domiciliary physiotherapist, occupational therapist, home help and meals-on-wheels service. Some or all of these agencies may be involved in the care of the patient in the community.

The support that the family and friends can provide is enormous, and close relatives and friends should be included when planning for discharge. To alleviate the usual anxieties caused by discharge, the nurse can offer relevant information about useful agencies which may be contacted in the community.

The patient should be reassured that all concerns and queries will be dealt with by his general practitioner and health care team, and if any further problems occur he will be referred back to the hospital for the appropriate care.

Patient education

Providing information to the patient and his family, in addition to education on all aspects of RA, is an essential part of his nursing care. This is by no means a simple procedure and many factors must be taken into account (see Chs 3, 5 and 6).

Patient information may be in the form of books, leaflets, posters and audiovisual aids, through patient–nurse interaction or through discussion with other RA sufferers.

It is important that the stage of the patient's own disease process is made clear. For a newly diagnosed patient, it would be inappropriate to discuss wheelchairs and stair lifts when it is more important that the patient has some knowledge about a 'flare-up'. Consequently, patient education and information must be tailored to the patient's specific needs.

Education of the rheumatoid arthritic can be divided into five main areas:

1. Prevention of joint deformity
2. Drug therapy and side-effects
3. The disease process
4. The use of aids to daily living
5. Available agencies.

Prevention of joint deformity

It is essential that everything possible is done to prevent joint deformity. The functional capacity of a deformed joint is reduced, consequently reducing the patient's quality of life.

The physiotherapist and occupational therapist are involved in this aspect of care. The physiotherapist introduces an exercise regimen aimed at strengthening the muscles around susceptible joints, particularly weight-bearing joints. She may advise on suitable recreational activities such as swimming and exercise classes.

The OT concentrates on providing joint protection. She makes resting splints to support the limb in the optimum position and will advise on the use of working splints, for example the futura splint. The OT can also offer advice about joint protection while the patient is carrying out activities of daily living, such as the use of gadgets to reduce the pressures exerted on affected joints.

The nurse must be able to reinforce the advice given to the patient and his family by being knowledgeable herself and being available to talk and answer any questions.

Drug therapy and side-effects

The patient should be well-informed about his drug therapy and the possible side-effects. Many of the drugs administered in the treatment of RA require careful monitoring. For example, patients taking the DMARDs will have monthly urine tests and frequent blood analyses to detect signs of toxicity. It is therefore important that the patient understands this need for monitoring.

Most rheumatology units provide information cards and booklets on all aspects of drug therapy which should be made available to every rheumatoid patient.

The disease process

The patient and his family may seek a prediction of the course of the disease and its prognosis. The nature of their questions is understandable; some of their concerns may be clarified, but it is an impossible task, as all concerned should be aware, to give definitive answers.

The patient is invited to take as much responsibility for his own treatment and care as possible, so that he feels he has some control. It is the role of the health care professional to direct the patient towards support groups and agencies which give the patient an opportunity to gain moral support from other sufferers.

The use of aids to daily living

The first disabled living centres were set up in the 1960s. Their role is to help the functionally disabled with every aspect of daily living. These centres have more than 15 000 pieces of equipment and aids to daily living available, ranging from simple suction egg cups to sophisticated electric wheelchairs (Clements 1987). Many of the aids are of a more modern design than is necessary, but patients find them to be of value. Some of the larger aids such as wheelchairs and walking frames are available from notable high street stores (see Ch. 10).

Patients should be informed of these centres so that they know of the variety of aids that may help them in their activities of living; alternatively, they may browse through the numerous catalogues on the market.

Agencies

The Arthritis and Rheumatism Council (ARC) and Arthritis Care are the two main agencies.

ARC produces a quarterly newsletter for its members with information on other rheumatoid diseases and advice to patients as well as information about current research. This agency produces several excellent information booklets for patients. Arthritis Care is a support group with local branches throughout the country. It offers help and support to patients and their families.

Informing patients about the various agencies available should be part of their ongoing education. Their introduction to these agencies enables them to interact with other sufferers and provides an ideal opportunity for fact-finding.

COMPLEMENTARY MEDICINE

As life changes in Britain, the general public have become more aware of health care, health promotion and the prevention of disease. In chronic diseases such as RA, patients are often looking for a cure, and some will turn to complementary medicine for a solution to their problem. Of course, as yet, too few people have consulted its different branches for a valid assessment of complementary medicine's successes to be made. (See Ch. 7 for further details of complementary therapies.)

DIET

Although there is no scientific evidence to prove the efficacy of a change in dietary intake in rheumatoid patients, many doctors would not disregard the benefits that a restrictive diet brings. Diet is certainly unique to each individual, and RA sufferers may experiment with different foods for many years before they feel comfortable with their dietary intake. Patients can often identify foods that disagree with them or trigger a change in their status quo. Some patients choose to remove red meat and/or dairy products from their diet.

SURGERY

Surgical intervention has a role to play in the management of local structural problems involving joints or soft tissue. Operative success depends on patient selection and performance of the most appropriate operation.

It is common for rheumatologists and orthopaedic surgeons to carry out combined clinics where there is an opportunity for thorough assessment. These clinics enable physicians and surgeons to discuss with the patient his present difficulties and the possible surgical treatment and expected outcome.

Some hospitals are fortunate in having clinical nurse specialists working alongside the medical team. This can be reassuring and very supportive for the patient and his family when the decision to accept surgery requires considerable thought and discussion about their fears and anxieties. It is also true that many patients have unrealistically high expectations and are often disappointed with the results. In addition to these important factors it is essential that the patient has a clear understanding of the postoperative period and the rehabilitation that will be required.

Assessing the patient's need for surgery is difficult: some will benefit more than others from embarking on a series of reconstructive operations. Every time a doctor asks the question, 'Is there a place for surgery in this patient's treatment?' he should also ask, 'Is there a case for leaving this patient alone?' (Soloman 1981).

The criteria used to decide on the need for surgery are:

- Pain
- Loss of function
- Joint instability
- Immobility
- Radiological joint destruction.

Common surgical procedures for rheumatoid arthritis are given in Table 11.10.

Specific preoperative nursing care plays an

Table 11.10 Operative treatment for rheumatoid arthritis

Soft tissue procedures	Bone and joint procedures
Synovectomy	osteotomy
Tenosynovectomy	arthrodesis
Tendon repair	excision arthroplasty
Nerve decompression	replacement arthroplasty

important part in preparing the rheumatoid patient for surgery. Using Roper's model, the nurse can assess her patient's specific needs.

The use of Roper's model with the preoperative rheumatoid patient

Assessment

Maintaining a safe environment (A) Loss of joint function will reduce the patient's ability to maintain personal hygiene. The patient must be aware of the need for a 6-hour period of fasting and receive the appropriate preoperative patient education. The presence of cervical spine involvement must be assessed by the physician.

Communicating (P) The patient must be given the opportunity to express his fears and anxieties both verbally and non-verbally. If a hearing device is worn it is quite usual to take it to theatre, and the theatre staff should be notified of this.

Breathing (P) Any preoperative chest problems will be identified.

Eating and drinking (A) The patient will be given nil by mouth for 6 hours prior to theatre.

Eliminating (P) Constipation or difficulty in micturition, especially when the patient is on bedrest, will be identified.

Dressing and cleansing (A) The patient's level of independence will be assessed.

Mobilizing (P) Mobilization should be unaltered prior to theatre. If a premedication is given, or a specific skin preparation carried out, the patient will be advised to remain on bedrest until theatre.

Controlling body temperature (N) Temperature on admission should be within normal limits.

Working and playing (N) In the preoperative period, watching television, reading and listening to the radio are all good forms of diversional therapy.

Sexuality (P) A change in body image is very distressing. However, the thought of forthcoming surgery to correct a deformity should be uplifting for the patient.

Sleeping (N) The patient's level of preoperative anxiety may be a problem and may influence his normal sleep pattern.

Dying (P) Some patients verbalize anxiety about their anaesthetic.

Specific preoperative problems and goals are identified in Table 11.11.

Care plan

1. Difficulty in maintaining hygiene needs and putting on theatre gown unaided:
- Maintain privacy at all times
- Assist with a wash at the bedside, or use the bath/shower
- Observe skin for any lesions or signs of pressure
- Dry skin well after washing
- Assist patient to dress in theatre gown, removing underwear and any prosthesis
- Care for mouth and teeth by offering/assisting to brush teeth
- Brush/comb hair as necessary.

2. Potential loss of skin integrity following skin preparation due to friable skin:
- Carry out a patch test if using a depilatory cream to detect any allergic reaction
- Avoid skin abrasions by using clippers for hirsute areas; and take great care when shaving or clipping as the rheumatoid patient has particularly friable skin.

3. Psychological needs and knowledge deficit due to impending surgery:
- Give the patient the opportunity to discuss his fears and anxieties by asking open questions
- Use non-verbal communication by:
  — sitting by the patient on the same level
  — leaning towards patient
  — maintaining eye contact
- Use opportune moments to talk in privacy, for example while attending to hygiene
- Listen attentively
- Provide the patient with all the information he needs to enable him to cope with his operation and the immediate postoperative period
- Involve the patient's family in all aspects of care and decision-making
- Suggest various means of relaxation and discuss the possibility of night sedation with the patient.

4. Unstable cervical spine:
- Ensure the patient understands the need for a cervical collar during the perioperative period
- Apply a soft, well-fitting cervical collar preoperatively.

5. Difficulty breathing postoperatively:
- Reinforce the physiotherapist's teaching programme
- Discuss with the anaesthetist the possibility that the patient may lie in the semirecumbent position postoperatively
- Allay any possible fears or anxieties that the patient may verbalize.

Implementation

The care plan will involve all members of the multidisciplinary team. The nurse will have the opportunity to spend some time with her patient, giving support and reassurance during the preoperative period. She should involve other family members as desired by the patient and try to create a calm relaxing environment. Although

Table 11.11 Identification of specific preoperative problems and goals

Problems	Goals
1. Unstable cervical spine with possible upper limb paraesthesia	The patient will be aware of the need to wear a cervical collar during the operation
2. Knowledge deficit and anxiety preventing normal sleep pattern	The patient will be fully conversant with his preoperative preparation as a result of patient education including a discussion on relaxation techniques and night sedation
3. Anxiety verbalized about breathing difficulties when lying flat postoperatively	The patient will receive preoperative chest physio and will be taught breathing exercises to prevent a postoperative chest infection. Positioning will be discussed.

inpatient facilities vary, it is comforting for the patient if his allocated nurse is able to accompany him to theatre. Ideally, the same nurse should also collect the patient.

Evaluation

The evaluation of the care plan will be carried out immediately after surgery. The nurse must be able to recognize her patient's needs and respond accordingly. This will most certainly involve the evaluation of pain and the need to provide pain management. This may require a number of interventions, such as changing position and relieving anxiety as the patient's pain is reassessed.

Postoperative nursing care

The problems identified here are only intended to be a guide for the practitioner to expand upon and develop further with her patient. When using the nursing process it is essential that the nurse does not forget that her patient is an individual with special needs.

Postoperative problems and goals

Table 11.12 outlines the identification of specific postoperative problems and goals.

Postoperative care plan

1. Difficulty in maintaining postoperative safety unaided:
- Maintain a clear airway
- Ensure that the patient receives the prescribed fluid replacement and that an accurate record is kept
- All vital signs should be recorded half-hourly immediately postoperatively.

2. Possible respiratory distress:
- Depending on the nature of the surgery, ensure that the patient is lying in either the lateral or semirecumbent position, enhancing good lung expansion
- Be aware that oxygen therapy may be required. An increased respiratory rate may be due to pain, chest infection or haemorrhage.

Table 11.12 Identification of specific postoperative problems and goals

Problems	Goals
Inability to maintain own postoperative safety	the patient will be able to maintain his airway assisted by good positioning; the patient is rehydrated; other vital signs will remain within normal limits; postoperative complications such as haemorrhage and joint dislocation will be prevented; uncomplicated wound healing; skin integrity will be maintained
Respiratory difficulty	the patient will have good lung expansion and will be well perfused
Neurological and circulatory impairment	colour, sensation and movement of extremities will be intact: early impairment will be detected and reported
Inability to maintain dietary intake due to: immediate postoperative recovery limited functional ability due to surgery	once fully recovered from the anaesthetic the patient will feel able to take and tolerate fluids and a light diet assistance will be offered with feeding and drinking if necessary
Difficulty with micturition due to reduced mobility	the patient will micturate within 12 hours after surgery
Poor wound healing due to RA and drug therapy	observe wound dressing for 'strike-through'; sutures will be left in place for a longer period than usual to allow wound healing; care for redivac drainage system
Compromised mobility due to surgery	a daily assessment will be made of the patient's potential risk of pressure sore development; the nursing care will reflect this score, therefore preventing loss of skin integrity
Difficulty maintaining body temperature	the patient's temperature will remain within normal limits
Postoperative pain	prescribed medication is given and its effectiveness observed; pain control will require reassessment; a pain chart may be a useful tool

3. Observation of the periphery following limb surgery:

Following surgery involving peripheral joints the limb will be elevated by the nurse. The upper limb may be elevated in a roller towel or on two pillows; this will depend on the degree of RA in the upper limbs. The lower limb may be elevated on a Braun frame or on two pillows. The foot of the bed may also be elevated.

- Test and record colour, sensation and movement of the periphery half-hourly immediately postoperatively
- Compare observations with the opposite limb.

4. Difficulty micturating:

- Ensure patient's privacy when using the bedpan or urinal
- If possible, allow patient to use commode or lavatory
- Encourage oral fluid intake
- Pain can inhibit micturition by increasing anxiety; therefore, ensure adequate pain relief is administered
- Use relaxation techniques.

5. Inability to maintain own temperature:

- Ensure an accurate preoperative assessment is available as a baseline for postoperative recordings
- Consider using a 'space blanket'
- Observe for haemorrhage.

6. Postoperative pain:

- Observe patient for non-verbal signs of pain or discomfort
- A pain scale may be a useful tool
- Monitor level, site and duration of pain
- Allow the patient to express his level of pain
- Allay any fears and anxieties
- Use relaxation techniques
- Assist the patient in changing his position
- Apply warmth or cold to the area
- Administer analgesia and monitor effectiveness, taking into consideration vital signs
- Evaluate analgesia and request changes accordingly; for example, changing from a regular 4-hourly injection to a continuous infusion, or using oral analgesic preparations

- Observe for signs of nausea and offer an antiemetic accordingly.

7. Limited mobility:

- Observe skin for any lesions or signs of pressure. Careful positioning is essential. The dependent patient should be lifted/turned well clear of the bed every 2 hours depending on his pressure score scale. Adapt this procedure if the patient has had major joint replacement surgery
- Use a 'monkey pole' if the upper limbs are unaffected with RA
- Use aids for the relief of pressure such as sheepskins and sheepskin bootees, etc. Bed cradles can be used but have a tendency to divorce the patient from his surroundings.

8. Difficulty washing and dressing:

- Assist with a postoperative wash and help patient to put on night attire
- Care for mouth and teeth, replacing dentures when patient is fully recovered from the anaesthetic
- Brush/comb hair as necessary
- Maintain privacy.

Implementation

A multidisciplinary approach is important. If possible, the allocated nurse should follow her patient through the whole procedure, from the preoperative stage to the postoperative period. This continuity instils confidence in the patient and can help to reduce his anxiety. The nurse must be adaptable to the needs of her patient and must act as his advocate, particularly over such issues as pain relief.

Evaluation

The plan of care should be revised or continued in the light of the evaluation. Evaluation is made at regular intervals by consultation between the patient and his nurse. Whenever possible, the goals that are set should be achievable. The aim of the multidisciplinary team is maximum independence for the patient within his own capabilities.

REFERENCES

Adams J C, Hamblen D L 1990 Outline of orthopaedics, 11th edn. Churchill Livingstone, Edinburgh

Aggleton P, Chalmers H 1985a Orem's self-care model. Nursing Times 81(1): 36–39

Aggleton P, Chalmers H 1985b Roper's activities of living model. Nursing Times 81:(7): 59–61

Arthritis and Rheumatism Council 1988 Rheumatism and the weather. ARC

Boyle J A, Buchanan W W 1971 Clinical rheumatology. Blackwell Scientific, Oxford

Boyle J A, Greig W R, Buchanan W W 1967 Twin studies in rheumatoid arthritis. World Medical Journal 14: 181

Clements S 1987 Aids to disabled living. Nursing Times 83(24): 54

Copeman W S C, Scott J T 1978 Historical. In: Scott J T (ed) Copeman's textbook of the rheumatic diseases, 5th edn. Churchill Livingstone, Edinburgh

Dieppe P A, Doherty M, MacFarlane D et al 1985 Rheumatological medicine. Churchill Livingstone, Edinburgh

Edmonds J, Hughes G 1985 Lecture notes on rheumatology. Blackwell Scientific, Oxford

Elliot M 1979 Nursing rheumatic disease. Churchill Livingstone, Edinburgh

Gunn C 1992 Bones and joints, 2nd edn. Churchill Livingstone, Edinburgh

Hickling P, Golding J 1984 An outline of rheumatology. Wright, Bristol

Holland C, Jayson M I V 1981 Rheumatoid arthritis. Medicine 1(10): 427–433

Jubb R, Consultant rheumatologist, Rheumatology Department, Selly Oak Hospital, Birmingham

Kane W J 1981 Current orthopaedic management. Churchill Livingstone, Edinburgh, p 333

Kraag G R 1989 Clinical aspects in rheumatoid arthritis. Triangle 28(12): 15–24

Morgan M 1986 The doctor-patient relationship. In: Sociology as applied to medicine. Bailliere Tindall, London

Olsen N J 1989 Assessment of disease activity in rheumatoid arthritis. Current Opinion in Rheumatology 1: 21–28

Pigg-Smith J S, Webb-Driscoll P W, Cantiff R 1985 Rheumatology nursing: a problem oriented approach. Wiley Medical, New York

Plewes J L, consultant orthopaedic surgeon, The General Hospital, Birmingham

Powell M 1986 Orthopaedic nursing and rehabilitation, 9th, edn. Churchill Livingstone, Edinburgh, p 544

Rideout E 1992 Caring for the patient with bone and joint disease. In: Royle J A, Walsh M (eds) Watson's Medical–surgical nursing and related physiology. Bailliere Tindall, London

Silman A J, Vandenbroucke J P 1989 Female sex hormones and rheumatoid arthritis. British Journal of Rheumatology 28: 1–173

Soloman L 1981 Surgery of the major joints in arthritis. Medicine 1(10): 451–456

Turner A, Foster M, Johnson S E 1992 Occupational therapy and physical dysfunction, 3rd edn. Churchill Livingstone, Edinburgh

Wood P H 1978 Epidemiology of rheumatic disorders. In: Scott J T (ed) Copeman's textbook of the rheumatic diseases, 5th edn. Churchill Livingstone, Edinburgh

Wright V, Haslock L 1984 Rheumatism for nurses and remedial therapists. Heinemann, London

FURTHER READING

Arthritis and Rheumatism Council – Reports on rheumatic diseases

Chesson S 1984 Social and emotional aspects of rheumatoid arthritis. Medical Education 914–915

Footner A 1989 Orthopaedic nursing. Bailliere Tindall, London

Gibbs H 1990 Behaviour problems. Nursing Standard 4(49): 52–54

Grennon D M 1984 Rheumatology. Bailliere Tindall, London

Hill J 1991 Assessing rheumatic disease. Nursing Times 87(4): 33–35

Judd M 1989 Mobility: patient problems and nursing care. Heinemann, Oxford

Kitson A L 1989 (project director) Standards of care – rheumatic disease nursing. RCN, Scutari, London

Mell J M H 1987 Manual of rheumatology. Churchill Livingstone, Edinburgh

Mell J M H 1988 Essentials of rheumatology. Churchill Livingstone, Edinburgh

Panayi G S 1980 Essential rheumatology for nurses and therapists. Bailliere Tindall, London

Powell M 1986 Orthopaedic nursing and rehabilitation, 9th edn. Churchill Livingstone, Edinburgh

Thomas F 1987 Restoring function to the arthritic hand. Nursing Times 83(3): 33–35

Warnes A (ed) 1989 Human ageing and later life: multidisciplinary perspectives. Edward Arnold, London

12

Other rheumatological diseases

Hilary Addison   Ninette Johnson

INTRODUCTION

There are some 180 conditions which can qualify as rheumatic disorders (Hickling & Golding 1984). This chapter covers the nursing care of just seven of these diseases – systemic lupus erythematosus, ankylosing spondylitis, gout, scleroderma, polymyositis/dermatomyositis and Sjögren's syndrome.

Rheumatic disease is a dreaded illness which conjures up pictures of disfigurement, disability and loss of independence. Although in recent years the prognosis has improved, sufferers do have to come to terms with chronic illness, recurrent or persistent pain and, possibly, other organ involvement.

Education is an important aspect of a comprehensive care programme for the patient and family. This can be achieved by the multidisciplinary or team approach. There may be emotional and social difficulties as a result of a chronic disease.

SYSTEMIC LUPUS ERYTHEMATOSUS

Systemic lupus erythematosus (SLE) is a rare rheumatological condition of unknown aetiology which can affect most or all of the systems of the body. It is most common in young women in the child-bearing years with a female to male ratio of approximately 9 : 1 (Morrow & Isenberg 1987).

The term 'lupus', from the Latin meaning wolf, has been used to describe ulcerative lesions on the face suggestive of the effect of being savaged by a wolf. Casenave and Clausit used the term lupus erythemaeux in 1852. The disease was previously known as 'disseminated lupus erythematosus' but is now termed 'systemic lupus erythematosus'.

Presentation

The disease begins most commonly with fever, fatigue, weight loss, joint and muscle pain. Other manifestations include skin rash, pleuritic chest pain, renal, psychological and neurological symptoms (see Fig. 12.1).

Laboratory tests used in the diagnosis of SLE

Urinalysis

Urinalysis may be carried out to detect proteinuria. Urinary tract infection can be excluded by sending a midstream specimen of urine for culture and sensitivity. If the result is negative then any proteinuria is indicative of renal involvement.

Haematology

Erythrocyte counts may be used to detect the presence of anaemia which can be due to chronic illness, iron deficiency or gastrointestinal bleeding. White cell counts that indicate leukopenia may be due to a flare-up of the disease. Detection of the presence of severe thrombocytopenia is important as it is life-threatening to the patient. A raised erythrocyte sedimentation rate (ESR) is indicative of disease activity but can also be a sign of infection.

Chemical pathology

Specific tests are for:

- antinuclear antibodies
- immunoglobulin
- anti-DNA antibodies
- autoantibody
- serum immune complex assay.

Skin biopsy

Biopsy of the rash shows histological changes which are typical of lupus.

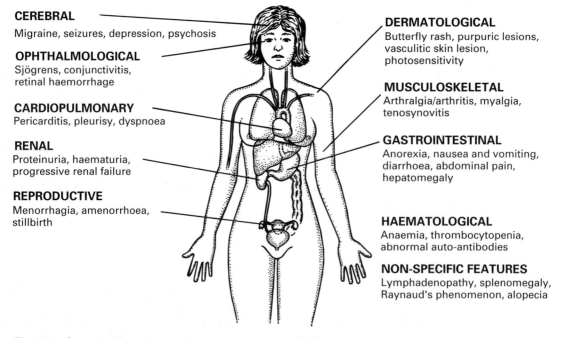

CEREBRAL
Migraine, seizures, depression, psychosis

OPHTHALMOLOGICAL
Sjögrens, conjunctivitis, retinal haemorrhage

CARDIOPULMONARY
Pericarditis, pleurisy, dyspnoea

RENAL
Proteinuria, haematuria, progressive renal failure

REPRODUCTIVE
Menorrhagia, amenorrhoea, stillbirth

DERMATOLOGICAL
Butterfly rash, purpuric lesions, vasculitic skin lesion, photosensitivity

MUSCULOSKELETAL
Arthralgia/arthritis, myalgia, tenosynovitis

GASTROINTESTINAL
Anorexia, nausea and vomiting, diarrhoea, abdominal pain, hepatomegaly

HAEMATOLOGICAL
Anaemia, thrombocytopenia, abnormal auto-antibodies

NON-SPECIFIC FEATURES
Lymphadenopathy, splenomegaly, Raynaud's phenomenon, alopecia

Fig. 12.1 Systemic effects of systemic lupus erythematosus (SLE).

Medical treatment

The medical treatment of SLE depends on the symptoms presented. There is no cure for this disease and it is difficult to predict which treatment will be effective for the individual patient. All treatment is aimed at suppressing the activity of the disease. Some patients do not require medication and others take medication only as needed or for short periods (see Table 12.1).

Counselling

One of the most important tasks of the professional caring for SLE patients is to develop good communication and a rapport with the patient. Counselling is a continuous process once the diagnosis has been made. Information about the disease and its possible associated problems is given. Handbooks and leaflets for patients about SLE, published by the Arthritis and Rheumatism Council and the Lupus Group (part of Arthritis Care), may be provided for patients to read and keep.

The patient should be encouraged to take an active role in his treatment; this could include learning to test his urine, taking and recording

Table 12.1 Medical treatment of systemic lupus erythematosus (SLE)

Severity of the disease	Medication/treatment
Mild SLE	analgesia anti-inflammatory drugs

SLE with specific problems	analgesia
	non-steroidal anti-inflammatory drugs (NSAIDs)
	slow-acting anti-rheumatic drugs (SAARDs)
	intra-articular steroids
	immunosuppressives:
	  high doses of oral corticosteroids
	  pulse high doses of IV steroid therapy
	cyctotoxic drugs:
	  azathioprine, chlorambucil, methotrexate IV or oral cyclophosphamide
	plasmapheresis:
	  sometimes used in the hope of removing autoantibodies from the circulation

his temperature and reporting any abnormality noted to the outpatient clinic.

Patients who also suffer from Raynaud's phenomenon are advised to avoid rapid changes of temperature and to wear gloves and socks when they go out in the cold. Where appropriate, patients should be advised to wear gloves when handling cold items, e.g. food from the freezer. Those who smoke are advised either to reduce the number of cigarettes they smoke or to give up the habit completely. This could reduce further circulatory impairment. Patients with Raynaud's have classical colour changes of their fingers and toes.

Skin involvement

Patients with photosensitivity should avoid strong sunlight as exposure to the sun can exacerbate the rash. Patients are advised to wear wide-brimmed hats. Barrier creams with sunscreen protection (factor 15 or higher) are recommended and should be applied frequently as a prophylactic measure. It should be stressed that there is more reflection of ultraviolet rays near water and snow.

Surgery

Surgical procedures may produce a flare-up of the disease. Surgery, if planned, should be carried out during periods of remission. This includes dental extraction.

Infection

Pyrexia may be due either to a flare-up of the disease or to infection. Infection may be masked by treatment for the disease. Identification of the presence of infection and its prompt treatment are important.

Family planning

Methods of contraception should be discussed with the rheumatologist/specialist. Most patients are able to take the contraceptive pill without complication. The intrauterine device is not recommended due to the increased risk of infection.

Pregnancy

Again the patient should seek the advice of her rheumatologist/specialist before planning a pregnancy. There is an increased risk of the disease flaring up during pregnancy and an increased risk of miscarriage. Regular and careful monitoring is necessary in order to detect early complications.

Case study: using an activities of living model for nursing the patient with SLE

Jane is a 40-year-old married woman with four children whose disease first presented 19 years ago as a facial rash with an ulcer on the side of her nose. She was sent by her general practitioner to a dermatologist who misdiagnosed her condition as a rodent ulcer. Six years later she was referred to another dermatologist, who correctly diagnosed her disease as systemic lupus erythematosus. Around that time Jane began to develop a feeling of unease about the diagnostic skills of the medical staff with whom she came in contact. Although she had no other symptoms of the disease she could not help worrying that the delay in diagnosis of her disease would make a difference to its progress.

Nine years later she developed Raynaud's phenomenon, with classical colour changes of her fingers and toes from white to purple to red, as a complication of her SLE. This was treated with a vasodilator drug to help to improve the circulation. A short time later she developed arthralgia, mainly in her knees and elbows.

Her disease remained stable for almost 6 years, after which she began to suffer from severe pain in her right shoulder, arm and leg after a bout of an influenza-like illness. This severe pain necessitated an admission to hospital where capsulitis of the right shoulder was diagnosed. This was treated with an intra-articular steroid injection with a good result. Blood tests showed that she had leukopenia and lymphopenia.

The arthralgia continued to make life difficult for her from time to time and non-steroidal anti-inflammatory drugs (NSAIDs) were tried as treatment. Unfortunately, she was unable to tolerate them as they caused skin rashes.

In the middle of the following year she was noted to have a dry mouth and she confirmed that she had had dry eyes previously. Sjögren's syndrome was diagnosed. (It is recognized that patients with Sjögren's syndrome tend to react adversely to drugs more commonly than do those with SLE.) She had patches of alopecia over various parts of her skin. There were no cutaneous lesions of the SLE type, but marked solar elastotic changes on her hands, forearms, upper arms and over the 'cape' region on her back (see Fig. 12.2).

Blood tests showed that she had strongly positive antinuclear antibodies (ANA) and positive rheumatoid factor. She was walking stiffly and painfully and found housekeeping increasingly difficult. She was treated with an intramuscular steroid injection and an antimalarial drug known to have good anti-inflammatory properties. She had become increasingly depressed and lost 2 stone in weight over a period of 6 months. By this time Jane had begun to suffer also from shortness of breath and pleuritic chest pain. She had 'crackles' at the bases of both lungs, and a chest X-ray showed areas of atelectasis, though thromboembolic phenomena could not be ruled out.

She subsequently had a venous quotient scan of her lungs. This is a ventilation and perfusion scan using Xenon gas breathed through a closed-circuit system with the result displayed on a television screen for the ventilation component. Using a radioactive isotope medium injected into a vein, the circulatory perfusion of the lungs is then displayed on the screen and recorded on an imaging film to indicate any abnormalities.

She was treated with systemic steroids with reasonable effect but the breathlessness and chest pain persisted. The steroids had the effect of making her

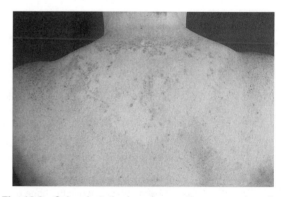

Fig. 12.2 Solar elastotic changes over the cape region of the back. (From Dr Michael Snaith and Mrs Brenda Hutton, with permission.)

cushingoid with increased facial hair and weight gain. At this time she was referred to a thoracic physician who diagnosed 'shrinking lung syndrome' caused by the SLE. She had an open lung biopsy which showed lymphocytic infiltration of the lungs with pleural fibrosis.

At the beginning of the following year Jane had a flare-up of her SLE when she had tender, swollen joints and increased breathlessness. Again she was treated with an immunosuppressant drug and systemic steroids, and felt markedly improved on this medication; 2 months later the immunosuppressant drug was stopped because a blood test indicated bone marrow suppression. Blood tests were repeated 1 week later and were again within an acceptable range so the immunosuppressant drug was restarted.

After 1 month had passed, her exercise tolerance was deemed satisfactory, although pleuritic chest pain persisted on occasion. Four weeks later her chest pain had become constant with nocturnal orthopnoea. She also complained of an abnormal sensation in her left foot which might suggest early sensory neuropathy. Her blood tests showed some neutropenia but no change was made to her medications.

Jane had the impression that the medical staff did not believe that her symptoms were giving her as much trouble as she described, and her confidence in them was once again undermined. (Sometimes the symptoms with which the patient presents in SLE are not indicative of how ill she feels.)

When Jane was seen in the outpatient clinic 3 weeks later she had gained weight but was suffering from acid reflux. Nausea would wake her at night and she occasionally vomited bitter fluid. She was treated with an H_2 blocker and an antiemetic and had barium studies the following month, which proved normal.

During another one-month check-up it was noted that she had gained 6 kg during the intervening period and so the dose of oral steroid was reduced. Her Raynaud's phenomenon had worsened 2 months later and this was again treated with a vasodilating drug.

When reviewed 6 months on, Jane had had several influenza-like illnesses which had exacerbated her breathing problems and had necessitated an increase in the dose of oral steroid again; it was hoped that this could be reduced as early as possible.

By the following autumn her lung function had improved and her breathlessness had decreased. She remained reasonably well until the next spring, when she again succumbed to influenza. This caused her joints to swell and become more painful again and a NSAID was prescribed. Over the summer her Raynaud's became a problem and she had a stronger analgesic prescribed for pain. The immunosuppressant drug and the NSAID were discontinued. At the time of this care study, her most recent problem requiring admission to hospital was neuropathy in her lower limbs, which may have been due to sensitivity to the NSAID.

Assessment of activities of living

Mobilizing She has difficulty climbing up and down stairs. At times she finds it difficult to keep the house clean and has to depend on her husband. She can walk for short distances only as the pain and stiffness in her joints and her breathlessness restrict her mobility. She has a wheelchair for use when going out but she does not like it.

Communicating She is nervous but reasonably articulate. She finds some questions easier to answer than others.

Breathing She becomes breathless on exertion. She smokes 20–30 cigarettes a day.

Eating and drinking She has a good appetite and has few food dislikes. Her fluid intake is approximately 1.5 litres per day. She enjoys an occasional alcoholic drink socially.

Eliminating She has her bowels open every other day and seldom suffers from constipation. She has occasional episodes of cystitis, particularly if she has not been very mobile.

Personal cleansing and dressing She often has difficulty getting out of the bath. She needs some help at times with dressing, in particular with underwear.

Controlling body temperature Because of the Raynaud's phenomenon, she has to make rapid changes of clothing due to sudden changes in peripheral body temperature.

Working and playing She worked until recently as a secretary but has had to give it up. Her disease has seriously curtailed her social activities and interests and she feels quite resentful about this.

Expressing sexuality She tries hard to wear attractive clothes and always puts on her make-up.

Sleeping Her sleep is often disturbed due to her

Table 12.2   Jane's care plan during her stay in hospital

Number	Patient's problem/need	Expected outcome	Action
1.	Pain and tingling sensation in both lower legs	For these sensations to diminish or resolve completely	Keep the bedclothes off her legs by using a bed cradle. Monitor the effect of medication in controlling them. Allow her time to express her anxieties about the condition.
2.	Breathlessness and chest pain	To control these to an acceptable level for her	Encourage her to reduce or give up smoking. Sit her upright with pillows to support her. Ensure that the medications are given and taken as prescribed. Refer her to the physiotherapist for chest and relaxation exercises. Ensure that she understands and maintains the exercise programme when the physiotherapist is not there.
3.	Generalized joint pain and stiffness	For these to be relieved by medication and support	Ensure that she recieves appropriate medications. Provide a pain chart for her to fill in so that the effectiveness of the medications can be monitored. Discuss with her the availability of a self-medication programme so that she can take her drugs at times most suitable for her. Refer her to the ward pharmacist for education and implementation of self-medication if she so wishes.
4.	Restricted mobility	For her to feel less dependent on others	Refer her to the physiotherapist for assessment and provision of any necessary walking aids and splints. Ensure that she uses the aids correctly and apply splints if necessary. Make sure that her locker and bed table are within easy reach and accessible. Provide a chair of appropriate height to make rising easier. Refer her to the occupational therapist for assessment with a view to providing aids at home, e.g. raised toilet seat, high chair or ejector chair, trolley to transport articles about the house.
5.	Difficulty in maintaining her personal hygiene	For her to feel refreshed and comfortable and able to attend to her intimate areas independently	Refer her to the occupational therapist for assessment and provision of any necessary equipment, e.g. bath board, bath seat, sponge on a stick. Encourage her to be as independent as possible and assist whenever she needs it with washing and bathing. Ensure that she is able to maintain her hygiene after toileting.
6.	Anxiety about her admission to hospital due to her previous misdiagnosis	For her to feel more relaxed and at ease during her stay	Provide information about the routines, layout and services available. Ensure continuous nursing care by the same nurses. Allow her to express her fears and concerns. Allow unrestricted visiting by family and friends. Point out the facility of being able to receive calls on the trolley telephone. Encourage her active participation in her daily care. Keep her informed about tests being carried out and the result of these tests.
7.	Difficulty sleeping at night	To improve her rest and comfort during her stay	Ensure that she has enough pillows to be supported comfortably. Try to keep noise levels to a minimum. If possible turn off lights which might disturb her. Offer her a hot drink to settle and when she is awake in the night. Encourage her to talk about any worries in the night as long as it does not disturb other patients.

breathlessness and efforts to find a comfortable position. She avoids taking sedation as much as possible.

Mental attitude (dying) She expresses anxiety about her future and what else the disease might do to her. She feels that the medical staff do not always believe her symptoms.

Table 12.2 is a summary of Jane's care during her hospital stay.

ANKYLOSING SPONDYLITIS

The name of this disease derives from the Greek 'ankylos', meaning bent, and 'Spondylos', meaning vertebra. Ankylosing spondylitis was known in antiquity and there is evidence of it in Egyptian mummies (Berry et al 1983).

Incidence and distribution

Ankylosing spondylitis (AS) used to be regarded as predominantly affecting males but with recognition of differences in clinical presentation in females, the ratio is likely to be as low as 2 : 1 males to females. The frequency of AS is governed by geographical variations, indicating the racial incidence of the HLA B27 antigen (Hollingworth 1988).

Pathology

AS is a seronegative arthropathy – i.e. the rheumatoid factor is not present in the serum; 95% of individuals with AS have the histocompatibility antigen HLA B27.

The disease tends to cause ascending involvement of the spine, with inflammation of the insertion of part of the annulus fibrosus into the vertebral body leading to eventual fusion of the spinal joints due to new bone formation (see Fig. 12.3). Costovertebral joint inflammation leads to restricted chest expansion. Thoracic spine involvement can lead to a fixed dorsal kyphosis which makes forward vision possible only by hyperextending the neck. Up to 25% of patients

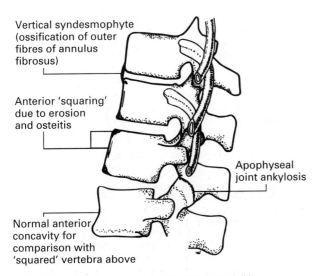

Vertical syndesmophyte (ossification of outer fibres of annulus fibrosus)

Anterior 'squaring' due to erosion and osteitis

Apophyseal joint ankylosis

Normal anterior concavity for comparison with 'squared' vertebra above

Fig. 12.3 Spinal changes in ankylosing spondylitis. (From Dieppe et al 1985, with permission.)

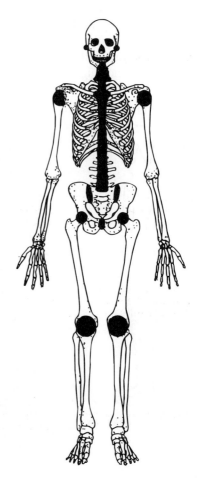

Fig. 12.4 Joint involvement in ankylosing spondylitis. (From Dieppe et al 1985, with permission.)

develop acute iritis which is associated with having the B27 antigen.

Women tend to present with peripheral arthritis and have less spinal involvement with a subsequently better prognosis. They are also prone to osteitis pubis if they have borne children (see Fig. 12.4).

AS can be complicated by aortitis and amyloidosis. Spondylitis associated with psoriasis and Reiter's syndrome can be misdiagnosed as AS.

Signs and symptoms

AS presents at around the age of 20 years with an insidious onset of pain and stiffness predominantly in the lumbosacral region. This is more evident in the morning and after resting. It is relieved by exercise but made worse by over-activity. Pain in the sacroiliac joints often radiates to the buttocks and thighs. Tiredness, weight

loss and low grade pyerxia are common symptoms of AS. Daily activities such as lifting and driving are made extremely difficult. Fixed flexion at the hips and knees causes the typical body flexion and bulging abdomen of the advanced AS sufferer (see Fig. 12.5).

Treatment

An exercise regimen is most important and ideally should be assessed and taught by a physiotherapist so that the individual patient can learn the exercises most appropriate for him. These exercises concentrate on extension and expansion, and the programme should be carried out twice a day, augmented by other regular exercises such as walking and swimming. Patients should be advised to have a firm mattress and to use only one pillow to give their spine good support and to encourage them to keep it as straight as possible. Pain and stiffness should be controlled

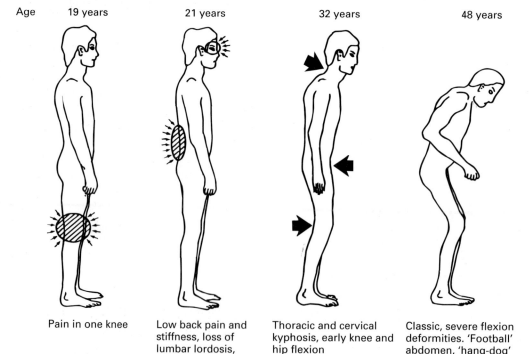

Age	19 years	21 years	32 years	48 years
	Pain in one knee	Low back pain and stiffness, loss of lumbar lordosis, attack of acute anterior uveitis	Thoracic and cervical kyphosis, early knee and hip flexion	Classic, severe flexion deformities. 'Football' abdomen, 'hang-dog' appearance, limited forward vision

Fig. 12.5 Classic progression of severe ankylosing spondylitis. (From Dieppe et al 1985, with permission.)

with non-steroidal anti-inflammatory drugs such as indomethacin.

Patients must be given a full explanation of the disease and be counselled by both medical and nursing staff on how to cope with any changes necessary at home and at work. They should be encouraged to involve their family because the cooperation of all concerned is vital for them to have a better understanding of the patient's needs. The occupational therapist and the social worker also should be involved at this stage because their advice on appliances, adaptations at home, services and benefits available can make the patient and his family feel more confident about the future.

As the disease becomes more advanced, surgery such as arthroplasty of the hips and/or shoulders might become necessary to allow the patient to maintain mobility and independence.

If these patients need to be admitted to hospital at any time, the nursing care should concentrate on maintaining their independence by referring them to other members of the multidisciplinary team for reassessment of their disabilities and needs.

If the patient is to be bed-bound for any reason – e.g. surgery – pressure area care should have a high priority due to the curvature of the spine; a pressure-relieving mattress may be required. Postoperative breathing exercises are also most important because of the patient's lack of chest expansion, predisposing him to chest infection.

GOUT

Gout is a systemic disease caused by the deposition of sodium waste in and around joints. It results from sustained elevation of blood uric acid levels (hyperuricaemia). Uric acid may accumulate within the joint to form tophi.

The disease is more common in men over the age of 40 years. It is rare for a premenopausal female to suffer from primary gout. A higher incidence is found in ethnic groups who have a high incidence of hyperuricaemia, such as the Maoris of New Zealand and other Polynesian races (Hart 1983).

Treatment

Acute attacks of gout are usually treated with non-steroidal anti-inflammatory drugs (NSAIDs) such as phenylbutazone 600 mg, with a gradual reduction over a few days, or indomethacin 150 mg, also gradually reduced over a few days.

Colchicine is another medication used to treat acute attacks; it is usually prescribed every 2 hours until the pain is relieved or until diarrhoea occurs. Local corticosteroid injection may have to be prescribed if the acute attack fails to respond to the oral medication.

Physical effects

The first attack usually affects one joint, namely the big toe. It becomes inflamed and very painful, often at night, and wakes the sufferer from his sleep. Fever is common.

Important aspects of the nursing care of the patient suffering from gout

As the patient is complaining of severe pain, it is important for the nurse to handle him with gentleness and quietness, taking extra care not to jolt the bed. The joint affected must be protected, i.e. if the big toe is affected a bed cradle should be used so that pressure from the bedclothes does not make it worse.

Medications must be given punctually, and the patient counselled on preventing further attacks by taking prescribed medications regularly. He should be advised to drink plenty of fluids to flush the urate through the kidneys. The importance of diet to control weight gain in order to maintain a low urate in the blood should be emphasized.

SCLERODERMA (PROGRESSIVE SYSTEMIC SCLEROSIS)

Scleroderma principally affects the skin; however, it may involve other organs such as the gastrointestinal tract, the heart, the kidneys and the lungs. In these cases it is termed progressive systemic sclerosis. Women are affected 3–4 times more often than men, in the age-group of 25–50 years (Morrow & Isenberg 1987).

In the early stages there may be inflammatory oedema and slight reddening but the long-term picture is of ischaemic atrophy and stiffening. Scleroderma is a term used for the skin lesion, which can be in plaques (morphes), distal (acrosclerosis or sclerodactyly, which implies involvement of hands and feet only), generalized or in 'sable cut' streaks (usually single).

Sclerodactyly is always associated with Raynaud's phenomenon and/or frank finger tip ischaemia. Early skin histology shows infiltration with lymphocytes around blood vessels. Later on there is dense fibrosis and loss of vessels.

The cause of scleroderma is unknown and it is often a progressive disease (see Table 12.3).

Presentation

An early symptom is an extreme sensitivity to cold (Raynaud's phenomenon) (see Table 12.3). The blood vessels constrict at times, and all it takes to trigger off the Raynaud's is for the sufferer to reach into the refrigerator. Another early symptom is swelling of the hands and feet, especially in the morning. Scleroderma also can cause joint inflammation. This may be accompanied by signs of pain, stiffness, swelling, warmth and tenderness. Muscle weakness can also occur.

Prognosis

Those suffering from a mild form of the disease may continue to lead a normal life. Progressive, severe forms lead to death from lung, heart or renal disease over a period of 5–10 years (Morrow & Isenberg 1987) (see Table 12.4).

Important aspects of the nursing care of patients suffering from scleroderma

As with other rheumatological conditions, education is an important aspect of nursing care. Patients will comply more easily with their treatment if they are involved in their own care.

Patients with Raynaud's phenomenon should be advised how to maintain good skin and to protect it from ulcerating. Patients should avoid exposure to cold by wearing suitable clothing and gloves, and should avoid strong detergents or other substances that irritate the skin. Other contributing factors which should be avoided include smoking and stress.

Patients with dysphagia should be advised about suitable drinks and foods, and told to eat slowly and chew food thoroughly. Drinking water will help soften foods. If reflux oesophagitis is present, the patient should be advised to eat small frequent meals and avoid drinking alcohol. It is also helpful not to lie flat but rather to sleep with the head resting on several pillows.

Table 12.3 Treatment of scleroderma

Systems affected	Treatment
Skin	drugs that may be used in the treatment of Raynaud's are prostacyclin infusion and a vasodilator; lubricant cream helps the dryness of the skin
Peripheral vessels (Raynaud's)	drugs as mentioned above; education on how to look after the skin (see care study on SLE)
Cardiac	pericarditis may respond to steroid therapy; coronary heart disease and congestive cardiac failure are treated with analgesia, diuretics and digoxin
Pulmonary	most rheumatologists use high doses of corticosteroid
Musculoskeletal	wasting and weakness of skeletal muscle may be helped by physiotherapy; tenosynovitis is treated by corticosteroid injection; arthralgia is controlled by non-steroidal anti-inflammatory drugs; myositis is treated with a combination of oral corticosteroids and immunosuppressive drugs such as azathioprine
Gastrointestinal	antacids, cimetidine and metoclopramide which stimulates the motility of the oesophagus can be effective
Renal	hypertension is treated by antihypertensive drugs; regular monitoring of plasma creatinine and urea are essential

Table 12.4 Physical effects of scleroderma

Dermatological	thickening and hardening of the skin; involvement of the face leads to a pinched, taut expression around the mouth
Peripheral vessels	Raynaud's phenomenon is present in 80% of patients with scleroderma; it is characterized by pallor followed by cyanosis of the extremities on exposure to cold; finger-tip tissue may be lost by major episodes of gangrene or by gradual atrophy starting with recurrent pitting of the finger pulp under the nail
Cardiac	pericarditis, pericardial effusion or cardiomyopathy
Pulmonary	pleural involvement is rare; if pulmonary fibrosis is present it causes dyspnoea; pulmonary hypertension may develop, resulting in cor pulmonale
Musculoskeletal	myositis; wasting and weakness of skeletal muscle which may be due to inflammatory changes; contracture of fingers, wrists, knees and elbows may occur due to the tightening of the skin and involvement of the tissues surrounding the joints
Gastrointestinal	oesophagitis; bleeding, ulceration and perforation; dysphagia due to diminished oesophageal peristalsis; dysphagia may result in aspiration of food into the bronchial tree causing pneumonia; mucostomia; hiatus hernia; inelasticity of the lips and cheeks may cause poor dental hygiene; incidence of dental caries is high; intubation during general anaesthetic can be a problem; large bowel hypomotility leads to constipation
Renal	involvement of the kidneys is rare but it is the most important cause of death in systemic sclerosis; hypertension
Nervous system	peripheral neuropathy; trigeminal neuralgia

Patients with a disfigurement will need psychological support and reassurance.

POLYMYALGIA RHEUMATICA

The term polymyalgia is derived from 'poly', meaning many, and 'myalgia', meaning painful muscles. The aetiology of polymyalgia rheumatica (PMR) is unknown. PMR usually occurs in those over 50 years of age, and it is more common in women than men in the ratio of 3 : 1. It may be associated with painful inflammation, especially of the blood vessels (arteries) of the skull; this is known as temporal arteritis (Currey 1980).

Treatment

Most patients respond to steroid therapy, the aim of which is to suppress symptoms. After a few weeks the dose may be reduced to the smallest possible amount; this may be guided by the result of ESR tests and the patient's progress.

Physical effects

Muscle stiffness and pain are worse in the morning and after exertion. The patient may have difficulty with the simplest activity such as dressing.

Loss of weight, general malaise and depression are the common complaints. Anaemia and low-grade pyrexia may also occur. If temporal arteritis is present, headaches are the main complaint.

Other symptoms that could be present are facial pain on chewing, tenderness and thickening of the temporal arteries and visual disturbance. The major complication of temporal arteritis is sudden blindness.

Important aspects of the nursing care of patients suffering from polymyalgia rheumatica

The aim of treatment is improvement of the patient's condition, mentally and physically.

Once the decision to give steroid therapy has been made, education of the patient and his family concerning the treatment is important. The dose, effects and side-effects of steroids should be explained. If available, a leaflet about steroid therapy should be given to the patient for future reference; the information in the leaflet should include details on when to take the tablets and who to contact in case of any problems. Patients should also carry a 'steroid card' in case of emergency.

SJÖGREN'S SYNDROME

Sjögren's syndrome can occur alone, or in

association with rheumatoid arthritis or other connective tissue diseases.

Incidence

Women are affected more frequently than men in a ratio of 9 : 1. Up to half of all patients with rheumatoid arthritis have Sjögren's syndrome and a third of patients with SLE are also affected.

Pathology

Sjögren's syndrome is typified by 'dry eye' or keratoconjunctivitis sicca. The mucosal surfaces of the lacrimal and salivary glands are progres-

sively destroyed, causing diminished or complete absence of secretions. Other organs and the musculoskeletal system can also be affected – e.g. the upper and lower respiratory tract, skin, stomach, vagina, lungs and muscles.

Signs and symptoms

Patients complain of fatigue, dry eyes, mouth and tongue. Hoarseness, dry nose, bronchitis, achlorhydria, dyspareunia, decreased sweating, pneumonitis and myositis are other examples of the effects of Sjögren's syndrome on organs and systems (Morrow & Isenberg 1987) (see Fig. 12.6).

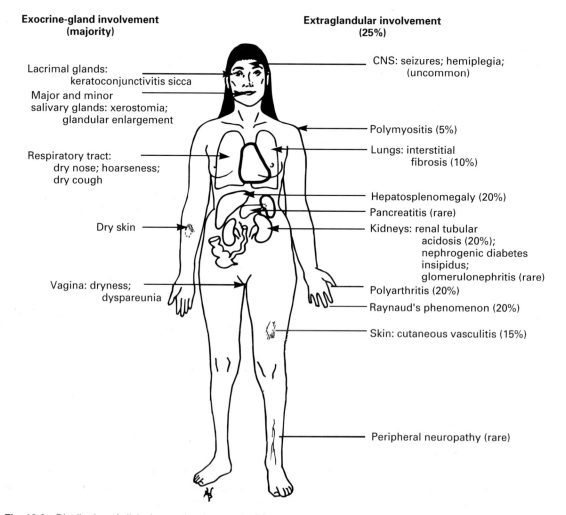

Fig. 12.6 Distribution of clinical organ involvement in Sjögren's syndrome. (From Dieppe et al 1985, with permission.)

Treatment

Sjögren's syndrome is usually a benign condition with treatment directed at symptomatic relief and prevention of damage to the eyes. Dry eyes are treated with methylcellulose eye drops, i.e. artificial tears. For dry mouth, patients are advised to increase their fluid intake and clean their teeth frequently; they are cautioned against the sucking of sweets containing sugar due to an increased susceptibility to dental caries. Patients should be advised to have regular dental check-ups.

Other symptoms of Sjögren's syndrome may require treatment with NSAIDs, corticosteroids or immunosuppressant drugs.

As Sjögren's syndrome is seen most commonly in association with another rheumatological disease, when the patient is in hospital with another disease the nursing assessment of the patient's needs or problems should take into account the patient's need to have drops instilled into his eyes and to have regular mouthcare. The patient should also be taught how to massage, or have massaged, his parotid glands before and after meals to encourage the production of saliva.

POLYMYOSITIS AND DERMATOMYOSITIS

Polymyositis is an inflammatory disease of muscle and is of unknown cause. The term dermatomyositis is used when the disease is accompanied by a characteristic rash: there is a heliotrope discoloration on the eyelids with a purple rash on the cheeks, forehead, shoulders, arms and upper chest (Berry et al 1983) (see Fig. 12.7).

Incidence

Polymyositis and dermatomyositis affect 8/100 000 of the population of Britain. People of all ages are affected but the disease usually peaks at the age of 50 years. Twice as many women as men are affected, especially when another connective tissue disease is present. Black people are affected more than Whites.

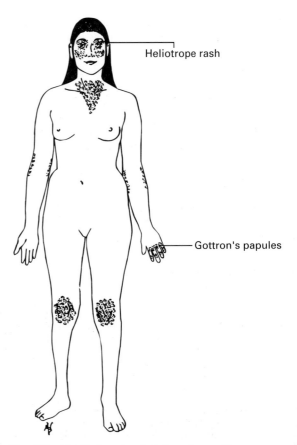

Fig. 12.7 Distribution of rash in dermatomyositis. (From Dieppe et al 1985, with permission.)

Pathology

Erythrocyte sedimentation rate (ESR) and serum gammaglobulin levels are raised in patients with myositis. Muscle biopsy shows that muscle fibres are abnormal; electromyography findings are also abnormal.

Clinical features

General malaise, loss of weight and pyrexia are common. Weakness and fatiguability of the proximal muscles, usually in the lower limbs at first, make climbing stairs and getting up out of a chair difficult. This progresses to the proximal muscles of the upper limbs, and brushing hair, hanging up washing and lifting articles off high shelves become difficult (Morrow & Isenberg 1987).

In the lower limb, the abductor muscles are affected more than the adductor muscles, and in the upper limb, the extensor muscles more than the flexors (Dick & Goodacre 1984). In some cases the muscles of the neck are involved, making the head feel heavy.

Muscle pain and tenderness are found usually only when there has been an acute onset of the disease; 40% of patients develop a transient, non-deforming, symmetrical arthritis affecting the fingers and wrists with occasional involvement of the elbows, shoulders and knees (Berry et al 1983). A positive rheumatoid factor is found in the blood in 50% of patients. Approximately 8% of cases are associated with underlying malignancy.

Treatment

The majority of patients with polymyositis and dermatomyositis can be treated, as outpatients, with corticosteroids. They may require immuno-suppressive drugs if corticosteroids fail or if prolonged treatment is necessary. Only those patients presenting with acute onset of myositis resulting in dysphagia or respiratory problems require admission to hospital for treatment. Exercise is most important to maximize the power of the affected muscles and to re-educate other muscles to cope with the extra burden. This may be carried out better in the formal setting of a physiotherapy department or hydrotherapy pool.

In the nursing assessment the individual's needs and problems which need to be high-lighted are those associated with respiratory difficulties and muscle weakness. Counselling should be offered to help the patient to under-stand the disease and to come to terms with it. Early referral to the physiotherapist, dietitian, occupational therapist and social worker is very important so that each can assess the patient and provide the treatment, aids to daily living and support appropriate to that patient.

REFERENCES

Berry H, Hamilton E, Goodwill J (eds) 1983 Rheumatology and rehabilitation. Croom Helm, London, p 34, 95
Currey H L F (ed) 1980 Mason & Currey's clinical rheumatology, 3rd edn. Pitman, London, p 120
Dick W, Goodacre J 1984 Introduction to clinical rheumatology, 2nd edn. Churchill Livingstone, Edinburgh, p 122
Dieppe P A, Doherty M, MacFarlane D et al 1985 Rheumatological medicine. Churchill Livingstone, Edinburgh
Hickling P, Golding J R 1984 An outline of rheumatology. Wright, Bristol, p 135
Hollingworth (ed) 1988 Mainsteam medicine – rheumatology. Heinemann, London
Morrow J, Isenberg D 1987 Autoimmune rheumatoid diseases. Blackwell Scientific, Oxford, p 49, 127, 257, 269, 337

FURTHER READING

Clark A, Allard L, Braybrooks B 1987 Rehabilitation in rheumatology – the team approach. Martin Dunitz, London
Dieppe et al 1985 Rheumatological medicine. Churchill Livingstone, Edinburgh
Hickling P, Golding J, 1984 An outline of rheumatology. Wright, Bristol
Mole J M H, Lee M 1987 Nursing care of rheumatic patients – principles and practice. Croom Helm, London
Panaye G S (ed) 1980 Essential rheumatology for nurses and therapists. Bailliere Tindall, London

USEFUL ADDRESSES

The Arthritis and Rheumatism Council
41 Eagle Street
London WC1R 4AR
Tel: 071–405–8575

The National Ankylosing Spondylitis Society
5 Grosvenor Crescent
London SW1X 7ER
Tel: 071–235–9585

British SLE Aid Group
25 Linden Crescent
Woodford Green
Essex

Lupus Group
Arthritis Care
5 Grosvenor Crescent
London SW1X 7ER
Tel: 071–235–0902

The Raynauds Association
112 Crewe Road
Alsager
Cheshire
Tel: 09363–2776

The Scleroderma Society
61 Sandpit Lane
St Albans
Herts
Tel: 0727–55054

Sexual and Personal Relationships of the Disabled (SPOD)
286 Camden Road
London N7 0BJ

RADAR
The Royal Association for Disability and Rehabilitation
25 Mortimer Street
London W1N 8AB
Tel: 071–637–5400

13

Bone tumours

Linda C. Russell

INTRODUCTION

This chapter describes the implications for an individual diagnosed as having a bone tumour. A brief description of the common types of tumours, their diagnosis and treatment is given. Finally, two case histories are presented to illuminate the specific nursing care required by individuals with a bone tumour. The first focuses on the problem-solving approach and nursing care of a young man undergoing limb salvage surgery, utilizing a metal endoprosthetic replacement; the second focuses on the effects of chemotherapy on a teenage girl.

For many people their worst fear is that of cancer; although great progress has been made over the years in the treatment of a number of malignancies, to many people cancer automatically means death.

Bone tumours are extremely rare and therefore many patients have multiple consultations prior to treatment – for example with the general practitioner, local orthopaedic consultant and/or oncology centre. Many people are treated at a local district general hospital as well as an oncology centre or a supraregional unit specializing in the treatment of primary bone malignancies, of which there are at present two in the country.

Multiple consultations take time; for the lucky ones this is a few weeks, for others many months. The reason for this delay is the difficulty in diagnosing bone tumours. The early symptoms of pain, which is often non-mechanical and worse at rest, followed by swelling, are well known, but there are many musculoskeletal aches and pains with which they can be confused, hence the diagnosis can be overlooked. The average time for an osteosarcoma to be diagnosed following the onset of symptoms is 3 months, and for Ewing's and chondrosarcoma almost a year (Grimer & Sneath 1990).

The nurse is very often in the unique position of being the first person to meet the patient and his relatives in the ward environment. It is essential to give them all a warm welcome and to familiarize them with their new surroundings. Careful consideration should be given as to where the patient is allocated a bed; for example, it would not be desirable to place an 18-year-old with a probable osteosarcoma next to someone of approximately the same age who is in hospital for terminal care.

The first objective is to provide a happy, friendly and inviting atmosphere on the ward. The nurse needs to build a relationship, based on trust, with both the patient and the family. The patient's knowledge of his condition, its prognosis and treatment will vary from person to person, but the nurse should try to allay his many fears. It must be stressed that there are various types of bone growth, both benign and malignant, and until thorough investigations and scans have been carried out a firm diagnosis cannot be made. Some patients will be only too willing to relate their life history; others are more reluctant. Those receiving cytotoxic drug therapy will be bald. Such problems tend to arise on oncological wards or specialized units more than on general orthopaedic wards, but they must be borne in mind when these patients are admitted.

In order to provide a systematic approach to nursing care the nurse needs to have a wide knowledge of the different types of tumour and their treatment. She must also have a full understanding of all investigations and why they are necessary. It should be remembered that it is always the nurse who forms the closest relationship with the patient and his family.

BENIGN TUMOURS OF BONE

Table 13.1 shows a classification of bone and soft tissue tumours.

Table 13.1 A classification of bone and soft tissue tumours

Tissue of origin	Benign	Malignant
Bone	osteoma	osteosarcoma
Cartilage	chondroma	chondrosarcoma
Fat	lipoma	liposarcoma
Fibrous tissue	fibroma	fibrosarcoma
Histiocytic	—	malignant fibrous histiocytoma
Muscle	myoma	leiomyosarcoma (smooth muscle) rhabdomyosarcoma (striated muscle)
Nerve	neurofibroma schwannoma	neurofibrosarcoma malignant schwannoma
Unknown	giant cell tumour	giant cell tumour Ewing's sarcoma

Osteoma

An osteoma is an innocent new growth arising from an osteoblast. It is uncommon, usually occurring in a long or flat bone as well as in the skull bones. It produces a small, rounded prominence upon the surface of the bone (Fig. 13.1), and may be composed of either hard, compact bone (ivory osteoma) or spongy bone (cancellous osteoma). It may be visible and palpable but

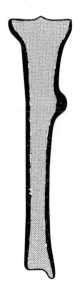

Fig. 13.1 Osteoma; it may occur on any bone, including those of the skull. (From Adams 1990, with permission.)

is otherwise symptom-free unless it involves the ear.

Treatment

It can be excised if symptoms necessitate this.

Osteochondroma

Osteochondroma, the most common benign tumour, which may also be called exostosis, is composed of a cartilage cap with underlying bone trabeculae. It protrudes from the cortex of bone, usually on a stalk, and originates from the growing epiphyseal cartilage plate. It will continue to grow until the cessation of skeletal growth. The growth can be single or multiple (the latter is known as diaphyseal aclasis), and produces a hard swelling near the joint. In severe cases it will interfere with skeletal growth, causing the patient to be deformed or dwarfed. Malignant change occurs in about 10% of patients with diaphyseal aclasia. Any increase in size of an osteochondroma after skeletal growth has stopped should be investigated to exclude malignancy (Fig. 13.2).

Treatment

Simple excision can be performed if the lump is symptomatic.

Chondroma

A chondroma is a new growth composed of cartilage cells, arising from the epiphyseal cartilage. There are two types:

1. Ecchondroma – the tumour bulges outwards; commonly found in flat bones, e.g. the ileum
2. Enchondroma – growth within the bone; commonest sites affected are the hands and feet (Fig. 13.3).

Pathological fracture is common because as the tumour expands the cortex is thinned.

Chondromata of the major long bones, caused by the failure of columns of epiphyseal cartilage to ossify, is referred to as Ollier's disease or dyschondroplasia.

A solitary chondroma can (rarely) undergo malignant changes and become a chondrosarcoma. This, however, usually occurs where major bones are affected, or in Ollier's disease.

Treatment

An ecchondroma can be surgically removed by simple excision, whereas an enchondroma will

Fig. 13.2 Osteochondromas; originating at the growth cartilage, they have migrated away from it with growth of the bone. Each is capped by cartilage. (From Adams 1990, with permission.)

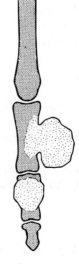

Fig. 13.3 Chondroma of two types: ecchondroma on proximal phalanx; enchondroma in middle phalanx. (From Adams 1990, with permission.)

need to be curetted. Following a curettage, conventional treatment would involve filling the resulting cavity with bone graft chips from the iliac crests. However, there is a new school of thought which states that there is no need to graft, for a number of reasons:

1. The graft is dead bone because it has no blood supply, and it does not add to the mechanical strength of the bone. Therefore, the patient will still need to be non-weight-bearing as no immediate strengthening is provided by the bone grafting.

2. For a large cavity, multiple donor sites will be needed. The donor site wound can be extremely painful; for example, the patient is often not able to wear a belt afterwards.

3. If there is no second incision, blood loss, haematoma formation and infection will all be reduced.

4. If the cavity is filled with bone chips this can obscure any recurrence.

Osteoclastoma (giant cell tumour)

This is an osteolytic tumour in the epiphysis of bone. It often produces expansion of the bone and can extend into the soft tissue. It commonly affects 20- to 40-year-olds, but is rare in patients whose epiphyseal plate is present. It affects the ends of long bones, and almost half the cases occur around the knee (Malcolm 1987). The tumour is very destructive and pathological fracture is common. The tumour extends up to the articular cartilage. A very thin outer shell is filled with a maroon-coloured vascular tissue with areas of haemorrhage and necrosis. It can be distinguished from a simple cyst by the age of the patient and the solid contents.

The symptoms experienced by the patient are pain and swelling; a tender, bony swelling can often be palpated (Fig. 13.4).

Treatment

Excision is possible if the tumour occurs in a bone that can be dispensed with, e.g. fibula or clavicle. Curettage and grafting have been the

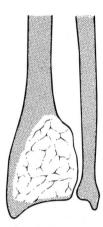

Fig. 13.4 Osteoclastoma (giant cell tumour) extending close up to the joint surface. (From Adams 1990, with permission.)

treatment of choice, although the tumour has a high rate of recurrence. If curettage is not possible, excision and implantation of a metal prosthesis is the most likely treatment (Fig. 13.5).

MALIGNANT TUMOURS OF BONE

Osteosarcoma

Epidemiology

Osteosarcoma is the second most common primary bone tumour, affecting three cases per million of the population (Price & Jeffree 1973). There are two main incidence peaks, the principal one during the second decade and a second, smaller, peak in late adult life. It is more common in males than females in the ratio 2 : 1.

Aetiology

There are no definite causes of bone tumours. However, there is an increased incidence for those who have been exposed to therapeutic irradiation. This can occur when radiotherapy has been used to treat a benign or malignant tumour within bone, or after therapy of an extraosseous tumour, e.g. carcinoma of the cervix, in which bone is irradiated within the treatment field.

In the older age range osteosarcoma often occurs secondary to Paget's disease.

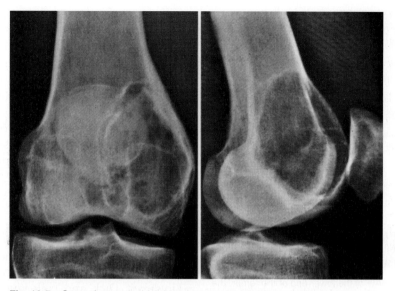

Fig. 13.5   Osteoclastoma which has destroyed most of one femoral condyle; it extends close up to the joint surface. (From Adams 1990, with permission.)

Site of origin

In most cases, osteosarcoma arises in the metaphysis of long bones, although it does occasionally originate in the diaphysis or epiphysis. The distal femur and proximal tibia are the most common sites, although many others can be affected, i.e. the proximal humerus, fibula, jaw, pelvis, spine, hands and feet (Fig. 13.6).

Signs and symptoms

Pain   At the beginning, there is very often a slight and intermittent pain which results from weakening of the bone, elevation of the periosteum by the tumour and possible minute stress fractures. The pain worsens as the tumour grows in size, causing soft tissue extension and possible nerve compression.

Swelling   This occurs as a result of soft tissue involvement. However, many patients do not complain of swelling as the metaphyseal masses are obscured by soft tissue. For very large masses there may be the added complication of venous engorgement.

Weight loss, pallor, fever and anorexia are all characteristic signs of advanced disease with multiple metastases.

Radiographic features

Radiographically, irregular destruction of the metaphysis with new bone formation can be seen. The cortex looks as if it has 'burst open' in multiple places. When new bone formation is seen at the boundary of the tumour under the

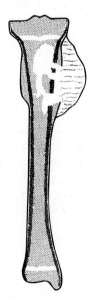

Fig. 13.6   Osteosarcoma, arising in the metaphysis and destroying the bone. (From Adams 1990, with permission.)

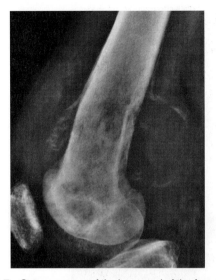

Fig. 13.7 Osteosarcoma of the lower end of the femur, the most common site of these tumours. The tumour has destroyed much of the lower end of the femur and has burst through the cortex into the soft tissues. (From Adams 1990, with permission.)

corners of raised periosteum, this is known as 'Codman's triangle' (Fig. 13.7).

Treatment

The introduction of adjuvant chemotherapy has made a more humane approach to surgery possible. Many centres around the world are now carrying out limb salvage techniques either by insertion of a metal endoprosthetic replacement or an allograft of bone, instead of amputation.

The role of surgery is to remove completely the tumour with a surrounding cuff of normal tissue of sufficient dimensions to prevent any recurrence. Local recurrence is dependent on the size of the margin resection and the grade of tumour. In the past it was thought that if amputation was the surgery of choice then recurrence would be nil, but this was found not to be so (Sweetnam 1973).

Limb salvage can be successful only if there can be a complete resection of the tumour and a resultant fully functional limb. There are, of course, instances in which salvage is not possible and the patient will need an amputation.

Although today there are very sophisticated scanning techniques, it is not until the tumour is exposed during an operation that the full extent of spread can be seen; hence, any patient needing an endoprosthetic replacement will need to sign a consent form for an amputation before going into surgery.

Endoprosthetic replacements can be custom-made for each patient, a process which takes 3 or 4 weeks. During this time the patient will receive preparative chemotherapy.

Allografts have been less widely used than endoprostheses because of the need to have a large bone bank available. One of the advantages of allografts is that they tend to improve with age, whereas if an endoprosthesis is used, there is an increased incidence of problems with time. However, Dick and colleagues (1985) reported a high rate of complications, including skin necrosis, wound infections, allograft reabsorption, fractures and non-union, in all patients receiving postoperative chemotherapy. Despite this, 60% of the survivors were judged to have a good or excellent result, which was encouraging and emphasized the need for further research and experience in this field.

Adjuvant chemotherapy is used both pre- and postoperatively. Usually three courses are given preoperatively. This shrinks the tumour and makes it less vascular and hence easier to remove surgically. Postoperative courses are given as a safeguard, so that cells left at the site of surgery are killed as are, it is hoped, any cells which have seeded elsewhere. The most common sites for metastases are the lungs and other bones (Fig. 13.8).

Chondrosarcoma

A chondrosarcoma is a malignant tumour which is derived from cartilage cells. It is slower growing than an osteosarcoma and therefore less likely to metastasize early, which means a better prognosis for the patient. It affects an older age range (40–60 years) and is more common in central sites of the body, e.g. pelvis, ribs and proximal ends of long bones. Chondrosarco-

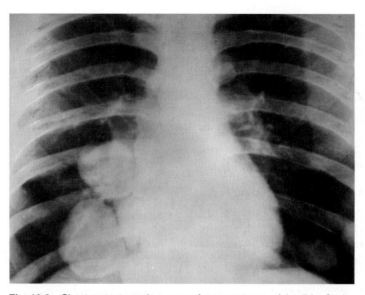

Fig. 13.8 Chest metastases in a case of osteosarcoma of the tibia. Such metastases are the usual cause of death. (From Adams 1990, with permission.)

mas can be subdivided into central/medullary and peripheral/juxtacortical according to the apparent site of origin.

Radiographically a medullary tumour shows as an erosion of the bone and may break through the cortex; a peripheral chondrosarcoma will show as a shadow in the soft tissue which grows away from the bone.

The tumour presents with pain and local swelling. The treatment of choice is excision and an endoprosthetic replacement, or amputation if the tumour is very extensive. This type of tumour shows little response to either chemotherapy or radiotherapy, although the latter can be used in palliative treatment.

Ewing's sarcoma

A Ewing's sarcoma is a highly malignant tumour of round cells of unknown histogenesis. It affects a young age group (5–20 years).

This tumour arises in the diaphysis rather than the metaphysis of bones. The most common sites affected are the femur and pelvis, although it can develop in any bones, including the skull (Fig. 13.9).

As with most bone tumours, the symptoms are pain and localized swelling. This tumour grows rapidly and it is not uncommon to have metastases on diagnosis. It spreads to other bones and to the lungs.

The patient's erythrocyte sedimentation rate

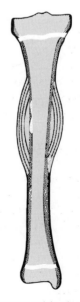

Fig. 13.9 Ewing's sarcoma arising in the diaphysis. (From Adams 1990, with permission.)

and white cell count may be raised and he may also present with general malaise, weight loss and pyrexia. The risk of pathological fracture is low except when a patient has received previous radiation.

Until approximately 10 years ago this tumour was nearly always fatal, but with the introduction of combination chemotherapy and radiotherapy the prognosis for these patients has improved considerably; the 5-year survival rate is 45–50%.

Treatment of a Ewing's tumour is the same as for an osteosarcoma but with the use of different chemotherapy regimens and with radiotherapy as an adjuvant to surgery if the margins of excision are not clear.

Multiple myeloma

This is a fatal malignant condition of bone marrow. It is characterized by multiple foci of plasma cells in the red bone marrow. It is disseminated though the skeleton via the blood stream and affects bones in which red bone marrow is abundant (Fig. 13.10). Plasma cells normally produce protein antibodies and in myelomatosis large quantities of protein can be detected in blood and urine.

The main symptom suffered by the patient is pain, which is widespread and characterized as a dull ache. The risk of a pathological fracture is high, particularly in the spine due to vertebral body collapse. Bone marrow destruction also leads to severe anaemia.

Investigations include Bence-Jones protein, blood samples for raised erythrocyte sedimentation rate, raised gamma globulin and myeloma band visible on electrophoresis. Sternal bone marrow puncture will confirm a rise in plasma cells.

The prognosis for these patients is poor, with no curative treatment. Chemotherapy will prolong life and radiotherapy can be given to local lesions to control pain.

Bone metastases

Metastasis is the term used to describe a secondary deposit of tumour (Fig. 13.11). If a primary breast cancer spreads to the bone, the tumour cells found in that bone will be breast cancer cells. Therefore, the treatment given to the secondary will be breast cancer treatment. Most

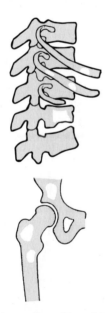

Fig. 13.10 Multiple myeloma. (From Adams 1990, with permission.)

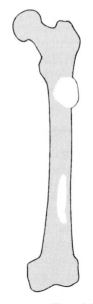

Fig. 13.11 Bone metastases. (From Adams 1990, with permission.)

cancers spread to distant areas by being transported in the blood stream. Because of this the bones which are prone to develop metastases are those that contain vascular marrow, e.g. vertebral bodies, ribs, pelvis and upper ends of the humerus and femur.

The tumours which commonly metastasize to bone are breast, prostate, lung, thyroid and kidney tumours.

Bone metastases can be very painful because sensory nerve endings are found in the periosteum. The pain experienced by these patients is very intense and the most effective treatment is palliative radiotherapy.

Metastases cause other potential problems. The risk of a pathological fracture is high. It can be treated by local splinting, internal fixation or a prosthesis.

Hypercalcaemia may develop when large amounts of calcium are released into the blood. Calcium is required to maintain the correct level of neuromuscular excitability. If levels become too high, messages sent by nerves to muscle will stop and the muscles will cease to function. Calcium levels can be lowered by prescribing drugs such as steroids or diphosphorates.

Metastatic spread is diagnosed by a bone scan and the main aim of treatment is to keep the patient comfortable and pain-free during the last stages of his life. This may require surgical intervention to treat pathological fractures or to prevent them.

INVESTIGATIONS AND DIAGNOSIS

Confirmation of a clinical diagnosis following thorough physical examination and history-taking is usually made by X-ray, which should show the early radiographic features described earlier in the chapter.

Computerized tomography (CT scanning)

A CT scan is an automated X-ray using a computerized image processor which produces cross-sectional images of any part of the body. A large number of very fine, low-level pulsed X-ray beams are used as probes. A xenon detector on the opposite side of the patient measures how much of each X-ray beam is transmitted through the body. To make an image of a particular slice of the body the pulsing X-ray source and the detector are rotated around the patient. The scan provides images of slices through the affected bone, giving a detailed examination of bone and the surrounding tissues, as the scan can discriminate between the densities of different tissues. This is primarily a non-invasive procedure, although contrast medium can be injected intravenously to enhance the scan. It is important to scan both the affected area and the chest, the latter to exclude chest metastases.

It is essential to explain to the patient both the procedure and the reasons why the scan is important; these are, to obtain a more detailed image of the size of the tumour and to check for spread of the disease to the lungs.

The scan is painless provided that the patient can lie flat and still in the tunnel of the machine. If pain prevents this, analgesia must be given prior to scanning.

Magnetic resonance imaging (MRI scanning)

MRI is a non-invasive diagnostic examination that uses a magnetic field and radio waves to depict the hydrogen density of tissues in the body. The image differentiates between tissues of differing hydrogen content (Zubay 1988).

MRI is more sensitive than CT scanning in diseases associated with increased water content, e.g. tumours, disc disease and cerebrovascular accidents. Images are produced over three planes: transverse axial (top to bottom), coronal (back to front) and sagittal (left to right).

Cortical bone lacks hydrogen atoms, thus making it possible to distinguish bone from soft tissue and bone marrow.

Visualization of the extent of soft tissue tumours, in addition to characterizing their histology (fatty tumours versus vascular tumours) and staging, is another application of MRI. It can be used in following the post-treatment effects of radiation/chemotherapy (Hendee & Davis 1985, Helms et al 1984).

The introduction of MRI is yet another major breakthrough in the diagnosis of malignant diseases. However, as with many scanners, it is expensive and at the present time not available at most hospitals.

The scanning process takes about an hour and the patient must be able to lie supine and very still; as the scan in each plane lasts 20 minutes there are opportunities to stretch and rest. Consideration should be given as to whether an analgesic or sedative should be given prior to the scan.

The patient will need no injection for the scan and it will be a painless procedure. As with any X-ray-type procedure a hospital gown will be needed and the patient must remove all jewellery, false teeth which contain metal, and any hearing aid, as any metal may alter the magnetic field and thus distort the image.

Contraindications

The following contraindications should be noted:

- Pregnancy
- Body size: maximum 136 kg or 52-inch girth
- Ferromagnetic bodies (e.g. iron, nickel and cobalt) – includes metal implants and prostheses
- Electronic implants (e.g. pacemakers)
- Patients requiring life support, unless they can be disconnected from oxygen and intravenous therapy for up to an hour.

Bone scan

A bone scan is a procedure which involves the intravenous administration of a radionuclide. Technetium-99m is the isotope of choice; it is labelled with a phosphate complex having an affinity for bone tissue.

Most of the total amount of radionuclide trapped by the skeleton will be taken up within the first 10 minutes. As the amount left in the

bloodstream will be quite high, the patient must be encouraged to drink at least 1 litre of fluid (e.g. water) to produce diuresis. Frequent visits to the toilet will reduce both the retained radioactivity in the bloodstream and the accumulated radiation dose to the bladder.

After a wait of at least 2 hours the examination can begin. The length of time this takes can vary from about 30 minutes to over an hour, the time depending on both the type of machine used and the number of images taken. Each image can take up to 6 minutes to acquire.

The film produced will be of the small X-ray type outlining the skeleton (Fig. 13.12). The images show the differential uptake of the radionuclide in bone tissue which is related directly to the bone's blood supply and level of turnover. Those areas, which have a richer blood supply and increased bone turnover, such as a bone tumour or the femoral epiphyses of a child, will accumulate more radionuclide, and areas such as the skull and the femoral shaft will accumulate less. In the case of the bone tumour this appears as an abnormal 'hot spot' and will probably be asymmetrical. Conversely, the epiphyseal 'hot spot' is both normal and symmetrical. Some bone tumours can, rarely, show as 'cold spots' – that is, areas of uptake less than normal bone.

There is no special physical preparation of the patient for the scan, but a full explanation of the procedure will help to put the patient at ease and reduce his fears. The application of a local anaesthetic prior to the radionuclide injection will reduce pain, and sedation can be given if necessary.

Following the scan the patient's excreta and blood will remain radioactive for about 24 hours. Any spills involving these will need to be dealt with carefully. Guidelines giving detailed procedures which must be adhered to will exist for each Local Health Authority.

Biopsy

The biopsy is the most important aspect of diagnosis. It is essential for radiographic exami-

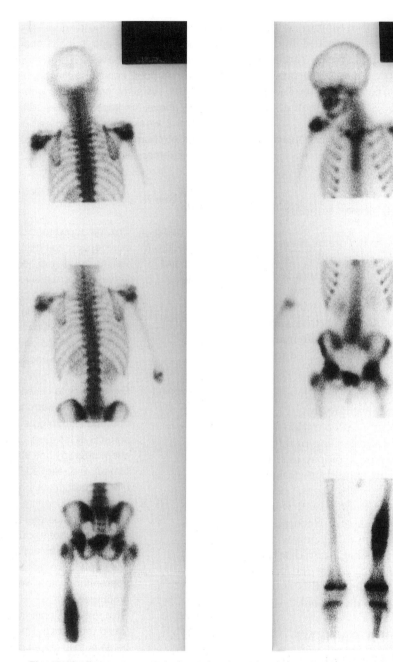

Fig. 13.12 Bone scan, anterior/posterior views showing marked increased uptake of isotope in relation to the mid-shaft of the left femur. No other area of abnormal skeleton activity identified.

nations to be carried out prior to biopsy for two reasons:

1. Difficulty in interpreting X-rays after biopsy

2. X-rays are required when planning how to carry out the biopsy.

The aim of a biopsy is to obtain an adequate and

representative sample of the tumour without producing complications which could interfere with subsequent treatment. Extreme care must be taken by the surgeon when performing an open biopsy so that, as far as possible, no un-involved compartment is contaminated with tumour cells.

The following types of biopsy are currently undertaken:

- Excision biopsy – tumour completely removed
- Incision biopsy – small piece of tumour removed
- Needle/core biopsy – small core of affected tissue obtained by a needle or drill
- Clearance biopsy – a small core of unaffected bone is taken either above or below the tumour. This is used to gauge the extent of spread along the bone. The aim is to ensure total removal of the tumour with safe margins so that the endoprosthesis will be fitted into healthy bone.

A full explanation of the operation is given to the patient before he signs a consent form.

Little specific preoperative preparation is re-quired, except shaving and cleansing of the skin if needed. The results of a bone biopsy may take 7–10 days to confirm. This should be explained prior to surgery.

Taking a sample of the tumour will weaken the bone, increasing the risk of a fracture. The patient in many instances will be non-weight-bearing on crutches. If possible, early discharge from hospital is encouraged, whilst the patient and family await the results, as this will be psychologically beneficial to the patient.

NURSING CARE OF A PATIENT UNDERGOING AN ENDOPROSTHETIC REPLACEMENT

Case study 1

Initial nursing assessment

David, a 24-year-old miner, has been admitted for endoprosthetic replacement of his right femur. He is accompanied by his wife and 2-year-old daughter. He has not worked since the diagnosis of osteosarcoma was made 12 weeks ago, but has been reallocated to an office job when he is fit. Throughout his life David has been in good health, so his diagnosis came as a bombshell. His symptoms started with pain and swell-ing just above his knee. He was referred and diag-nosed in 2 weeks, and up to now he has had three courses of chemotherapy. His pain is now controlled on Coproxamol 4-hourly.

David's problem	Nursing intervention
Fear of being separated from his wife and daughter	Provide accommodation on site for both; encourage full use of open visiting hours and help David to leave the ward environment to be with them. His wife can assist with his basic needs such as washing and dressing. Involve the social worker for advice on any benefits and travel allowances they may be entitled to.
Fear of losing his leg	Explain fully to David why he must sign a consent form for both operations; reinforce the positive aspects of his care, i.e. chemotherapy has shrunk the tumour and relieved his pain; show him the prosthesis and how it works; introduce him to another patient who has had the same surgery. Do not exclude the possibility of amputation. Let him talk through his fears. If appropriate, show him a video on amputees.
Pain and immobility	Give regular Coproxamol p.r.n. as David requests it. Encourage him to be as mobile as possible, non-weight-bearing on his crutches. Physiotherapist to visit prior to surgery to discuss exercises and how quickly after surgery he will be able to get up.
Fear of the actual operation	Allow David to discuss his fears. Explain all procedures and the preoperative preparation he will

require. Introduce him to the anaesthetist and recovery nurse so that he can question them too.

Post-surgery problems

Pain in his right leg	Intravenous Omnopon via a pump for 24 hours; intramuscular Omnopon p.r.n. progressing to oral analgesia. Position David comfortably in bed, well supported on pillows. Encourage plenty of rest and relaxation.
Immobility due to surgery	David will be on bedrest for 2 days, so that he stays in a neutral position. Gentle knee flexion, abduction and adduction exercises using a sliding board will be supervised by the physiotherapist from day 2; 48 hours after the operation David can begin mobilizing, partial weight-bearing with crutches. Hyperextension of the knee must be taught, as his quadriceps are still weak. This means 'locking' his knee back when putting weight through it. By 2 weeks after surgery he will be full weight-bearing on two sticks. Straight leg raising can be attempted at 2 days (success usually after about 1 week). The nurse should also supervise and encourage mobility alongside the physiotherapist. Prior to discharge David should be walking well unsupervised with two sticks. He should be able to straight leg raise and get up and down stairs.
Potential failure of his wound to heal	Remove Redivac drain 48 hours post-operation. Explain that the wound is closed with dissolvable sutures and the skin with an Opsite dressing. Observe the wound for any oozing and signs of infection. Make 4-hourly temperature recordings. Soak off Opsite dressing in the bath or shower 2 weeks after surgery, when the wound should be healed and dry. Provide a letter outlining infection risks and the need for antibiotic therapy with a contact number.
Difficulties of continuing rehabilitation at home	Advise David to be up and about as his health and strength allow him. Give him a contact phone number on discharge. Physiotherapist will give him a list of exercises to be practised at home. He must not lift heavy weights, jump, twist or play any sports, except swimming or cycling. He will be readmitted 6 weeks after surgery for 1 week of intensive physiotherapy.

Preoperative preparation

The psychological preparation of these patients for surgery is more complex than their physical preparation. Some patients will have waited for as long as 3 months for surgery, during which time they may have been non-weight-bearing on crutches, trying to make the best of their life, with constant hospital visits for chemotherapy.

The patient's first hurdle is to come to terms with signing the consent form, which they are required to do for either a prosthesis or an amputation. This is necessary because until the surgeon has exposed the tumour, he cannot be certain that he can perform the replacement surgery, and an amputation may be required. Even with the most sophisticated scans there may still be unforeseen problems, as discussed earlier in the chapter.

The question of when to tell the patient about the possibility of an amputation is controversial. Some will advocate that the patient be informed when the diagnosis is confirmed and the plan of treatment is discussed. Others feel that the patient and family have enough to contend with at this time – the patient's cancer, his fear of dying, chemotherapy and radiotherapy – which can give the patient a negative frame of mind, and that limb preservation surgery in the future gives him a goal towards which to work. For the unlucky ones for whom limb preservation fails, the nursing implications of caring for an amputee who is not adequately prepared for his altered body image are immense.

Each endoprosthesis is made to measure for the individual. This is done by taking measured X-rays called protocol films, which are sent to the bioengineer.

The operation and postoperative recovery period must be discussed with the patient and relatives. This should include a visit from the nurse, who will explain what lines and drains the patient may have on waking up, and from the anaesthetist to discuss premedication, night sedation and the method of anaesthesia. The emotional preparation is just as important as the physical and the nurse is the key provider of this (see Ch. 17).

Physically the patient must be infection-free and his skin in good condition. A dental check is made and any oral sepsis eliminated. The patient and relatives will benefit from their mutual involvement in the preoperative preparation and from the relatives being able to accompany the patient to theatre.

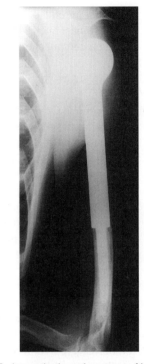

Fig. 13.13 Endoprosthetic replacement of left proximal humerus.

Postoperative care

The postoperative recovery time is relatively short. The patient will be home 2 or 3 weeks after surgery if the recovery period is free of complications. An endoprosthetic replacement in the upper limb will require an even shorter stay in hospital (Figs 13.13 and 13.14).

The priorities of postoperative management for the nurse are pain control, mobility and wound care of the patient.

Pain

Removal of the tumour will have eliminated the patient's intense pain, especially the patient with a pathological fracture. He will still experience varying degrees of pain but this can be controlled with opiates progressing to oral analgesia. It is important to keep the patient pain-free so that he can tolerate physiotherapy.

Mobility

The aim of limb salvage surgery is to provide

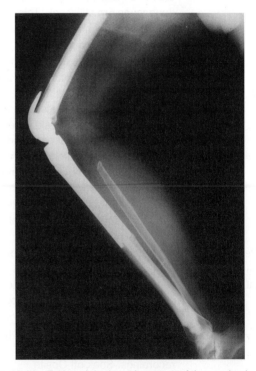

Fig. 13.14 Endoprosthetic replacement of the proximal tibia, lateral view.

the patient with a fully functional limb. Early mobilization is one of the principal priorities of postoperative care. Lower limb surgery patients will be slightly restricted until their drains are removed at 48 hours, after which they will be mobilized, partial to full weight-bearing with crutches. For proximal femoral replacements 2 weeks' bedrest is advised. This is necessary as the muscles cannot be reattached to the prosthesis but are sewn to each other. Bedrest will allow healing to take place and the patient to regain control of the limb. The leg tends to fall into external rotation and the nurse must ensure that it is kept in a neutral position with the aid of a knee flexion piece and sandbags. The principles of nursing care for these patients are the same as for a total hip replacement. It is the responsibility of the nurse to ensure that the patient is fully aware of the prescribed limitations imposed on him by hospital staff and the reasons for maintaining them.

The patient receiving an endoprosthesis of the upper limb is able to ambulate relatively quickly. His arm is immobilized in a sling and gentle physiotherapy is begun. Early mobilization is advocated for all patients but intensive physiotherapy is not started until 6 weeks post-surgery, by which time the patient will have left hospital. The patient is readmitted for a week's stay which includes gym sessions twice daily and hydrotherapy. This admission, although it is hard work, is relatively pressure-free and provides time for patients to relax mentally. Many patients say chemotherapy is more bearable during this time, because they are more active between treatments; some of them even go back to work part-time.

Wound care

A vacuum drain will be in situ for a minimum of 48 hours. Opsite can be used for wound closure in preference to skin sutures. This has the following advantages: it allows maximum observation as the whole wound is visible; a cosmetically more acceptable result is achieved; and the patient is happier as the scar is less noticeable.

Strict asepsis is essential and all nursing interventions to prevent infection are initiated. Intravenous antibiotic cover is required if infection is suspected. If infection does occur the prosthesis can become loose and may need revising, or, at worst, the limb may have to be amputated.

On discharge, advice is given regarding the need for antibiotic cover for any systemic infections or prophylactically for dental treatment and surgery.

PREPARATION FOR CHEMOTHERAPY
Case study 2

Initial nursing assessment

Julie, an 18-year-old, has been admitted for her first dose of chemotherapy. Biopsy results have confirmed an osteosarcoma of her proximal tibia. Julie has agreed to take part in a trial and is to receive six courses of chemotherapy at 3-weekly intervals. She is accompanied by her father as her mum has to look after her younger sisters. Julie is waiting for her 'A' level results and hopes to go to university to study English. She enjoys swimming, reading, fashion and socializing with her friends.

Julie's main worry on admission was that she would be bald when she left the ward in 4 days' time. Reassurance was given that although her hair would fall out, it would not happen overnight. It had been arranged that the hairdresser would visit and help Julie to choose a wig which she would be able to take home. Being a follower of fashion she had already discussed other alternatives, for example hats, scarves and turbans, with her friends.

Hospital visiting was not restricted except by Julie herself. Her dad was with her constantly and they both wanted to be independent and control as much of the care as possible. This was encouraged by allowing them to fill in the oral section of the fluid balance chart, the importance of which was discussed. They were both happy for Dad to help with the washing, dressing and bed pans. This posed few problems; it was explained that many of the drugs used were carcinogenic, hence the importance of following the safe handling of cytotoxic drugs policy. (Each district should have its own guidelines formulated from the regional policy.) For them, this meant Dad wearing the gloves and aprons provided when handling bed pans or vomit bowls. Julie's name was written on them and the nurses carried out the necessary tests and measurements on them.

Chemotherapy

Before Julie was given cisplatinum and doxorubicin she was hydrated with 3 litres over 6 hours of a saline solution with added potassium, magnesium and calcium – the electrolytes which would be lost through excessive urine output. Fluid was also given continuously so that Julie didn't have to bother with eating or drinking if she was feeling sick. Unfortunately some patients are very nauseated even if antiemetics are given.

Generally, the next part of the treatment, siting the cannula, is considered by many patients to be the worst. Some treatment centres will use central lines but this is not advocated by all because of the increased incidence of infection. Time should be spent on choosing a vein as doxorubicin is a vesicant drug which can easily cause phlebitis and extravasation (Feldstein 1986). Nurses working in oncology units are more experienced in cannulation of these patients, hence the necessity for the extended nursing role. The patient will be more at ease with someone they know and trust. Many patients fear admission for chemotherapy for a number of reasons, so if they can start their treatment immediately, it will be psychologically beneficial for them.

Throughout Julie's course of treatment the nurse closely observed the cannula site for signs of phlebitis. An emergency pack for the treatment of extravasation was close at hand should it be needed.

Once the chemotherapy has started the main problem for a patient is boredom. Julie was non-weight-bearing on crutches, making it impossible for her to get up and walk, but she could sit out in a chair or wheelchair. Her dad watched television and played cards with her and this helped to take her mind off the treatment and its possible side-effects. Distraction techniques often help prevent nausea and vomiting and time passes more quickly.

On completion of treatment Julie was given a contact telephone number which could be used 24 hours a day. It is more effective to encourage the family to phone if they have any problems at home rather than give them a long list of the side-effects

Julie might experience. Blood forms are also given for postchemotherapy checks. The white cell count is most important, in order to monitor neutropenia. Julie will swing from feeling ill to feeling well to feeling ill again, when her white cell count is low. A patient once described the post-treatment state as 'like having a terrible hangover for a week!' A provisional date for the next treatment is made, providing Julie's blood results have returned to normal.

Chemotherapy is the term used to describe the administration of cytotoxic drugs. The length of treatment varies according to the type of tumour being treated. It is essential that, before the start of any treatment, a full explanation of what chemotherapy entails is given to the patient and his relatives.

The initial counselling session is very important. Each patient will have his own worries, for example, a father may worry about his children's reaction to his loss of hair, whereas an 18-year-old youth will want to know, 'Can I have a drink with my mates?' It is important to focus on the patient's anxieties and not to generalize too much.

There are several investigations the patient will need to undergo before starting cytotoxic drug therapy and these can be a good initial focus for a counselling session. Blood samples should be taken for a full blood count, urea and electrolytes, and liver function. The results of these first tests are a baseline for future reference. The patient should be made aware that the drugs affect not just cancer cells but all cells in the body and blood cells are the most affected; hence the necessity of numerous blood samples.

The patient's kidney function should also be checked. This can be done by obtaining a 12- or 24-hour urine collection and accompanying blood sample. Urine creatinine and serum creatinine are measured and a creatinine clearance given. This is an accurate check of kidney function, which is an essential baseline to have as many of the drugs administered are excreted in the urine via the kidneys.

Other organs, too, can be affected and need monitoring; for example cisplatinum causes high-frequency hearing loss; thus, a hearing test is required. Doxorubicin causes cardiomyopathy, necessitating an echocardiogram.

The importance of these tests should be explained in such a manner as not to worry the patient unduly. Careful follow-up and a repetition of the investigations will be performed so that side-effects can be picked up at the earliest possible opportunity and adjustments made to the dosage of cytotoxic drugs to prevent permanent damage.

Alopecia is a side-effect of many drugs and can be one of the most distressing as it alters body image. Ice packs, which cause vasoconstriction of the vessels in the scalp, are advocated at some centres with varying degrees of success. The patient can find this an extra burden during treatment and poor results prove to be discouraging. Time should be taken by the nurse to counsel the patient over hair loss, and a hairdresser should be involved at an early stage to give advice on the style and colour of available wigs.

Cytotoxic drugs can cause infertility in both men and women. It is essential that the possibility of sperm banking be discussed before chemotherapy is started. This again will depend on the individual, but even if he is not in a steady relationship or planning a family immediately it may be too late after treatment, and this must be stressed.

At this early stage it is wise not to bombard patients with information but to allay anxieties and offer more time for further discussion. Patient booklets (e.g. *Chemotherapy – your questions answered*, published by the Royal Marsden Hospital), videos and other patients who are carefully chosen are good sources of information. If possible, all these tests and investigations should be carried out during the patient's initial visit. This ensures that as soon as the biopsy results are confirmed, chemotherapy can be started immediately as time is precious.

PRINCIPLES OF CHEMOTHERAPY

The introduction of adjuvant chemotherapy has improved the prognosis for many patients. To fully understand the principles of the use and actions of these drugs the nurse must be familiar with the cell cycle (Fig. 13.15).

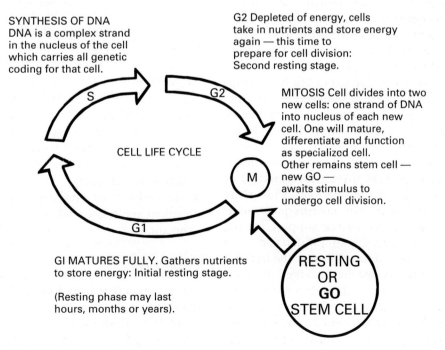

SYNTHESIS OF DNA
DNA is a complex strand in the nucleus of the cell which carries all genetic coding for that cell.

G2 Depleted of energy, cells take in nutrients and store energy again — this time to prepare for cell division: Second resting stage.

MITOSIS Cell divides into two new cells: one strand of DNA into nucleus of each new cell. One will mature, differentiate and function as specialized cell. Other remains stem cell — new GO — awaits stimulus to undergo cell division.

CELL LIFE CYCLE

S

G2

M

G1

RESTING OR GO STEM CELL

GI MATURES FULLY. Gathers nutrients to store energy: Initial resting stage.

(Resting phase may last hours, months or years).

Fig. 13.15 Diagram of cell cycle.

Cells reproduce when they receive a stimulus, usually because another cell has died. When cells reproduce, two cells exist where there used to be one. One cell goes on to mature and carry out a designated function; the other usually remains a stem cell. This stem cell will rest until it receives another stimulus to reproduce. The cell cycle is the process which all stem cells undergo in order to reproduce themselves.

Cytotoxic drugs are categorized by their action on the cell cycle. Phase-specific drugs are toxic to cells only in a named phase, and cycle-specific drugs kill cells in more than one phase or in unknown phases. However, chemotherapy will not kill cells which are in the G_0 (resting) phase. Combination chemotherapy entails a number of drugs which all have different actions on the cell cycle.

At the present time a 100% cure rate has not been achieved for any malignant bone tumour. Therefore the chemotherapy courses used are still trial regimens. Since September 1986 most patients with operable osteosarcomas have been entered into a trial run jointly by the Medical Research Council (MRC) and the European Organization for Research in Cancer (EORTC). This trial is designed to compare cisplatinum and adriamycin with a long-term regimen using high-dose methotrexate and other drugs.

The term 'trial', when used in connection with chemotherapy, has a major impact on patients. The subject must be broached carefully and diplomatically. Patients are not obliged to enter the trial and this must be emphasized. If they agree to participate in the trial they will be selected at random by the computer to receive either the short course, which involves six treatments, three preoperative and three postoperative; or the longer one, which lasts a year with many more cycles of treatment at more frequent intervals. The nurse must provide support for patients and relatives without influencing their decision. Many would happily enter the trial if it could be guaranteed that they received the short course! If they decide not to enter, they can choose which regimen they follow – a very difficult decision to make; the shorter course is more appealing in terms of time spent on therapy, but a year of treatment could possibly give a better chance of survival. Unfortunately no-one knows the answer.

When the regimen has been decided upon, the nurse should have a further counselling session with both patient and family to discuss the frequency, effects and implications of treatments, both during the treatment and after the patient's return home.

The handling of cytotoxic drugs

The reconstitution of cytotoxic drugs is very dangerous and guidelines are laid down for the safety of those handling them. Today, in many centres, all the mixing is done by the pharmacist in a special airflow cabinet to reduce the possibility of contamination. Great care should be taken wherever these drugs are handled as many of them are carcinogenic or teratogenic, as well as having irritant effects on the skin, eyes and mucous membranes (Green 1983). All units administering these drugs should have a local policy which includes guidelines for dealing with spillage, for the disposal of contaminated linen and for the treatment of extravasation.

Cisplatinum and doxorubicin are commonly used for the treatment of osteosarcoma. The action of these two drugs and their side-effects are given below.

The key factors when nursing a patient on chemotherapy are:

- The preventative measures taken where possible to stop side-effects occurring
- Immediate intervention when unpreventable side-effects do occur
- Most importantly, constant support for patient and relatives both in and out of hospital.

Cisplatinum

The action of this drug is not fully understood. It interferes with some of the components which make up strands of DNA. It is described as a class III cell cycle non-specific drug. Side-effects include:

- Nausea and persistent vomiting
- Diarrhoea at higher doses
- Nephrotoxicity, which necessitates prehydration (3 litres in 6 hours), forced diuresis with mannitol during treatment, and strict monitoring of fluid balance
- Bone marrow depression, especially white blood cell formation
- Cranial nerve damage (auditory nerve) leading to tinnitus and deafness
- Hyperuricaemia.

Doxorubicin

This is classed as an 'antimitotic antibiotic'. It works by distorting DNA in both cancer and normal cells. This distortion prevents mitotis (cell division) from taking place. Side-effects include:

- Red flush, local reaction and phlebitis in sensitive veins
- Red urine (the drug is excreted in the urine)
- Alopecia, i.e. total hair loss
- Cardiotoxicity, which causes cardiomyopathy
- Nail pigmentation
- Bone marrow depression
- Nausea and vomiting.

CONCLUSION

Nursing patients with bone malignancies can be very rewarding but also extremely stressful. It is impossible to avoid emotional involvement with such patients. As nurses we must provide support for each other as well as for patients.

Much research has analysed stress levels suffered by nurses working in oncology, all of which draws the same conclusions:

- All staff coming into contact with the families will be under pressure.
- Every action possible must be taken to minimize stress levels by:
  — promoting effective communication between peer groups
  — making allowances for 'off' days
  — providing emotional support during the grieving process.

Research carried out in a paediatric oncology ward has looked at many aspects of stress management, specifically time management and altering nurses' shift patterns as a way of reducing stress (Roscoe & Haig 1990). For example, long shifts should be discouraged as nurses may become overtired and more stressed themselves, decreasing their ability to cope with stressful situations.

It must also be remembered that there will always be success stories, too. Many patients do recover from this type of extensive surgery and treatment and live long, happy and fulfilled lives which include marriage and having a family.

Advances in surgical techniques and cytotoxic therapy are being made all the time. The future looks optimistic that the prognosis for all can be improved. Until then 'nurses can bring a permanent change of perspective for patients suffering with cancer. Their new awareness can also improve the care they give to cancer patients' (Lyall 1988).

REFERENCES

Adams J C, Hamblen D L 1990 Outline of orthopaedics, 11th edn. Churchill Livingstone, Edinburgh
Dick H M, Maunin T I, Mnaymneh W A 1985 Massive allograft implantation following resection of high grade

tumours requiring adjuvant chemotherapy treatment. Clinical orthopaedics 197: 88–95
Feldstein A 1986 Direct phlebitis and infiltration. Nursing 86 (Jan): 45

Green J A, Macbeth F R, Williams C J, Whitehouse J M A 1983 Basic medical oncology. Blackwell, Oxford, p 160

Grimer R J, Sneath R S 1990 Diagnosing malignant bone tumours. Journal of Bone & Joint Surgery 72B: 754–756

Helms C, Moon K, Genant H, Chafetz 1984 Magnetic resonance imaging – skeletal applications. Magnetic Resonance Imaging 7(9): 1429–1435

Hendee W, Davis K 1985 Magnetic resonance imaging part 2 – musculoskeletal applications. Contemporary Orthopaedics 11(3): 45–58

Lyall J 1988 Life after cancer. Nursing Times 84 (11): 26–29

Malcolm A J 1988 Osteosarcoma, classification, pathology and differential diagnosis. Seminars in orthopaedics 3(1): 1–12

Price C H G, Jeffree G M 1973 Metastatic spread of osteosarcoma. British Journal of Cancer 28: 515–524

Landsdown R, Pike S, Smith M Reducing stress in the cancer ward. Nursing Times 86(38): 34–37

Sweetnam R 1973 Amputation in osteosarcoma. Journal of Bone Joint Surgery 55B: 189–192

Zubay R L 1988 Understanding magnetic resonance imaging from a nursing perspective. Orthopaedic Nursing 7(6): 17–22

14

Hip and lower limb problems

Jan McCall

INTRODUCTION

This chapter aims to give a broad picture of caring for the hospitalized patient with lower limb problems, with the exception of paediatric care, trauma and rare conditions of the lower limb which are outside the scope of this book. The aim is to offer a practical baseline of principles on which the nurse can build and adapt in order to meet her patient's individual needs.

Major social, scientific and technological changes have provided fresh challenges for health care workers, not least for the orthopaedic nurse who cares for the patient with lower limb problems. The major advancement of implant surgery has improved and prolonged life for many people. Such advancements, together with new ideologies in nursing practice, have given rise to major changes on the orthopaedic ward and in the community.

Hip replacements are more commonplace than total knee replacements, but with technological and engineering advancements the practice of such surgery is rapidly increasing. Many conditions affecting the lower limb are now prevented by good health education and changes in lifestyles. Technological advances such as magnetic resonance imaging aid accurate diagnosis of conditions at a much earlier stage. Many treatments are now quick and relatively easy due to such inventions as the arthroscope and laser, giving rise to the term 'band-aid' surgery. Day surgery units and outpatient work are thriving, and for the numerous inpatients undergoing major surgery, many of whom are now from an older age group, the average length of stay has been greatly reduced. However, compared with other nursing specialities, patients with orthopaedic problems are still hospitalized for a considerable length of time. This has the advantage for the orthopaedic nurse of giving her time to develop a closer relationship with her patient. Together with the nurse's specialist knowledge and skills this relationship will be the foundation of therapeutic nursing care.

Problems which affect the patient's lower limbs often limit physical function and cause pain, anxiety, loss of social function, possible unemployment and changes in body image. An understanding of normal function, disorders and treatment together with relevant research-based nursing knowledge, will enable the orthopaedic nurse to provide rationalized care.

THE KINETIC CHAIN OF THE LOWER LIMB: STRUCTURE AND FUNCTION

The kinetic chain of the lower limb consists of the whole lower limb, including the foot and its joints, the ankle, knee and hip joint, and is the system that everyone depends on for ambulation.

The hip joint

The hip joint is one of the most stable joints in the body and yet it allows movement in all directions – i.e. flexion, extension, abduction, adduction, circumduction and rotation. The head of the femur, the longest bone in the body, is covered by a layer of cartilage; it fits into the acetubulm (cup) at the side of the pelvis (innominate bone) forming a ball and socket joint (see Fig. 14.1).

In order for one to stand, the hip needs to be extended; in order to sit, flexion of the hip is required. A combination of flexion and extension is involved in normal walking. During walking, forces acting across a normal hip joint consist of total body weight plus the pull of the abductor muscles, gluteus medius and minimus, which works out at an average load of 2.5–3 times the

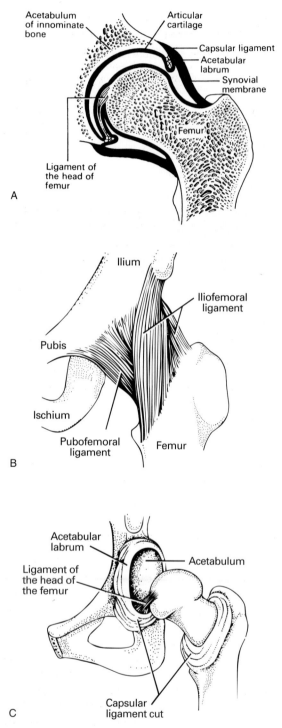

Fig. 14.1 The hip joint, anterior view: A. Section; B. Supporting ligaments; C. Head of femur and acetabulum separated to show components. (From Wilson 1990, with permission.)

body weight on each hip. Therefore, the head of the femur needs to be almost spherical in shape with very smooth articular cartilage in a near perfectly matching acetabulum to distribute the forces applied through it. However, since the weight-bearing surface is extremely small and takes so much strain it is understandable that the hip joint is the site of many mechanical problems.

The knee joint

The knee joint is the largest joint in the body. It is a complex, major weight-bearing joint and is of great importance in walking and posture.

The knee consists of two joints: the tibio-femoral and the patellofemoral. The two condyles of the femur articulate with the two condyles of the tibia; the patella articulates with the anterior aspect of the femur between the two condyles. The knee, therefore, is not a true hinge joint, although it acts in a way which is similar to a hinge. The knee joint is an extremely stable joint. The capsule is strengthened by ligaments and strong muscles such as the quadriceps. The joint also contains two semilunar cartilages otherwise known as menisci. All of these structures work together to allow the movements of flexion and extension with rotation of the tibia on the femur. Like the hip joint, the knee joint takes the entire body weight (see Fig. 14.2).

The ankle and foot joints

The ankle is a hinged joint formed between the lower end of the tibia on the medial side, the lower end of the fibula on the lateral side and the talus below. Although the ankle takes the whole body weight it is strengthened only by ligaments, including the medial and lateral ligaments. Dorsiflexion allows the foot to be raised upward and plantarflexion allows a downward movement. The foot, regardless of its size or shape, also has to bear the total weight of the body. The hindpart of the foot comprises the talus, calcaneus (heel), navicular, cuboid and three cuneiform bones. The forepart of the foot consists of five metatarsals and the phalanges

of the five toes. The foot is supported by a multiplicity of tendons (see Fig. 14.3).

ORTHOPAEDIC CONDITIONS OF THE LOWER LIMB

It is hardly surprising that breakdowns, disorders, deformities and dysfunctions occur within such essential and complex joints.

The hip joint

Arthritis in the hip joint is common. Some rare conditions give rise to arthritic changes in the hip but the most common types of change are due to degenerative joint disease such as osteoarthritis and arthritis related to rheumatoid diseases (see Chs 10, 11 and 12).

Pain is one of the major presenting problems, closely followed by limited mobility due to joint contracture. Such joint changes are often confirmed by X-ray or imaging.

Non-operative measures for these conditions include:

- Weight reduction (in obese patients the hip will have to carry a greater load than it is mechanically capable of handling)
- Reduction in activity or specific exercises to stretch out flexion contractures of the hip
- Anti-inflammatory and analgesic medication
- The use of walking aids such as a stick on the opposite side to the affected hip to relieve mechanical stress
- Other supportive measures such as heat.

Surgical intervention includes arthrodesis, osteotomy, pseudoarthrosis and arthroplasty.

An arthrodesis is a fixation/fusion of the joint in a functional position. An osteotomy involves a division of the femur between the trochanters in order to alter the line of weight-bearing. A pseudoarthrosis involves excising the head and neck of the femur; this leaves a gap which eventually fills with fibrous tissue. These procedures are seldom performed nowadays because, while the pain is reduced, little improvement is made in the patient's mobility.

A far more common procedure is arthroplasty;

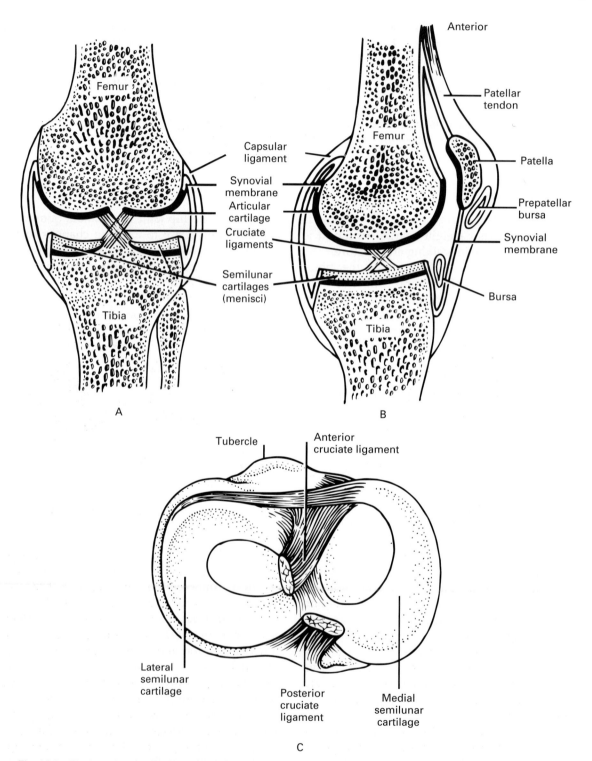

Fig. 14.2 The knee joint: A. Section viewed from the front; B. Section viewed from the side; C. Tibia viewed from top. (From Wilson 1990, with permission.)

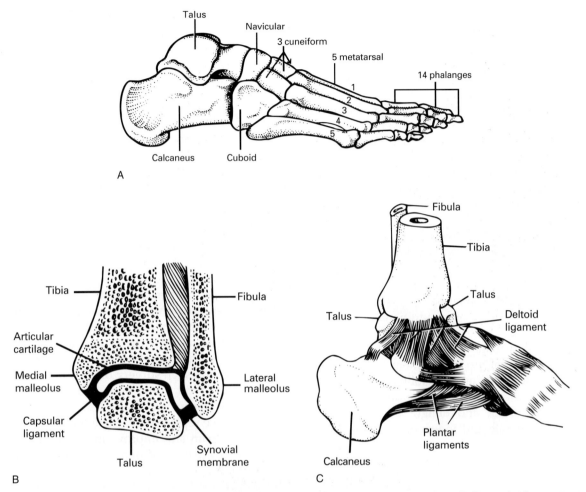

Fig. 14.3 The foot and ankle: A. Lateral view of foot; B. Section of left ankle view from the front; C. Supporting ligaments of the ankle, medial view. (From Wilson 1990, with permission.)

in fact, total hip replacement is one of the most common orthopaedic operations currently undertaken (Smith 1989).

Hip replacement is major joint reconstruction for a degenerative disease and should not be entered into lightly. It requires serious thought and planning on the part of the patient, his family and the multiprofessional team. While it is a very successful operation in most cases, there are risks, possible complications, disadvantages and contraindications.

Many types of prosthesis for total hip replacement have been designed over the years. Surgeons develop their own preferences and work with a bioengineer, biomechanic, metal-

lurgist and scientist in the search for technological excellence. Both the femoral head and the acetabulum are replaced during a total hip replacement arthroplasty. Virtually all of the early replacements were made from stainless steel. However, it soon became apparent that many people had a reaction to steel. Research into biocompatibility (the way the patient accepts a foreign implant) with other metals and alloys is still going on. Another biocompatibility hazard used to be the material known as methylmethacrylate, a cement-like substance which held the components in place (Royce 1988). Recent developments in engineering have led to prostheses that do not require cementing.

John Charnley is perhaps the most renowned name connected with hip replacements. He designed a low friction arthroplasty, believing that a small head meant less friction and, therefore, less wear. He filled the large space that was left in the acetabulum with plastic. The Charnley total hip prosthesis is one of the most commonly used types of prosthesis today (see Fig. 14.4).

Revision of a total hip replacement should only ever be necessary if the original implant fails for some reason. Occasionally this may happen due to such complications as deep wound sepsis, loosening of the prosthesis or trauma to the hip or surrounding structures. The surgical procedure for revision is very similar to that of the initial arthroplasty, but removing the original prosthesis can be extremely difficult. Complicated reinforcement may be required and so bone grafting may be necessary. Thus, a revision carries its own additional risks and considerations.

The orthopaedic nurse caring for patients undergoing total hip replacement is able to act as carer, educator and rehabilitator, playing a key role in the health care team and sharing the patient's wonder and delight as he becomes pain-free, mobile and independent. In order to effectively assess and care for the patient, she must have an understanding of the functions of the hip, the disease process and the operative measures (see Table 14.1).

Table 14.1 Total hip replacement: surgical approaches and nursing implications

Approach	Description	Implication
Anterior	patient's leg is externally rotated and abducted to dislocate the head of the femur anteriorly	keep patient's ankles together if possible to prevent postoperative dislocation
Lateral	the greater trochanter is cut off before the hip is properly exposed and then wired back on at the end of the procedure	avoid undue stress on the hip and use abduction wedge such as a Charnley
Posterior	the hip is adducted and internally rotated to dislocate posteriorly	use abduction wedge

The knee

Total knee arthroplasty has a lower rate of success than total hip arthroplasty (Harburn 1989). Long-term results are still being monitored as the life of the current prosthetic devices appears to be around 10 years, which means that performing such surgery on a young person may severely limit future options if the implant fails for any reason.

A total knee replacement is usually performed to decrease pain and improve mobility and stability. There are many different types of prosthesis available on the market (Fig. 14.5 illustrates the Oxford total knee prosthesis) and they fall into three main categories: non-constrained, partially constrained and totally constrained. The

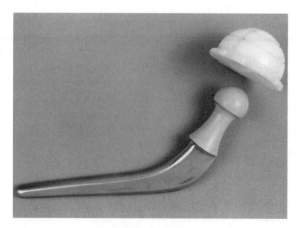

Fig. 14.4 The Charnley total hip prosthesis.

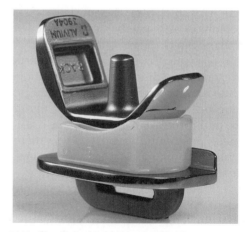

Fig. 14.5 The Oxford total knee prosthesis.

surgeon will decide which type is the most suitable for the patient from the patient's history and circumstances, and from radiographs and studies of leg alignment which indicate where and how the body weight is passing through the knee.

A total knee replacement, like all surgery, is not without risks. Crenshaw (1987) believes that between 10 and 15% of patients will develop early complications such as haematomas and necrosis of the skin. Thrombotic problems such as deep vein thrombosis are also a major concern but are often diagnosed at an early stage when treatment can be given effectively (see Ch. 5). Other complications include failure of the prosthesis, loosening, malalignment and fractures.

Revision of total knee replacements is necessary in 10–13% of cases. Pain, instability, wear and loosening are the most common reasons for revision.

The ankle and foot

The majority of everyday foot problems develop from biomechanical causes and many can be treated by a chiropodist. Other foot problems commonly arise from congenital deformities such as talipes equinovarus (club-foot) or flat feet. Footwear such as high heels or platform shoes can give rise to foot complaints, as can occupational factors. Structural and functional problems may be reflected in the posture and the behaviour of the foot on weight-bearing, and symptoms, therefore, can occur in the knee, hip and lower back (Neale & Adams 1985). Pain and disability are probably the two most common complaints of individuals with foot problems. Metatarsalgia is the term given to pain in the interphalangeal joints. Surgery does not always improve such pain (Sutherland Muckle 1986) and, in fact, any foot surgery may cause it. For this reason careful consideration should always be given before surgery is undergone for purely cosmetic reasons.

There are numerous medical conditions affecting the complex structure of the foot (see Table 14.2).

Hallux valgus

Hallux valgus is a painful lesion of the first metatarsal head, more commonly known as a bunion (see Fig. 14.6). In advanced stages the whole structure of the forefoot becomes affected, and due to an alteration in gait can cause not only a painful toe but an aching foot, ankle and knee. This condition is more common in women, obese people and during pregnancy (Neale & Adams 1985). Conservative treatment includes using special footwear or orthoses, or having steroid injections. Surgery is performed to remove the exostosis and correct valgus deformity. An oestotomy or arthrodesis of the first metatarsophalangeal joint may be carried out. Since 1904

Table 14.2 Some common orthopaedic conditions of the adult foot

Condition	Site	Description	Treatment
Hammer toe	common in the second toe	the metatarsophalangeal joint is extended and the interphalangeal joint is flexed to a right angle; a corn often forms over the affected joint	conservative strapping, operative arthrodesis or filleting
Morton's neuroma	usually in the webbed space between the third and fourth toe	neuroma which causes sudden sharp pain and burning sensation	surgical removal
Hallux valgus	first metatarsal head of hallux	hallux abducted and axially rotated; commonly known as bunion	can require arthroplasty (see text)
Ingrown toenail	commonly hallux	can be caused by cutting the nail too short or leaving a sharp corner	surgery to remove the sharp piece of nail piercing the skin
Foot instability	due to trauma, disease, disorder, structural or congenital deformity		corrective surgery; can require triple arthrodesis

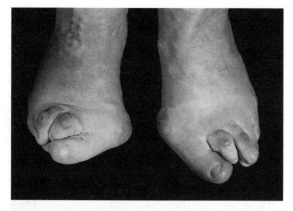

Fig. 14.6 Hallux valgus.

when Keller first described this treatment, there have been nearly a hundred variations (Bartell 1985) by people such as Akin, Silver, Chevron and others. Keller's operation renders the hallux flail, so fixation is achieved with a 'K' wire in order to maintain alignment. The patient needs a special shoe or slipper for a few weeks postoperatively.

Other joints

Other foot surgery includes the triple arthrodesis procedure, usually performed for major instability in the foot. This procedure fuses the talocalcaneal, talonavicular and calcaneocuboid joints.

Arthritis commonly attacks the foot. However, total joint replacement of the ankle for arthritis of the foot is fairly rare. A number of prostheses have been developed, mostly comprising high density polyethylene for one joint surface and stainless steel for the other. However, conservative treatments such as weight reduction, support and rest are more common. This may be due to the fact that foot surgery carries the risk of many complications including:

- delayed or non-union of the bones
- infection
- fibrosis
- adhesions
- avascular necrosis
- haematoma.

Such complications have many implications for nursing care, and the orthopaedic nurse should observe 'colour, sensation, mobility, warmth and pedal pulse' for their signs and symptoms. For example, even slight friction and pressure can cause inflammation and may well lead to infection, or the medial dorsal cutaneous nerve may be impaired resulting in paraesthesia of the hallux. Her knowledge should extend to such detail and she should be able to identify and act on such potential problems, hence her need to understand and appreciate 'normal' function. Burnip (1991) points out how shameful it is that so many nurses cannot justify why they are making observations or describe how they should act on the outcomes.

There is no doubt that foot disorders cause much pain, deformity, inconvenience and many mobility problems. The nurse can help to minimize these problems by educating her patients in foot care (see Fig. 14.7).

THE OUTPATIENT

Rehabilitation is a creative process beginning with preventative care, continuing throughout hospital treatment and involving adaptation by the individual to a new life (Craig 1989) (see Fig. 14.8).

Assessment often begins in the outpatient department, which may be the patient's first experience of the hospital. The initial assessment may take either a few minutes or, it is hoped, much longer, but this will depend on circumstances. Many patients with lower limb problems will have waited and suffered at home for some time before their outpatient appointment (Laing & Taylor 1982). The Royal College of Nursing (1988) provides guidelines on how nurses can make this waiting time a positive experience for the patient: by helping to prevent a deterioration in his general health and well-being, by allaying his fears and anxieties, and by reassuring and giving him support. Such guidelines also apply from the time the patient is seen in the outpatient department until his admission for treatment. By providing health education and aids to living the nurse can improve the patient's quality of

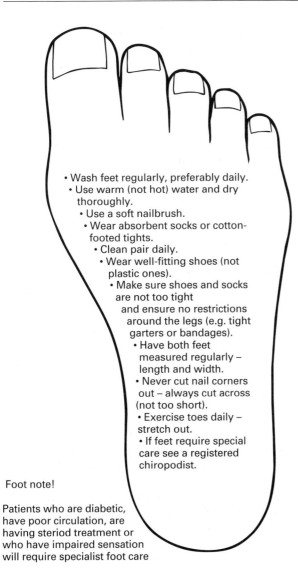

• Wash feet regularly, preferably daily.
• Use warm (not hot) water and dry thoroughly.
• Use a soft nailbrush.
• Wear absorbent socks or cotton-footed tights.
• Clean pair daily.
• Wear well-fitting shoes (not plastic ones).
• Make sure shoes and socks are not too tight and ensure no restrictions around the legs (e.g. tight garters or bandages).
• Have both feet measured regularly – length and width.
• Never cut nail corners out – always cut across (not too short).
• Exercise toes daily – stretch out.
• If feet require special care see a registered chiropodist.

Foot note!

Patients who are diabetic, have poor circulation, are having steriod treatment or who have impaired sensation will require specialist foot care

Fig. 14.7 Adult foot care.

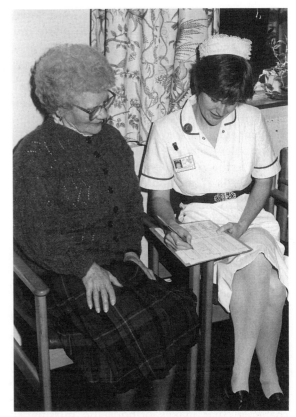

Fig. 14.8 The outpatient.

life. Care of preadmission patients also reduces the likelihood of preventable cancellation of surgery on admission: for the patient who has developed a pressure sore, has an infected toe-nail or mouth, or is malnourished or obese, there is a greatly increased risk of infection, immobility and other postoperative complications (see Ch. 2).

In the outpatient department the nurse's function is to provide nursing care, but in reality she still carries out many non-nursing functions (Out-Patients Report, 1990). There, she has the opportunity to establish a good nurse/patient relationship when she assesses the patient's physical, psychological, social and spiritual needs, using her skills and knowledge to seek out his understanding of his condition, expectations, needs and problems. The nurse also acts as the patient's advocate by helping him to maintain his dignity, answering his questions, giving him information and advice, allowing him to talk, reassuring him and ensuring his comfort, safety and well-being. She liaises closely with her medical colleagues, as a member of the multidisciplinary team, to ensure that accurate information is transmitted.

PRINCIPLES OF NURSING CARE
Introduction

The general principles involved in nursing individuals with problems of the hip and lower limbs that should be evident in each ward, unit or team are the following:

- A nursing philosophy
- A system of delivery of care which allows an interpersonal relationship to develop between the patient, nurse and the patient's family
- A named nurse for each patient
- A problem-solving , individualized approach such as the nursing process
- Standards of care and quality measures which are monitored and acted upon
- A model of nursing which complements/ enhances the ward's philosophy – many orthopaedic wards work to a model of independence
- Care which reflects physical, psychological, social and spiritual needs.

These principles should be used as a guide and as a baseline for practice (see also Ch. 3). Details of nursing care are determined by individual patients and their unique situations; for example, not all patients having the same lower limb surgery will have the same pain. It is this challenge that makes orthopaedic nursing so exciting, dynamic and innovative.

The principles of care discussed in this chapter pertain to patient-centred problems, but it is also important to appreciate that patients' problems cannot be seen in isolation. For example, pain, information-giving and anxiety are very closely connected, as are comfort, pain and sleep. The skilled orthopaedic nurse looks for such connections in order to provide more effective care.

Reducing pain

Pain is an extremely common problem for patients with lower limb problems and it is the main presenting symptom of most patients (Royce 1988) (see also Ch. 7). It may arise from the patient's medical condition – for example, joint destruction, inflammation, muscle atrophy, spasm etc. – or from interventions to help the patient, such as splinting, exercises, positioning, forced immobility, surgery and its complications. In view of its causes preventing pain,

although highly desirable, may be an unrealistic goal for patient and nurse at times. The aim of nursing care should be to achieve pain control which is acceptable to the patient.

The effective management of pain begins preoperatively with a baseline assessment which is carried out by the nurse and other multidisciplinary team members (Ketchin 1989).

The nurse must ascertain the nature and causes of pain in the patient, and discover the factors which affect his perception of pain and the action he takes to alleviate it, i.e.:

1. What coping mechanisms does he use?
2. What aggravates the pain?
3. What relieves it?
4. Where is its location?
5. Where is the distribution?
6. Where is the radiation?
7. Is it worse at rest?

Answers to these questions provide vital clues to the cause of pain. For example:

- A knee joint filled with blood or fluid can cause pain at rest
- Nocturnal pain is often a characteristic of osteoid osteomas
- An aching hip may suggest a haematoma
- Sudden pain in the hip may be the result of dislocation
- Acute pain in the calf may indicate a deep vein thrombosis and in the chest a pulmonary embolism.

The nurse should also be aware of less obvious areas of pain, for example:

- The patient with arthritis who has aches and pains in non-operative joints, possibly due to increased work for those joints or to positioning
- The muscle spasm postoperatively
- The back pain from having to remain relatively supine
- The wound dressing that is too tight
- The sore infusion site
- The distended bladder in the patient who is unable to pass urine
- The crippling stomach ache of the patient who has had a total hip replacement and is suffering from flatulence.

The orthopaedic nurse can take preventative, educative and practical measures to help alleviate such problems.

Preventative measures

The nurse can ensure that:

- Analgesia is given prior to physiotherapy or an uncomfortable dressing change
- Muscle relaxants are prescribed
- The patient is in a good and comfortable position.

Educative measures

Informing the patient of his condition, treatment and expected outcomes helps to reduce his pain and anxiety (Boore 1978). The nurse should encourage the patient to help actively in the control of his pain by allowing him to administer his own medication (Bird 1990). The nurse should discuss the patient's expectations with him in order to plan a strategy of care and pain management. Many patients believe that surgery will relieve their pain and, indeed, this is often the case for major joint replacement (Haworth et al 1981); however, the patient who is undergoing 'minor surgery', for example to a toe, may not realize how painful a procedure this can be.

The patient's anaesthetic should also be discussed and explained. Is he going to have an epidural or spinal anaesthetic, and does he understand the procedure and its implications? The United Kingdom Central Council (1990) has made it quite clear that the nurse must ensure that the patient has such an understanding, and she must act as his advocate.

Practical measures

There are numerous practical ways in which the nurse can help to alleviate pain:

- Changing the patient's position
- Careful handling of the joints
- Administration of analgesia
- Complementary approaches such as relaxation, distraction and massage

- Removing or reducing the cause of pain (e.g. removing the tight dressing)
- Reducing the inflammation.

Reducing anxiety

Admission to hospital generates anxiety in most individuals, and this can intensify the pain experienced (Thompson 1988). The patient's anxiety level is not necessarily proportional to the severity of the surgery, as there will be many other factors affecting it.

Often intervention is non-specific; but it is important that the patient receives honest factual information in an understandable form and this depends on the nurse's interpersonal and communication skills and the extent of her knowledge.

Providing information

Information-giving is a very important aspect of care for patients undergoing lower limb surgery. Not only does it reduce anxiety and aid recovery but it is also a patient's right to have such information. Without it the patient cannot be involved as an active partner in care, give informed consent or exercise his right of choice. Information-giving is important at all stages of care, but particularly prior to admission, prior to surgery or any invasive procedure and prior to discharge, as the patient must be prepared for these events.

Before the patient's admission, it is essential for the nurse to inform him verbally of admission and postoperative routines, and follow this up with a clear and simple letter or leaflet that the patient and his family may keep for reference (Fig. 14.9). Details should include:

1. What to bring with him
2. How long he may be in hospital
3. What to expect
4. By whom he will be seen
5. Where in the hospital he should go on admission
6. Where to park
7. Which ward he will be on
8. What will happen during surgery

Ref: THR/adm   Hospital name, address,
                                                telephone number and who
                                                to contact for further information

Dear

Following your consultation with (consultant's name) at your recent out-patient appointment a date has been set for you to have your total hip replacement operation at this hospital.

The date scheduled for admission is (date time am/pm). Please would you let me know as soon as possible if this is acceptable to you.

Patients are usually admitted one or two days prior to hip surgery. This allows time for various examinations and investigations to be carried out, all of which are necessary for your treatment and will be fully explained and discussed with you. This time also allows you to meet the various members of staff who will be caring for you and provides the opportunity for you to ask questions. Your Consultant will have explained much of the plan to you and may have given you a leaflet but if you have any concerns or worries please feel free to ask. We are here to help you.

After your operation you will spend some time in our recovery unit before returning to your ward. On average most patients are in hospital between 7 and 10 days. A full assessment and instructions will be given to you before you leave. You should expect to be off work for at least . . . weeks and you will need someone at home to help you when you are discharged.

I have enclosed a patient's booklet which tells you more about the hospital facilities, parking, visiting, what to bring etc.

I look forward to hearing from you.

Yours sincerely,

Fig. 14.9 Preadmission letter for total hip replacement patients.

9. What is expected of him after surgery
10. The exercises, the drains and infusion.

The patient should be encouraged to ask questions and discuss his concerns.

Information-giving commences in the outpatient department, where there should be documentation (which could be in the form of check-lists) to record this. Such a structured process, including a planned teaching programme, helps to prevent the provision of fragmented, incomplete, inaccurate or overwhelming information.

Once the patient is admitted to hospital, visits by staff such as the anaesthetist, physiotherapist and occupational therapist may be appropriate. The patient must be given time to ask questions and be reassured. Information on aspects of care such as equipment and procedures should be offered, and the disease process, specific treatment and plan of care discussed. Giving information is very often synonymous with informed consent, which is not the same as written consent. Most nursing actions require informed consent, but few need written consent.

Many patients may be familiar with the concept of joint replacement, but the nurse needs to ensure that the patient has knowledge of the operative procedure, the surgeon's approach and the expected outcome. It is often from this exchange of information that potential problems can be identified and preventative measures taken to reduce risk.

Teaching is a valuable form of information-giving, and planned teaching programmes can be used for instruction on self-medication, discharge planning and preoperative preparation (see Fig. 14.10).

Such programmes do not replace the care plan, although they may be incorporated into it, nor the preoperative check-list, although they could be combined with it. Setting a clinical standard on preoperative information-giving is a good way of ensuring that such care is always offered.

Knowledge or skill	Checked
Patient has seen a prosthesis	
Patient states an understanding of his condition	
Patient can explain operative procedure	
Time has been allowed for discussion, teaching and questions	
Patient understands the importance of positioning postoperatively	
Patient understands the importance of movement postoperatively	
Patient can explain the importance of deep breathing	
Patient can explain the importance of leg exercises	
Patient can demonstrate how to perform deep breathing	
Patient can demonstrate how to perform leg exercises, independently and using equipment	
Patient can state the desired frequency of exercises	
Patient can demonstrate how to lift	
using a monkey pole	
using other lifting aids	
with a Charnley wedge in situ	
to use a bedpan	
Patient can demonstrate how to roll with a wedge in situ	
Patient has discussed plan of care with nurse	
Problems, goals and nursing action have been recorded on the care plan	
The patient can explain the postoperative 'procedure' (drains, infusions, wound care etc.)	
The management of pain has been discussed and planned	
The patient understands the pain chart to be used	
The patient has been seen by the physiotherapist	
The patient has visited the gym	
The patient can demonstrate how to walk with a frame/other walking aids	
The patient has had an opportunity to talk to another patient who has undergone similar surgery	
Supportive literature has been given to the patient	
The patient's relatives have been involved in the plan	
All aids etc. required are readily available	
Comments:	
Date: Signed:	

Fig. 14.10 Preoperative teaching programme evaluation/check-list for patients having a total hip replacement.

Information-giving is an aspect of nursing which is expanding due to public expectation and societal changes; with innovative practice it is becoming an exciting and challenging part of the nurse's role.

Promoting mobility

Virginia Henderson (1966) considered that the need to move and maintain desirable postures was fundamental to all people. Immobility is often thought of as a complete lack of movement, but frequently it refers to limited or decreased mobility (see Chs 5 and 6).

The patient who suffers from lower limb problems may have limited mobility for a variety of reasons including:

- pain
- stiffness
- spasm
- deformity
- postoperative protocol (e.g. positioning)
- bedrest
- immobilization of a limb in a cast or splint.

Early postoperative mobility is beneficial (Pugh 1989), and patients who have undergone total hip replacement surgery may be out of bed as early as the second postoperative day. Chapter 5 gives more detailed information on the complications of impaired physical mobility.

Assessment of the patient's mobility should begin preoperatively in the outpatient department to obtain a baseline and to identify problems. Preventative measures include specific exercises to strengthen muscles, advice on a weight-reducing diet and the provision of mobility aids such as walking frames or sticks.

Preoperatively the patient is often fairly mobile, so without thorough preparation before, he may be surprised to find that he is restricted postoperatively.

Postoperative care is very dependent on pre-operative preparation. The frightened, nervous and helpless patient will be reluctant to move – will his stitches burst? Will the hip dislocate? The nurse should aim to motivate the patient to move by setting minor, achievable mobility goals rather than unrealistic major hurdles; for example, by encouraging the patient to move in bed, stand out, or take a couple of steps. The patient who has undergone foot surgery may need to hang his feet over the side of the bed first as he may experience a throbbing pain prior to heel-walking. Besides practical preoperative preparation, such as advising the patient to visit the gym preoperatively, there are many other ways in which the nurse can help the patient, for example by liaising very closely with the physiotherapist and developing a plan of care in collaboration with the patient and physiotherapist.

The patient's requirements for initial mobilization

1. The patient requires adequate sleep, rest and nutrition in order to have enough energy for exercise.
2. The patient's pain must be under control.
3. The patient requires knowledge and understanding of what is expected of him.
4. The patient should understand the importance of movement.
5. The patient must be motivated to move.
6. The patient must be able to move.

Nursing implications for patient's initial mobilization

The nurse should aim to meet the patient's needs for initial mobilization as stated above and offer positive reinforcement, encouragement and support. She should have knowledge of the surgery undertaken and its implications; for example, the patient should avoid extreme hip flexion in the case of total hip replacement. She should ensure that the patient's safety and comfort are maintained by addressing the following questions:

1. Does he have suitable footwear – not sloppy or slippery – and are his toes protected?
2. Does he have clothing which is not trailing (too long a dressing-gown or a hanging hem)?
3. Is the bed/chair the right height for the patient?
4. Is he 'attached' to any drips or monitors?
5. Does he have aids to mobility?
6. Can he use equipment/walking aids safely and correctly?
7. Is the splint or cast properly maintained and in a correct and comfortable position?
8. Is the environment safe (no wet floors, rugs or obstacles)?
9. Are the bed brakes on?

Ideally the nurse encourages the patient to move but there are times when she has to assist him. The care plan should clearly state how to move the patient, what method of lift to use, what aids are used and how many nurses should help. The move should be recorded when completed, as should the patient's education regarding mobility.

The nurse should ensure that the patient uses aids to mobility safely and correctly. For walking frames, crutches and sticks:

- The hand grip and size should be checked.
- The height and weight of the aid should be considered.
- The type of aid should be appropriate; it would be of little use for a frail old lady with rheumatoid arthritis to have underarm crutches.
- The nurse should escort the patient until she assesses that the patient is competent and happy to walk alone.
- The single stick is held in the hand on the opposite side to the affected joint.

- Small slow steps are taken.
- The feet are kept parallel, with the body upright.

Some of the many other aids to mobility used for patients with lower limb problems include:

- A kinetic knee machine (see Fig. 14.11)
- Slings and springs for gentle bending of the knee.

Knee immobilizers or long-leg casts may be used for patients undergoing repair or constructive surgery to the knee; casts may be used for foot surgery. All patients undergoing lower limb surgery will require some form of physiotherapy.

It is usual for patients who have undergone knee surgery to have the limb elevated initially. This may be done by using frames such as the Braun's frame or by elevating the foot of the bed. The nurse must remember to lower the bed while the patient is using a urinary bottle or bedpan.

A postoperative knee exercise programme may initially keep the knee in extension, with quadriceps exercises encouraging tightening of the quadriceps muscles by 'pulling' the knee-cap. Following this, straight leg raising (SLR) may commence, followed by gentle bending increasing to an ultimate 90° flexion of the knee if possible.

Patients who have undergone hip replacement surgery will need to keep flexion to a minimum in order to prevent dislocation and muscle contracture. A Charnley wedge may be used to keep the hip abducted (see Fig. 14.12). (Further information for total hip replacement patients can be found in Fig. 14.15.)

Promoting a positive body image

Surgery of the lower limb may prove to be a welcome relief from distressing symptoms for most patients, but they still also need to accept their altered body image – from the immediate postoperative period when they are adorned with drips and drains and white gowns to the time of their complete recovery when they have a scar and may no longer be disabled. The nurse is ideally placed to help the patient cope with this. However, although preadmission and preoperative preparation may help to ready patients for their course of treatment and care, preparation for their change in body image is an aspect of nursing still under discussion:

1. Do nurses allow patients to wear their own clothes?
2. Are the theatre gowns modest?

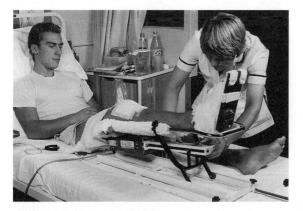

Fig. 14.11   Kinetic knee machine.

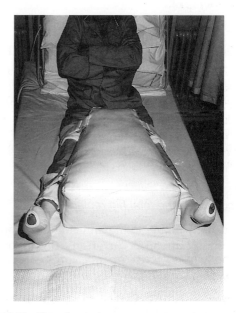

Fig. 14.12   Charnley wedge.

3. How does the patient feel about having a Charnley wedge jammed between their legs?

4. How does the patient feel about having to use a walking frame?

Many patients undergoing lower limb surgery will feel apprehensive, bored and depressed, and in this way undermine their own self-esteem. The nurse can do much to counteract these feelings by involving patients (and their families) in their own care – ensuring that there are tasks for them to do on the ward and that group activities are encouraged – and by showing understanding and being constantly empathetic with them.

Ensuring adequate nutritional intake

Nutrition is an important aspect of care for the patient undergoing lower limb surgery. Recent studies have shown that many hospitalized patients are undernourished (Coates 1985). This has major implications for the orthopaedic nurse and providers of health services. Not only do patients require an adequate caloric intake to aid sound healing, but a balance of calcium, Vitamin D and protein is essential in preventing bone disorders.

Preventing complications

A general anaesthetic and any type of lower limb surgery has potentially serious complications, including shock and haemorrhage. The importance of preoperative assessment, education and preventative care by the orthopaedic nurse cannot be stressed enough. In addition, she must be able to recognize signs of complications and act on them accordingly.

Dislocation of the total hip replacement

This usually occurs in the immediate postoperative phase but can occur at any time (Footner 1987). The patient experiences sudden pain; the affected limb may be in external rotation and is seen to be slightly shorter than the other leg. The affected hip may appear swollen. Occasionally the hip lies in internal rotation. An X-ray confirms dislocation, which must then be reduced.

Correct positioning in mobilization, which ensures that the hip is not flexed beyond 90° or abducted, is the most effective way to prevent dislocation.

Infection

The control of infection is very important in implant and deep bone surgery. Its incidence has been greatly reduced over recent years, largely due to better anaesthetics, better instruments, clean air theatres, improved clinical practices, advanced surgical techniques and the use of prophylactic antibiotics. The nurse must be very vigilant in monitoring for signs of infection, such as a sudden raised temperature and a reddened suture line. However, oozing of the patient's wound, a common occurrence following a total hip replacement, is not always a sign of infection as it can occur through fatty breakdown.

After a total hip replacement the thigh is often oedematous; this may result in an increased tendency to develop blisters from surgical tape. Irritation of the suture line should also be avoided; and the prevention of other infections such as those of the chest and urinary tract is of paramount importance. In all cases the nurse must demonstrate a sound knowledge of wound healing and wound care as good nursing practice is essential in controlling infection. Further information on this topic can be found in Chapter 8.

Deep vein thrombosis

Deep vein thrombosis (DVT) is a significant problem for patients undergoing lower limb surgery. Brown (1983) and Cruess and Rennie (1984) suggest that it exists in up to 50–70% of all surgical cases, many of which are asymptomatic and diagnosed with venograms and scans (see Ch. 5 for further discussion of this).

Physiotherapy and early ambulation are the most effective preventors of DVT; elastic stockings and/or anticoagulant therapy, or intermittent calf compression boots, are also sometimes used.

The orthopaedic nurse must always be on the alert for the classic signs and symptoms of DVT such as calf pain, raised temperature and groin tenderness. The clinical practice of the nurse, based on knowledge of the proven methods of prophylaxis, will have a direct bearing on the recovery of the patient (Drinkwater 1989).

Pressure sores

As with all hospitalized patients, the nurse should assess the risk of the patient developing pressure sores (see also Ch. 5). The length of operation, position on the table, immobility, drugs, nutritional status, mobility status and weight are some of the factors that should be considered (see Fig. 14.13). Examples of patients who are more at risk include those with rheumatic diseases who may have very frail skin, those with osteoarthritis who are often obese, and those taking courses of steroids. Specific risk areas for pressure sores in people who have undergone lower limb surgery include the heels, knees and sacral regions although, of course, other areas may be affected. Good nursing practice – correct positioning and lifting, avoidance of trauma, maintenance of dry and clean skin, straightened bed clothes, early ambulation and the use of preventive aids – helps to dramatically reduce the risk of this preventable complication.

Paralytic ileus

As the gut is situated very close to the hip joint, it

Patient's Name:

PRESSURE AREA RISK ASSESSMENT

Ring scores in table, add total

Build/weight for height		Risk areas visual skin type		Sex, age		Special risks	
Average	0	Healthy	0	Male	1	**TISSUE MALNUTRITION**	
Above average	1	Dry	1	Female	2		
Obese	2	Oedematous	1	0–5 yrs	2	Terminal cachexia	8
Below average	3	Clammy	1	6–45 yrs	1	Cardiac failure	5
CONTINENCE		Tissue paper	2	46–64 yrs	2	Peripheral vascular disease	5
		Discoloured	2	65–74 yrs	3		
Complete/ catheterized	0	Broken/spot	3	75–80 yrs	4	**NEUROLOGICAL DEFICIT**	
Occasionally incontinent	1	**MOBILITY**		81 yrs+	5		
		Fully	0	**APPETITE**		e.g. Diabetes, CVA, MS, paraplegia, motor/ sensory	4–6
Incontinent (urine only)	2	Restless/fidgety	1	Normal	0		
Incontinent (faeces only)	2	Apathetic	2	Poor	1	**MAJOR SURGERY/ TRAUMA**	
		Restricted	3	NG Tube/fluids only	2		
Doubly incontinent	3	Inert/traction	4	NBM/anorexic	3	Above waist	2
		Chairbound	5			Below waist/spinal	5
						On table 2 hrs	5
Score: 10+ at risk, 15+ high risk, 20+ very high risk						**MEDICATION**	
						Steroids, cytotoxics Anti-inflammatory	4

Pre-operative score: _____ Date: _____
Post-operative scores: _____ Date: _____
_____ Date: _____

Fig. 14.13 Pressure sore risk calculator.

is aggravated during hip surgery and this may result in a paralytic ileus. It is, therefore, important that the nurse ensures that the bowel sounds are present before commencing the patient on oral fluids. Fluids should be increased gradually as tolerated.

A girth measurement may be useful in some circumstances – but the nurse should be aware that an increase in measurement (distension) may be due to urinary retention.

Other complications

Other complications of lower limb surgery include:

- haematomas
- necrosis of skin
- poor wound healing (especially in the knee where the skin is stretching)
- constipation
- muscle wasting.

The nurse can prevent these, by being vigilant in her observation of vital signs, dressings/drains, and neurovascular status (especially pedal pulse for knee and foot surgery).

Ensuring a safe discharge

Each patient will require a systematic, yet individualized, documented plan for discharge that can be used from the 1st day of admission, or ideally prior to admission, until after discharge. In the 1990s discharge is occurring much earlier due to advances in surgery and care and a demand for hospital beds. Preparation is essential, as leaving the 'security' of the hospital can be extremely frightening for the patient.

Everyone recovers at his own rate. The nurse and the multidisciplinary team – physiotherapist, occupational therapist and doctor – must ensure by assessment that the patient is well prepared and ready and able to go home.

The patient should be actively involved in his discharge planning so that together he and his nurse can identify problems and clarify the care required. Check-lists/programmes are very

useful for this (see Fig. 14.14); plans should consider the following:

- What is the expected date of discharge?
- Has this been discussed with the patient and his family?
- Does the patient require assistance with daily tasks (bathing, dressing, feeding, toileting)?
- Which services are required (for example, community or social services)?
- What medication is required? Can the patient self-administer?
- Has the patient an acceptable understanding of his care?
- What exercises are required? Can the patient perform them?
- What follow-up is required? Does the patient have an appointment? Can he get to it?
- Does the patient know who to contact in an emergency? Has he the telephone number? Has he a telephone or a helpful neighbour?
- Has he or can he have access to community resources?
- How will he get home?
- Will someone be at home?
- Does he need special aids – raised toilet seat, walking aids, bath mat, etc.?
- When can he return to work?
- Does the patient have to lift at home?
- Does he have stairs?
- Is there a long walk to the shops?
- What are his individual concerns – loneliness, boredom, pain?
- Is the wound well healed?
- Has the patient been given information on metal detectors (implants will set off detectors)?
- Has the patient been assessed by a physiotherapist, occupational therapist and doctor?

The patient needs much information and support to ensure a safe and effective discharge. Written and verbal advice should be given. Booklets/pamphlets explaining the dos and don'ts or the exercises to be undertaken (see Fig. 14.15) are extremely useful as they act as a reference source and a reinforcement of previous instruction. Specific advice should be written down; the surgeon may want the patient who has to have dental work carried out the follow-

Discharge plan	Patient's name:	Check:

Expected date of discharge:
Support services required:
                arranged:
Transport arrangements:
Someone at patient's home:
Outpatient appointment made:
Notification to GP:
Drugs to take home:
         collected:
Special aids required:
Wound clean and dry:
  sutures removed:
Patient seen and assessed by Doctor:
                               Nurse:
                               Physio:
                               OT:
                               Other:
Home visit:
Relative seen:
Patient satisfaction questionnaire given:		

Patient education/information programme prior to discharge Patient has been given time to discuss discharge. Patient demonstrates knowledge and understanding of the condition and operation. Patient can explain the activities he is able/unable to perform. Patient can demonstrate safe mobility and transfers. Patient demonstrates knowledge of community resources available. Patient understands the potential for triggering metal detectors. Patient can state the date, time and venue of his follow-up appointment. Patient can state the number of who to contact in an emergency, or if concerned. Patient has knowledge of any medication necessary. Patient can safely demonstrate how to administer any medication. Patient has received leaflet on guidance and exercises. Patient, family and multi-professional team (including community) are happy with discharge plan. Discharged: Signed:		

Fig. 14.14 Discharge form for the total hip replacement patient.

ing month to be put on prophylactic antibiotics to reduce the risk of infection.

By planning in advance the nurse is able to address these issues. Advice on dieting, sleeping and sexual habits should be offered and much time should be set aside for the patient to ask questions and express fears. This also enables the nurse to assess and suggest practical measures such as the use of:

- A bath mat to avoid slipping
- A towel or a pair of tights hooked around the bath taps to help the patient sit up
- Bags of sugar on the patient's feet for leg exercises.

Ideally the nurse, patient and occupational therapist should visit the patient's home before discharge to check his home circumstances and

INFORMATION FOR PATIENTS WHO HAVE HAD A TOTAL HIP REPLACEMENT

Following a total hip replacement special care should be taken to protect the joint to allow time for healing and strengthening.

Certain movements place undue stress on your hip and these should be avoided. This information is designed to help you over the next few months and you should also follow the advice and exercises given to you by the physiotherapist and occupational therapist. Either therapist, your doctor or your nurse will answer any questions or concerns you may have. Please feel free to ask.

DO NOT BEND to such an extent that the angle between your body and your operated hip is less than 90°.

DO NOT FLEX YOUR HIP to more than 90°.

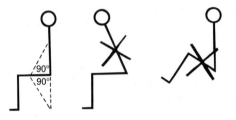

Think about this when you are dressing, picking things up, using the toilet, getting up from a chair, getting in and out of a car, the bed or the bath and having sexual intercourse. Remember to practise the other points the therapist has taught you, using the aids supplied to help you. Try to avoid low seating and beds.

DO NOT TWIST ROUND.
DO NOT CROSS YOUR LEGS. You must not cross your operated leg over the midline of your body.

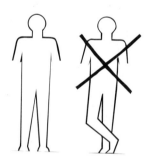

At first it may be best to sleep on your back. If you place a pillow between your legs this will prevent you from crossing your legs. Later you may sleep on the unoperated side with a pillow between your legs and after a few months you should be able to sleep on the operated side.

When **climbing stairs** remember to lead with your unoperated leg going up and your operated leg coming down.

Check with your doctor before you start **driving a car**.

Usually **sexual intercourse** may be resumed 6-8 weeks after the operation if you are progressing well. You and your partner's position should take into account the principles of not twisting, crossing the legs, flexing the operated hip or bending your body too much.

Your doctor will advise you about your **employment** depending on the type of work you do.

A total hip replacement is a major operation. You must allow adequate time, rest, nourishment and exercise during your convalescence. If, once home, you require further information please contact ....

Fig. 14.15 Information for patients who have undergone total hip replacement.

Topic: Anxiety

Care group: Patients with lower limb problems

Standard statement: The patient's anxiety is reduced by providing a safe secure environment, information and therapy.

STRUCTURE
- Each patient has a named nurse with orthopaedic knowledge.
- The ward philosophy and booklet are available for the patient to see.
- Other information on lower limb conditions, health education etc. is also available.
- There is a flexible working pattern on the ward.
- There is open visiting.
- There is a specialist aromatherapy/massage nurse available within the hospital.
- Walkmans, tapes, televisions, radios and books are available to each patient.
- Interpreters are available on request.

PROCESS
- The nurse introduces the patient to the ward environment, philosophy, staff, other patients.
- The nurse offers literature as available and appropriate.
- The nurse assesses the patient's perception and causes of anxiety.
- The nurse offers appropriate measures to review these, e.g. pain control, referral to outside agency.
- The nurse utilizes the patient's own coping mechanisms and maintains the patient's 'usual' routine as much as possible.
- The nurse employs anxiety-reducing measures such as massage, relaxation and diversional techniques.
- The nurse reassures the patient, giving open and honest information and creating an atmosphere of trust.
- Time is given for the patient to express anxiety.

OUTCOME
- An acceptable balance between social interaction and privacy is maintained.
- The patient will express and/or demonstrate a lower anxiety level.
- The patient will state that he is well informed of his condition and care.
- The patient will express control of his anxiety level.

Adapted from work undertaken by the Standard Care Plan Group at the Nuffield Orthopaedic Centre, NHS Trust

Fig. 14.16   Standard of care: anxiety.

Topic: Pain control

Care group: Adults who have had lower limb surgery

Standard statement: The patient's pain levels will remain within acceptable limits.

STRUCTURE
- A skilled and knowledgeable nurse is allocated to the patient.
- Pain charts are available for use on the ward.
- Assessment sheets and care plans allow for pain assessment and management.
- Equipment such as ice, massage oils and analgesics is available on the ward.
- National, district and local drug administration guidelines are available.

PROCESS
- The nurse assesses the patient's perception of pain and contributory factors.
- The nurse allows the patient to express feelings about pain.
- Appropriate measures for pain relief are selected and planned with the patient and carers.
- Care is documented on the care plan and pain charts.

Fig. 14.17   Caption see overleaf.

- The nurse settles the patient in a comfortable position.
- The nurse employs anxiety-relieving measures such as massage, relaxation, deep breathing and diversional/distraction therapy.
- The nurse utilizes the patient's own coping mechanisms.
- The nurse uses external pain measures such as ice, heat, compression and elevation.
- The nurse gives open, honest information.
- The nurse administers prescribed medication in a correct and safe manner.
- The nurse ensures that the patient has analgesia before physiotherapy, uncomfortable dressing changes etc.
- The nurse eliminates pain factors such as tight dressings, uncomfortable splinting, sore infusion sites etc.
- The nurse evaluates and documents the outcomes of actions taken.
- The nurse ensures the correct use of splints and braces.
- Spiritual support is considered and privacy offered.
- The nurse refers to a pain specialist if required.

OUTCOME
- The patient has an understanding of the cause and nature of his pain.
- The patient receives prompt and appropriate pain relief measures.
- The patient has relieved or decreased pain.
- The patient expresses a sense of control over measures used to control/relieve his pain.
- Within 30 minutes of administering analgesia the patient will express that he is more comfortable. Patient's behaviour will support statement.

Adapted from work undertaken by the Standard Care Plan Group at the Nuffield Orthopaedic Centre, NHS Trust

Fig. 14.17 Standard of care: pain control.

Topic: Mobility

Care group: Patients who have had lower limb surgery

Standard statement: Each patient will realize his full mobility potential.

STRUCTURE
- Each patient has a named nurse with orthopaedic knowledge.
- A physiotherapist and occupational therapist are available.
- Documentation is available relating to assessment, planning, implementation and evaluation of care.
- Patient information leaflets are available on the ward.
- Aids to mobility are available from the physiotherapy department.
- Each ward has a lifting and handling facilitator available for teaching and advice.
- A gym and hydrotherapy pool are available for patient use.

PROCESS
- Assessment of the patient's degree of mobility is made on admission and reassessed daily.
- Care planning takes into account the expected degree of mobility.
- The nurse discusses with the patient the plan of care and explains the causes of restricted mobility.
- The nurse encourages and utilizes the patient's existing mobility and coping mechanisms.
- The nurse educates the patient and carers in the safe and correct use of walking aids, splints etc.
- The nurse encourages the patient to be as independently mobile as is practicable/possible.
- The nurse works with other members of the multi-professional team in the prevention of possible musculo-skeletal complications and the promotion of mobility.
- The nurse takes appropriate action to prevent the complications of bedrest.
- The nurse ensures that a physiotherapist's and occupational therapist's assessment has been carried out and care prescribed on care plan.

Fig. 14.18 Continued on page 305.

OUTCOME
- The patient will maintain his optimum level of mobility within the limitations of treatment.
- The patient will suffer minimal complications caused by restricted mobility.
- The patient will utilize aids to enhance his mobility.
- The patient's mobility will increase to a safe and optimum level.
- The patient states confidence with his range of mobility.

Adapted from work undertaken by the Standard Care Plan Group at the Nuffield Orthopaedic Centre, NHS Trust

---

Fig. 14.18 Standard of care: mobility.

assess how he will manage by carrying out a trial run, which will also boost his confidence.

SUMMARY

Many patients suffering from lower limb conditions never reach the stage at which treatment is required (Roberts 1988), though in some cases treatment may be required but not provided until the condition becomes crippling and unbearable. Much needs to be done in future nursing practice to ensure that this suffering is addressed and prevented.

One method of maintaining and improving care is through the development of quality monitoring and enhancing initiatives such as standards of care systems. Examples of these, related to patients with lower limb problems, are given in Figures 14.16–14.18.

REFERENCES

Bartell L 1985 Bunionectomies. Orthopaedic Nursing 4(1): 21–28

Bird C A 1990 Patient self-medication. Surgical Nurse 3(1): 22–26

Boore J 1978 A prescription for recovery. Royal College of Nursing, London

Brown P 1983 Clinical teaching opportunities. Nursing Mirror June 8: 33–36

Burnip S 1991 Why do nurses take blood pressures postoperatively? Surgical Nurse 4(2): 15–19

Coates V 1985 Are they being served? Royal College of Nursing, London

Craig C 1989 Mr Simpson's hip replacement. Nursing 3(44): 12–19

Crenshaw A B 1987 Campbell's operative orthopaedics, 7th edn. C V Mosby, St Louis, MO

Cruess R L, Rennie W R J 1984 Adult orthopaedics. Churchill Livingstone, Edinburgh

Drinkwater K 1989 Management of deep vein thrombosis. Surgical Nurse Feb: 24–29

Farrell J 1982 Illustrated guide to orthopaedic nursing, 2nd edn. J B Lippincott, Philadelphia

Ferguson T 1961 The aftercare of the hospital patient. British Medical Journal 1: 1242–1244

Footner A 1987 Orthopaedic nursing. Bailliere Tindall, London

Harburn R 1989 Total knee arthroplasty and revision. 18 CONA 11: 2

Haworth R, Hopkins J, Ellis P, Acriyd C, Mowat A 1981 Expectations and outcome of THR. Rheumatology & Rehabilitation 20(2): 65–70

Hayward J 1975 A prescription against pain. Royal College of Nursing, London

Henderson V 1966 The nature of nursing. Collier MacMillan, Ontario

Ketchin V J 1989 Approaches to pain management. Surgical Nurse Feb: 1–22

Laing W, Taylor D 1982 Hip replacement and the NHS. Office of Health Economics, London

Lorimer D (ed) 1993 Common foot disorders, 4th edn. Churchill Livingstone, Edinburgh

Pugh J 1989 Mobility in the post-operative phase of care. Surgical Nurse 2(5): 15–19

RCN 1988 Guidelines for nurses caring for patients awaiting major joint replacement. Royal College of Nursing, London

Roberts F 1988 Milly's hip replacement. Nursing Times 84(8): 42–45

Ross J S, Wilson K J W (eds) 1990 Foundations of anatomy and physiology, 7th edn. Churchill Livingstone, Edinburgh, p 385, 387, 371, 388

Royce C L Jr 1988 Primary care orthopaedics. Churchill Livingstone, New York

Smith C 1989 Total hip replacement. Nursing Times 85(46): 28–31

Sutherland Muckle D 1986 An outline of orthopaedic practice. Wright, Bristol

Thompson C A 1988 Perception of pain. Surgical Nurse Oct: 6–8

UKCC 1990 The code of professional conduct for nurses, midwives and health visitors. United Kingdom Central Council, London

Value for money unit 1990 The role of nurses and other non-medical staff in out-patient departments. EL(90) P/44

NHS Management Executive Report, London

Webb C 1985 Sexuality, nursing and health. John Wiley, Chichester

World Health Organisation 1979 Formulating strategies for health for all by the year 2,000. WHO, Geneva

15

Shoulder and upper limb problems

Deborah Wheeler

INTRODUCTION

In common with other orthopaedic patients, many of those who present either in hospital or to their general practitioner with non-traumatic disorders of their shoulder or arm tend to be older than those who suffer trauma. As with other areas of the body, these joints are affected by constant use, although to a lesser extent than the weight-bearing joints of the leg. However, several of the joints of the upper limb, such as the shoulder, wrist and hand joints, are more complex in their anatomy and physiology than comparable joints of the lower limb, such as the hip or foot. This can cause the patient presenting with a disorder of the upper limb to experience a wide range of problems which may not all be immediately apparent to the nurse.

The loss or limitation of use of one or both of the upper limbs will have a profound effect on the quality of life of any patient and will greatly restrict his normal activities. This chapter and the nursing care described within it will therefore be based around Orem's self-care model for nursing, focusing on the return of the patient to independence. Orem devised her model around people's need to practise self-care in everyday life, calling these aspects of daily living universal self-care requisites, and considered how these self-care requisites are affected by both the ageing process (developmental self-care) and illness (health deviation self-care) (see Table 15.1) (Walsh & Judd 1989). She viewed nurses as working with patients in a wholly compensa-

Table 15.1 Orem's self-care model

Universal self-care requisites:
   maintenance of a sufficient intake of air
   maintenance of a sufficient intake of water
   maintenance of a sufficient intake of food
   provision of care associated with elimination processes
     and excrements
   maintenance of a balance between activity and rest
   maintenance of a balance between solitude and social
     interaction
   prevention of hazards to human life, human functioning
     and human well-being
   promotion of human functioning and development within
     social groups in accordance with human potential,
     known human limitations and the human desire to be
     normal
Developmental self-care requisites
Health deviation self-care requisites:
   human structure
   physical functioning
   behaviour

tory, partly compensatory or supportive/educative role, according to the patient's own self-care abilities. Therefore, this model would seem appropriate when planning care for any patient who has a mobility problem, given that disabilities of the shoulder and upper limb will impinge on a patient's overall mobility.

Care plans have been included to illustrate the problems experienced by patients with disorders of the joints of the arm. Although they have been related to specific procedures, many of the problems illustrated are the same for any patient undergoing surgery to that part of the arm.

ASSESSMENT

When assessing any patient with an upper limb problem, there are a number of factors the nurse will need to consider in terms of his self-care abilities. Principally, she should assess what movement he currently has, and whether this is likely to improve or deteriorate in the future. She should then consider how this lack of movement is affecting the patient psychologically, and how well he can rest and relax, for example, when he is in pain and discomfort. It is important for the nurse to assess what effect any lack of mobility has on other self-care requisites, such as the ability to prepare a meal or get dressed. She

should also assess the social setting in which the patient is living, or to which he will be discharged, and how this will affect his ability to be self-caring within the limits of his mobility (Walsh & Judd 1989) (see Table 15.2).

It can be easy for the nurse to lose sight of the fact that the patient with a disabled upper limb, who is able to walk unaided, will still have mobility problems. The *Oxford Illustrated Dictionary* defines mobility as 'freedom of movement', and this should apply equally to all limbs. The patient's inability to move his arm joints through their normal range will affect his lifestyle. Many patients express surprise at how dependent they are on a particular arm, and any surgery will initially compound their inability to perform what would seem simple, everyday activities. Orem (1980) stresses the importance of including the family and significant others in a patient's care, and this is especially appropriate when orthopaedic patients with long-term problems have been relying on their support and help with everyday needs.

In addition to assessing a patient's physical needs, nurses now have to deal with his raised expectations of health care. Diers (1981) comments on how the public's understanding of health and health care has increased as a result of its exposure to the mass media. Patients are no longer automatically compliant, neither will they tolerate ill-prepared explanations, but will often expect to understand why following a prescribed treatment is necessary or important.

TECHNOLOGY

Technological advances, some of which will be dealt with in this chapter, have served to raise

Table 15.2 Patient mobility and self-care assessment

a. What movement does the patient have?
b. Is this likely to improve or deteriorate in the future?
c. What are the psychological effects of any lack of
    movement?
d. Is the patient able to rest and relax?
e. What effect has the lack of movement on other self-care
    activities?
f. How does the patient's home setting affect his self-care
    abilities?

many patients' expectations of health care. Those for whom no direct cause of their problem can be found, or for whom there is no 'quick cure', may have difficulty in adjusting psychologically to their disability and this may stretch the skills of the nurses caring for them.

Equally, technological advances now mean that patients are being treated for a much wider range of diseases than previously, and there is pressure on nurses to obtain sufficient knowledge to provide care for all these patients. An example of this within orthopaedics is shoulder arthroplasty; this procedure is now being performed in an increasing number of centres, and yet comparatively little has been written about it in comparison to hip or knee replacements. This chapter will aim to rectify some of these omissions. The focus will, however be on the surgical care of patients with shoulder and upper limb problems, and the reader should refer to Chapters 10 and 11 for further information regarding the non-surgical care of patients with osteo- or rheumatoid arthritis.

PRINCIPLES OF NURSING CARE

The overall principles of care are similar for all patients with upper limb problems and so will be discussed in general first.

Loss of independence

Current demographic trends have led to a greater proportion of the population surviving to ages when degenerative diseases, many of which are orthopaedic in nature, are more widespread. The older person may already have other pathology present which impinges on his degree of independence, but the loss of function of one of his arms may precipitate a period of total dependence.

Much of the current focus and provision for disabled people is aimed at those who have lost the use of their lower limbs, and yet a person depends equally on the use of his upper limbs. Many elderly people, especially women, live alone, having outlived their partners, and so loss or limitation of the use of an arm seriously affects their ability to cope in such areas as preparing meals and washing and dressing. The *Standards of Care for Orthopaedic Nursing* (Royal College of Nursing 1990) stress that nurses must be sensitive to these needs and ensure that each patient is helped to cope by being involved in his own care and by being able to make informed choices. The nurse should also remember that the patient may depend on the use of an aid, such as a walking stick, for his mobility. Any disorder of his arm may leave him unable to use it and so deprive him of his independence.

The role of the multidisciplinary team in maintaining a patient's independence cannot be underestimated. Nursing care of these patients should be geared towards actively preparing them for self-care and liaising with other disciplines to ensure that they are fully assessed and all their needs are met.

Psychological needs

Limitations on their independence such as those described above are likely to affect patients psychologically in two areas. First, they will feel frustrated by their inability to carry out what are generally regarded as simple everyday tasks. This may make them feel resentful of the disorder which has disabled them, and embarrassed at having to ask for help to perform these activities, especially when they are of a personal nature. Second, their incapacity may leave them feeling bored and unable to fill their hours with their usual activities involving the use of their hands and arms, such as knitting, sewing, gardening or 'DIY' tasks. Some people find it difficult to adjust to their limitations, especially if they have led a very full life. In addition, they may find it difficult to obtain adequate help and support if there are no outward signs of their disability, such as walking with a limp or using a stick, as their disability may not easily be accepted as valid by outsiders.

The nurse, as patient advocate, has a valuable role to play in the community in helping the disabled patient and family to cope with the prejudices and attitudes of the rest of society.

Physical needs

So far the psychological effects of loss of independence for a patient with an upper limb problem have been discussed. However, the patient will naturally meet a wide range of physical difficulties, which the nurse will assess as a priority.

Nutrition People with a disorder of their arm or shoulder may have difficulty in maintaining a sufficient intake of both water and food. They may be able to walk to the shops but not manage the journey home with heavy bags of shopping. In these days of supermarket shopping, relatively few shops offer a home delivery service, and so the patient may be dependent on others to do his shopping for him. It should also be remembered that fresh foods, such as fruit and vegetables, weigh more than convenience packet foods, and so even those patients who are able to carry their own goods home may not be purchasing food which is nutritionally balanced.

Food preparation can be equally difficult. Loss or limitation of the use of one or both hands can make apparently simple tasks, such as opening tins or packets or peeling fresh vegetables, almost impossible. Disability of the shoulder can make lifting items down from cupboards unmanageable, or can leave the patient unable to manoeuvre dishes in or out of the oven. He may find lifting a kettle or saucepan difficult, and risk injury if the contents are hot.

Even when food is prepared for him, a patient may still be unable to cope. Cutlery may be difficult to manipulate for anyone with disability of the hand or wrist, and patients may be unable to exert sufficient pressure to cut their food into manageable pieces. It can be embarrassing for an adult to admit that he cannot cut up his own food and requires someone to do it for him. The nurse should be aware of the aids available, such as large-handled cutlery and plate guards, and should ensure that the patient is referred to the appropriate agencies, such as occupational therapy, for assessment and help with these problems (see Ch. 5).

Elimination The patient with an upper limb problem may find elimination difficult, as a result of factors discussed above. In addition, an insufficient intake of fibre and fluids and a lack of exercise may leave him constipated.

While the patient with hand and arm disability may have no difficulty in getting to the bathroom to use the toilet, he may be unable to unfasten buttons or zips. This problem may be compounded in the older patient by an urgent or frequent need to urinate, as a result of such disorders as prostatism. In this situation, it may be acutely embarrassing for the patient to ask for help. Equally, it may be awkward for him to clean himself after opening his bowels. Shoulder problems may make it difficult for the patient to reach his anus, or hand problems may leave him unable to grip the toilet tissue. Having to request help with such a personal function may result in loss of dignity for the patient, and the nurse must deal with the situation with tact and understanding.

Dressing and personal hygiene General personal hygiene is likely to be difficult for a patient with an upper limb disability. Disorders of the hand and wrist may make it awkward for him to turn taps on or off, or to soap and rinse a flannel or sponge in order to wash. It can also be difficult for a patient to manoeuvre himself in and out of a bath if he is able to take little or no weight through his arms. Equally, a person with a shoulder disability may be unable to reach certain parts of his body in order to wash. If he has little or no shoulder movement, it may be difficult for him to wash the axilla of the affected arm. This may result in the patient having what is, for him, unacceptable body odour, or, especially in hot weather, reddened or sore skin of that axilla and perhaps even excoriation.

The patient may also have difficulty in dressing. Buttons and zips are awkward to fasten when there is loss of fine hand movements. Shirts, blouses and jumpers may be impossible to put on unaided when the patient has impaired shoulder mobility. Many of these problems can be overcome by the nurse encouraging the patient to learn new techniques for dressing, and by suggesting devices, such as the use of velcro, to replace zips and buttons. Replacing small buttons with larger ones can help, and there is a range of dressing aids available to assist the patient.

Motivation and dignity In order to motivate the patient towards self-care, he should be encouraged to undertake as much of his own care as possible, especially in relation to such areas as personal hygiene, nutrition and elimination. However, he should not be expected to carry out more than he can manage, and a full nursing assessment will establish realistic goals, with the need for nursing intervention clearly and appropriately identified. The patient's relatives and friends should be involved as much as possible.

The nurse will need to liaise with the occupational therapist to educate the patient in the use of appropriate aids. By working with the physiotherapist, the nurse can ensure that unaffected joints and limbs maintain their normal range of movements.

It is most important for the nurse caring for a patient with a disability of his upper limb to help him maintain his dignity and self-esteem. In situations where the patient requires help with simple everyday tasks, the nurse's most valuable skills are tact and understanding, treating the patient at all times as an intelligent human being, recognizing that his wishes are of paramount importance and ensuring that his feelings are treated with respect.

Loss of function

The reader should refer to Chapter 5 for more information on mobilization.

Much of the loss of independence previously described will be attributable directly to the loss of function of the affected joint. There may be one or more causes of this (see Table 15.3):

1. Pain can be a severely limiting factor in that if movement of a joint causes pain, the natural reaction will be to avoid that movement.

Table 15.3 Reasons for loss of joint function

Pain
Joint destruction
Muscle atrophy

2. Certain disease processes such as osteoarthritis will eventually destroy the joint surfaces, and so movement may be limited due to the joint surfaces being roughened and unable to move freely.

3. Disuse of a joint or limb will cause muscle atrophy and may limit joint mobility by loss or disruption of the mechanism of movement.

The first two causes – pain and the disease process – may be resolved by medical or surgical intervention. However, the third cause, muscle disuse, is treated during the period after surgery. Here the nurse works with the physiotherapist and occupational therapist, reinforcing the techniques and exercises they teach the patient.

The overall aim of any period of rehabilitation must be determined by the patient's needs and expectations. It should be realistic and relevant to the patient; for example, a 70-year-old lady is unlikely to require circumduction following a shoulder arthroplasty, whereas a 25-year-old man undergoing a repair for anterior dislocation of the shoulder may wish to continue bowling for his local cricket team.

Equally, the nurse needs to be aware of the important movements in each joint for normal function; for example, medial rotation is necessary at the shoulder for a person to lift his hand to his mouth, and the ability to oppose the thumb is essential for grip. This knowledge may be gained from anatomy books (see also Ch. 4).

Rehabilitation exercises of the arm can be divided into three categories:

1. Passive movements
2. Active assisted exercises
3. Strengthening exercises.

Passive movements

These exercises are used to help maintain the patient's range of joint movements and to preserve the joint's gliding mechanism. They also help to prevent the development of adhesions or soft tissue contractures.

Initially they are carried out by the physiotherapist, but may subsequently be performed by a nurse, relative or friend, or by the patient himself who will move the affected limb with the unaffected arm.

Active assisted exercises

These may begin as early as the first postoperative day if this is permitted by the surgeon. They are designed to allow the affected muscle to work partially and may again involve the use of the unaffected arm or of pulleys and other aids.

The programme of exercises is planned by the physiotherapist to meet the individual patient's needs; other methods, such as use of the gymnastic ball, pendulum exercises for the shoulder and hydrotherapy may also be included (Fig. 15.1).

Strengthening exercises

In order to reduce the risk of further injury, these exercises commence much later in the patient's rehabilitation programme, when the soft tissue structures around the joint have healed. Since many patients have less pain in their arm and may even feel stronger following surgery, they do not realize how easily they can injure the healing tissues.

Strengthening exercises taught by the physiotherapist include the use of isolated isometrics on each muscle in turn. Latex straps are a new

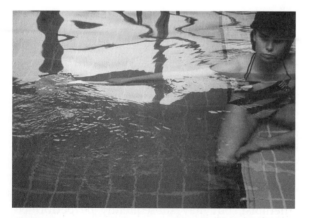

Fig. 15.1 Hydrotherapy.

aid used in strengthening exercises, especially of the shoulder; each strap has graded resistance, and by pulling against it the patient can dynamically exercise the joint. Once the joint has become well strengthened, a piece of bicycle inner tube may be used, especially for fit men.

The use of biofeedback is increasing in orthopaedic centres. It is commonly used in the treatment of unstable shoulders for habitual dislocation or for abnormal movements.

The occupational therapist's treatment complements that of the physiotherapist in helping the patient regain the use of the affected arm. The patient's programme is individually designed to include relevant functional activities. Those activities that the patient will carry out at home and work are incorporated into the programme. Preoperatively, the occupational therapist assesses the patient's use of each arm, establishes hand dominance, and notes any compensatory movements the patient may have adopted to avoid pain. The patient is also assessed for his potential ability to cope at home postoperatively; for example, he may be increasingly disabled for an initial period by having one arm immobilized in a foam wedge. Aids and adaptations are supplied only as necessary. Some patients may need extra assistance if they have lower limb problems and are unable to take any weight through their hands or arms for a time, leaving them unable to use any crutches or walking aids.

The nurse's role as educator is not limited to passing on new knowledge and skills, but also includes changing attitudes and assisting the patient and family to adjust to a new way of life where necessary (Footner 1987). This may include working with other professionals, such as occupational therapists, to help the patient to use new aids or pieces of equipment and to educate the patient's family in this as well. Any health education needs, such as losing weight or giving up smoking, should be identified, information volunteered, and support given as part of the overall care of the patient. Information may also include details of statutory organizations and voluntary groups who may provide additional help and support.

Pain and discomfort

Although the management of a patient's pain has been dealt with extensively in Chapter 7, it is worth further consideration here, as nursing research continues to show that nurses are often ineffective in dealing with their patients' pain. Over 10 years ago, McCaffery stated that pain is what the patient says it is. Postoperative pain is variable; each patient must be assessed individually by the nurse.

Although many nurses will think immediately of drug therapy when a patient complains of pain, there are a variety of other approaches available to them. Ensuring that the patient's arm is properly supported and that the patient is in a comfortable position helps initially. Use of a roller towel, for example, may result in shoulder and neck discomfort if it is not applied correctly and the patient's arm is inadequately supported. Good elevation minimizes the development of oedema and so helps to reduce pain.

The use of a heat pad may help an area which is aching and tense. Conversely, many patients with acute inflammation of an area may find relief from the application of an ice-pack; this should not, however, be placed directly against the skin, and should be changed at regular intervals as it becomes warm.

Other members of the multidisciplinary team may be involved in pain management – especially physiotherapists, who see it as one of their main roles. They have a range of skills which may be of value to the patient, including the use of ultrasound and shortwave diathermy.

The main consideration for the nurse must be to keep the patient comfortable at all times. Pain prevents the patient from cooperating with his personal care and disrupts his sleep, thus increasing his tiredness. Medical advice should be sought if the patient complains of any new areas of pain. Controlling their pain helps patients to remain motivated in maintaining their self-care and in their subsequent rehabilitation.

Complications of surgery

As with any other form of surgery, the orthopaedic nurse observes the patient postoperatively for any signs of complications from the surgery to his arm. These fall into three broad areas: neurological impairment, vascular damage and oedema.

Whatever the observations, it is vital that they are carried out formally and recorded. With individualized care and recent trends towards primary nursing, it is likely that one nurse will be carrying out the observations over a period of time. However, she will not be present 24 hours per day, and those replacing her need to be aware of previous data. Use of a chart to document the observations helps to ensure continuous assessment (see Table 15.4).

Neurological impairment

The nerves supplying the arm divide out from the brachial plexus into four main branches:

- the musculocutaneous nerve
- the radial nerve
- the ulnar nerve
- the median nerve.

Table 15.4 Neurovascular observations

Sensation
Movement
Colour
Warmth
Comparative radial pulses

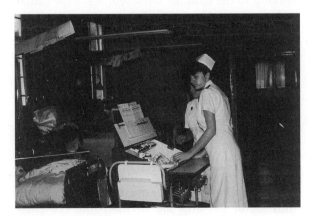
Fig. 15.2 Pain relief.

They can be damaged during surgery by either direct trauma or undue pressure. Nursing observations are aimed at detecting whether any trauma has taken place and preventing any further deterioration.

The focus of any nursing observation is to assess the motor and sensory function of the affected arm. This is generally done by evaluation of the movement and sensation of the fingers, care being taken to assess each finger in turn. These observations should also be carried out preoperatively in order to establish a baseline, as those patients with an arm disorder such as carpal tunnel syndrome are likely already to have an altered neurological status, which may or may not improve immediately post-surgery. Some patients may complain of altered sensations in their hand, such as 'pins and needles' or numbness, but others may assume that this is to be expected, and so the nurse should specifically question them about this.

Where possible, wrist movement should also be assessed, with the nurse being aware that flexion is controlled by the ulnar nerve and extension by the radial nerve. Damage to or compression of either will impair wrist mobility. It should also be remembered that the ulnar nerve lies superficially at the elbow, and so care must be taken to ensure that the arm is well supported along its length.

Vascular damage

In conjunction with any assessment for neurological impairment of the hand and arm postoperatively, the nurse evaluates the vascular status of the limb. As with neurological impairment, any damage may be caused by direct trauma during surgery, or by undue pressure.

Nursing observations therefore focus on the perfusion of the distal part of the arm, several points being taken into consideration. The colour of the hand and fingers should be assessed: an adequate blood supply will be indicated by a pink colour. Any cyanosis or blanching should be noted and reported immediately. It is not always easy to assess the skin colour of patients who have dark skins, so it can be useful to assess venous return in the nail bed. This is done by applying pressure to one of the finger nails until it blanches. On release, the nail bed should immediately regain its pink colour and any sluggishness would indicate a less than acceptable vascular flow to the hand.

The temperature of the limb can also be a useful guide to circulation, as a well-perfused arm will feel warm to the touch. However, several factors need to be taken into consideration when assessing the warmth of a limb:

1. The patient's main body temperature should be noted, as someone who has an oral temperature of 35.5°C, which is not uncommon immediately following a general anaesthetic, is unlikely to have warm extremities.
2. The outside air temperature is also a factor, as an exposed limb is unlikely to feel warm to the touch in cold weather.
3. Both hands and arms must be assessed in order to judge whether the limb is unduly cool. Any difference in temperature between the two limbs would alert the nurse to potential problems.

Pulses are also indicative of vascular flow within a limb. As with the skin temperature of the arm, it is important that the nurse compares the pulses in both arms for strength. The most common site for this observation is the radial pulse, and both pulses should be felt simultaneously. This observation is generally carried out only for surgery to the upper arm or shoulder, as any surgery to the hand or wrist will leave the radial pulse inaccessible due to dressings or splints.

Oedema

Oedema is a natural response of the body's tissues to any trauma, be it accidental or intentional, such as surgery. The inflammatory response provoked by surgery results in changes in the permeability of the blood vessels and increased vascular flow, allowing leakage of plasma into the tissues (David 1986), which causes swelling of the arm. As in the leg, the muscles of the arm are divided into compartments by bands of fascia. Although the skin and tissues of the forearm are relatively elastic in nature, these layers of fascia are inelastic and so will not expand to accommodate any swelling. As a result, pressure within the muscle compartments of the arm will increase, causing compression of the soft tissues and structures of the arm. This, therefore, can potentially compromise the blood flow within the arm, or prevent efficient conduction by the peripheral nerves.

In order to prevent gross oedema of the arm, therefore, it is necessary to elevate it following surgery for a minimum of 24 hours to assist lymphatic drainage. However, this is not possible with certain shoulder operations where the arm may be held close to the chest wall in a body bandage, and so extra vigilance is required from the nurse for these patients. Practical methods of elevation of the arm are discussed in the next section.

With oedema in mind, all rings and jewellery must be removed from the affected arm prior to surgery, to prevent constriction of the fingers. Some female patients may be distressed by the need to remove their wedding ring should their left hand or arm require surgery, and so it is vital that the nurse explains tactfully why this is necessary.

Joint stiffness

Immobilization or disuse of joints over a period of time can lead to a degree of stiffness, particularly in patients whose arms are immobilized in a sling for a long term. The nurse needs to be aware of this as potential problem and to ensure that, where possible, any patient with an immobilized arm puts the unaffected joints of that arm through a normal range of movements at least twice per day in order to retain the elasticity of the joint capsule, especially in the shoulder.

Immobilization and elevation

As discussed in the previous section, the arm is immobilized and elevated postoperatively in order to prevent the development of complications. Immobilization allows resting of the surrounding soft tissues to aid healing and prevent dislocation of any prosthesis. It also allows the arm to be held in the optimum position following surgery. Elevation helps to prevent or reduce oedema, and so prevents the development of neurovascular complications and reduces pain. This section outlines some of the common forms of immobilizing and elevating the arm and shoulder postoperatively. Further details of the principles of immobilization are discussed in Chapter 6.

Roller towel

The patient's arm is held in a roller towel attached to a stand at the side of the bed. This method may be used for immobilization of the shoulder in abduction following surgery or, more commonly, to achieve high elevation of the hand (see Fig. 15.3).

Application   The nurse should slip the towel up to the axilla, with the patient sitting towards the appropriate side of the bed, not in the middle. The height of the stand should be adjusted so that the upper arm is supported horizontally. The pole of the stand should be incorporated into the towel. Three safety pins are then required and should be placed as follows:

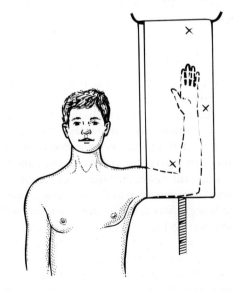

Fig. 15.3   Elevation of arm using roller towel; X marks position of safety pins.

- one in the crook of the elbow
- one lateral to the forearm at wrist level
- the third at the top of the roller towel to prevent it from slipping off the stand.

The nurse needs to check that the height of the stand is altered according to the patient's position, i.e. whether he is in bed or sitting in a chair. The patient's shoulder should be comfortable and to help, the nurse can place a pillow under the upper arm for added support. This also reduces pressure on the ulnar nerve at the elbow.

Broad arm sling

Slings are used to give comfort and support to an injured hand or arm and to spread the weight of the arm evenly across the neck and shoulders. When resting in a broad arm sling, the patient's elbow is flexed at 90° and is supported across the chest (see Fig. 15.4).

Application With the patient standing and supporting the affected arm, the nurse should place the triangular bandage across his chest, with the small angle of the triangle pointing towards the elbow and the long edge of the bandage towards the unaffected arm. The affected arm should be placed across the patient's chest, on top of the bandage, with the elbow flexed at 90°. The bandage should then be folded upwards from below the arm, and tied in a reef knot on the same side of the neck as the affected arm. A reef knot should always be used as this ensures a strong weight-bearing tie. The edges at the elbow should be tucked in and held with a safety pin. Padding may be placed under the sling at the neck to prevent chafing and rubbing.

It is important to ensure that the hand is supported by the sling and not hanging out, as this may predispose the patient to oedema of the hand and will cause pressure and rubbing at the wrist from the edge of the bandage. Exercises for the fingers, wrist, elbow and shoulder should be demonstrated to the patient as appropriate, to be carried out every few hours. The patient and his relatives should be aware of the purpose of the sling and should be able to reapply it themselves if necessary, as it is functional only if properly used and applied.

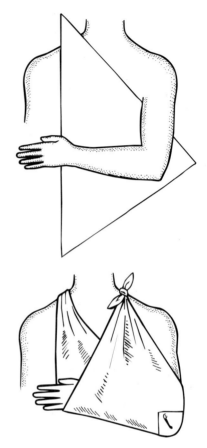

Fig. 15.4 Broad arm sling.

High arm sling

This sling maintains the hand at the level of the shoulder, ensuring high elevation and reduction of oedema following surgery (see Fig. 15.5).

Application With the patient standing and supporting the affected arm, the nurse should flex the patient's arm so that the tips of the fingers rest on the opposite shoulder:

- The triangular bandage should be placed as for a broad arm sling, only with the bandage on top of the arm, not under it.
- The bandage should then be folded below the arm upwards underneath the arm to encase it, and tied behind the patient's shoulder with a reef knot.
- The corners of the bandage at the elbow should be tucked in and secured with a safety pin.

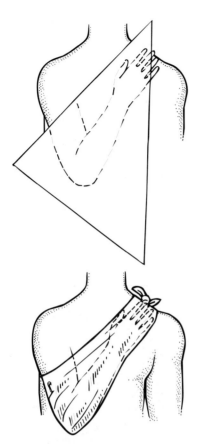

Fig. 15.5 High arm sling.

As with the broad arm sling, the patient needs to be taught relevant exercises for the joints of the arm and hand to prevent any loss of function through disuse. It is also important that the hand is held in position by the bandage to maintain elevation and support, and the patient should be made aware of the need to readjust the sling should the hand slip out.

Collar and cuff

This is used more commonly for support than for elevation. It is supplied as a roll of foam strip covered by a stockinette, and so can be cut to the length required. It fulfils the same function as a broad arm sling and can be applied in a variety of ways as demonstrated in Figure 15.6. Care should be taken to ensure that the parts encircling the arm are loose enough to prevent constriction and to allow ease of removal and reapplication by the patient.

Body bandage

This is a method of immobilizing the shoulder and upper arm following surgery, providing a good position for healing and aiding patient comfort (see Fig. 15.7).

Application   This must be carried out by two persons, with the patient sitting on a stool to allow ease of access:

- One person holds the arm in the required position to prevent further injury and ensure the position is maintained during application of the bandage.
- The nurse should wash and dry the axilla on the affected side carefully without abducting the arm, and also the area beneath the breasts for female patients. This checks the integrity of the skin prior to application of the bandage, ensures optimum cleanliness while the areas are accessible, and helps the patient to feel more comfortable.
- Pads should then be placed wherever two skin surfaces come into contact, i.e. in the axilla, in the flexure of the elbow, underneath the hand, and, for female patients, beneath the breasts.
- The arm is placed across the body with the palm resting on the opposite clavicle.
- A 15-cm woolroll bandage is then applied from the front smoothly around the trunk in one direction, and in spiral turns around the shoulder.
- 15-cm crêpe bandages are applied in the same way and fastened with zinc oxide tape.
- The procedure is repeated two further times to give a total of six alternating layers of wool and crêpe bandage.
- The hand and fingers must be visible, to allow their neurovascular status to be checked.
- The bandage is then encased with 10-cm elastoplast, or a layer of plaster of Paris may be applied.

The bandage may be left in place for between 1 and 6 weeks and changed as necessary, at which times the skin condition can be checked.

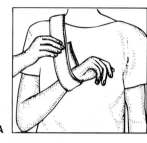
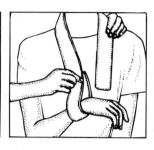
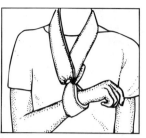

1. Take approx. 75 cm of Collar 'n' Cuff and place arm in required position.

2. Support the wrist with one end of the Collar 'n' Cuff, the other end being taken round the neck.

3. Bring the two ends together and fasten with tie provided, ensuring sufficient room for the hand to be withdrawn from the Collar 'n' Cuff.

Excess tie can be cut off and cut edge tucked into the Collar 'n' Cuff to make a neat finish.

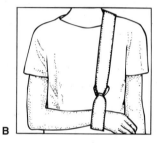
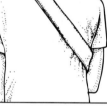

1. To support an arm in a balanced position, often in conjunction with forearm casts, take approx. 1.5 m of Collar 'n' Cuff and tie one end around the wrist.

2. Take the Collar 'n' Cuff around the neck and over the opposite shoulder, bringing it across the back of the patient.

3. Bring the loose end through, and over the arm at the elbow.

4. Secure and tie behind, again ensuring there is sufficient room for the arm to be removed from the Collar 'n' Cuff.

Fig. 15.6 Collar and cuff. A. To fit as a traditional sling. B. To support the arm in a balanced position. (From Seton, with permission.)

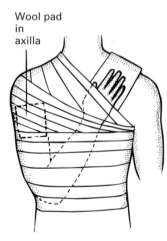

Fig. 15.7 Body bandage.

The patient should be taught appropriate finger exercises, and also taught to look for any abnormalities of colour, warmth and sensation in the affected hand; these should be reported immediately to senior nursing or medical staff.

Abduction wedge

This is a method of immobilization of the shoulder which allows the patient to be ambulant (see Fig. 15.8), unlike the roller towel which tends to limit the patient's independence. Splints, such as the aeroplane splint, are now being used less frequently; the use of a foam wedge is much more comfortable for the patient because it is lighter to wear; it is also more

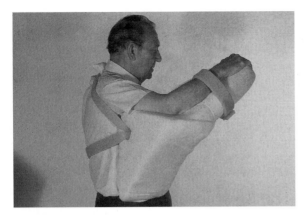

Fig. 15.8 Abduction wedge.

effective in maintaining lateral rotation of the shoulder. Patients may be discharged home wearing these, which helps them to preserve their independence and shortens their hospital stay.

Scarring

The assumption is often made that the rest of the wound heals at the same rate as the skin wound. David (1986) points out that biologically this is not so; the healing process continues for some time, with the realignment of collagen, shrinking and a change in colour. External scar tissue can, in fact, reduce skin flexibility and limit mobility, extension and full movement at joints. Consequently, care of the wound is needed after the initial healing phase. Movement improves the flexibility of skin scars by orienting the collagen fibres; the nurse should recognize the importance of exercises and start them, in conjunction with the physiotherapist, as soon as possible.

Minimizing scarring demands skilful prevention of damage to the wound. Scars on the arm are often not covered by clothing, and the nurse should ensure that any scars, however minor, are cosmetically acceptable to the patient. It is worth noting that the skin over the upper arm and clavicle appears to heal less easily than the rest of the arm, and while surgeons avoid this area whenever possible, good wound care helps to minimize any adverse effects.

Any irritation of the healing tissue may in-

duce chronic inflammation, which could lead to wound breakdown and a resultant unsightly scar. This is especially true of surgery in the shoulder area, and may be particularly pertinent for women, as bra straps may cause friction against the wound. Ideally the patient should stop wearing a bra for the first few weeks following surgery, but if this is unacceptable, the bra strap needs to be well padded; a sanitary towel may prove useful for this.

Lifting and handling the patient

It is often difficult for a patient whose arm is elevated or immobilized in any way to maintain a comfortable position in bed. His ease of mobility is restricted and positions such as sitting in bed are awkward for him to achieve without help. A tendency for the patient to slip down the bed causes friction and may result in pressure sores from shearing force, and so he will need assistance in adjusting his position at regular intervals.

Research has indicated that some of the nurses at greatest risk from back injuries through lifting are those who work on orthopaedic wards (Rogers & Salvage 1988). Lifting or handling a patient with an immobilized arm may not immediately appear as difficult for the nurse as, for example, handling a patient following total hip replacement. However, lifting a patient who has undergone shoulder surgery may preclude the use of most of the conventional lifting techniques taught to nurses.

The most important maxim for a nurse to remember when moving a patient is to lift only when absolutely necessary. The lift and its degree of difficulty should be assessed, and the patient never lifted by only one person. A patient following upper limb surgery is generally able to use his unaffected arm to assist himself to move. Attaching an aid such as a 'monkey pole' to the patient's bed and teaching him how to use it may preclude the need for the nurse to actively lift at all. Equally, patients should be shown to bend their knees and push with their heels to move themselves up the bed when necessary.

Not only is lifting hazardous for nurses

but also, if badly carried out, it may cause the patient pain and possibly further injury. To hold someone around his shoulder following surgery is painful, and reinforces the need for nurses to educate patients to enable them to move independently.

Assistance from the nurse should focus on supporting the patient at his affected side to prevent loss of balance.

Information-giving

Many patients are anxious about their admission to hospital, which may be partly because they lack procedural information. Many hospitals now send patients information booklets which explain hospital routines, and surgeons are beginning to conduct preadmission clinics. It is unfortunate that few nurses are involved in these, as they are an ideal opportunity for the patient to meet ward nurses, who can carry out an initial nursing assessment.

On arrival at the ward, the nurse should answer any of the patient's questions accurately and honestly. It is also valuable for nurses to volunteer information, as the patient may be unable to identify all the gaps in his knowledge. Information-giving should not be limited to the time of the patient's admission, but should continue during the whole of his stay. The nurse should make time to listen to any of the patient's fears or worries (Hayward 1975, Boore 1978). Once she has established a relationship with him, he will be more likely to share any worries he may have and ask questions about his treatment and care.

The nurse's role in the giving of information also encompasses passing information about the patient on to other relevant members of the health care team, and acting as the patient's advocate. This can be achieved by making an accurate assessment, maintaining the patient's care plan, evaluating the care given, and sharing this with other members of the health care team in addition to the patient and his family.

The national *Standards of Care for Othopaedic Nursing* (Royal College of Nursing 1990) emphasize that all patients should be able to make informed decisions about their care and future health, and that they should be satisfied with their levels of independence in self-care activities. It is therefore apparent that these goals can be achieved only if the nurse volunteers and shares information with the patient. His active involvement in care planning will increase his understanding and motivation, so that he is more likely to cooperate fully and cope positively with his admission and care.

THE SHOULDER

The shoulder joint is classified, like the hip, as a ball and socket joint (see Fig. 15.9). However, unlike the hip, it relies mainly on muscles and soft tissues for its support. These muscles allow the complex movements of the shoulder joint, which has the greatest range of movements of any joint in the body. Surgery will naturally affect the function of these muscles and weaken the supportive soft tissues, which must then heal before the beneficial effects of the operation can be felt.

Shoulder arthroplasty

This is a growth area in orthopaedics, following the successes in the past 20 years of hip and knee

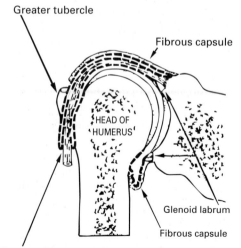

Fig. 15.9 Anatomy of the shoulder joint. (From Smith et al 1983, with permission.)

joint replacements, and the procedure is now being performed in an increasing number of centres (see Fig. 15.10). It is an elective procedure which is carried out to relieve pain which may be limiting shoulder function.

However, although patients expect the procedure to reduce their pain and improve the function of their shoulder joints, they may not be prepared for the necessarily prolonged rehabilitation period. Rehabilitation following shoulder arthroplasty may take as long as 6 months to a year before the patient regains full, normal, pain-free shoulder movements. It is therefore important that patients are made aware of this, so that their expectations of the surgery are realistic.

Preoperative considerations

Assessment of the neurovascular status of both arms is essential to provide a baseline for postoperative observations. Hand dominance should also be noted; if the dominant arm is the one requiring surgery, then it is often useful at this stage for the patient to begin practising self-care activities using his non-dominant hand, to help him improve his coordination.

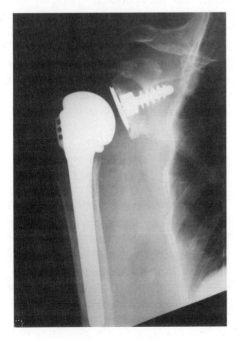

Fig. 15.10 Total shoulder replacement.

The physiotherapist generally meets the patient at this point to begin teaching him the exercises which will be carried out postoperatively. Deep breathing exercises are also important, as many patients will initially have their arms immobilized in body bandages which will restrict their chest movements.

The need to remove all jewellery, especially rings, prior to surgery because of the possibility of postoperative oedema should be emphasized.

Skin preparation will depend upon the surgeon's instructions. The debate over shaving has intensified in recent years. The general effect of shaving is to damage the epithelium and produce an environment in which skin flora such as *Staphylococcus aureus* can become established (David 1986). Consequently, any shaving should be carried out as near to the time of the operation as possible to reduce colonization and avoid an increase in the infection rate. Even in skilled hands a safety razor may cause minor skin abrasions, and many surgeons now advocate clipping the hair or using a depilatory cream. Whatever method is used for removing body hair, good general hygiene is essential, and the nurse should ensure that the axilla is thoroughly washed.

Postoperative care

Air Orthopaedic patients will require the same nursing care as that given to all patients after a general anaesthetic. Special attention should be given to their airways as initially they will be nursed flat on their backs, and then in a semirecumbent position when fully conscious. Deep breathing exercises are commenced if their arms are immobilized in a body bandage, as their chest movements will be restricted.

Water The patient will be able to drink when he is fully conscious. All items should be placed within reach of his unaffected arm so that he can retain some independence. An intravenous infusion may be in progress; some anaesthetists insert this into the patient's foot, so that the use of his unaffected arm is unimpeded.

Food When the patient is eating, he will need assistance with food: a pork chop and peas can be difficult to eat with one hand! Food should be cut up into portions which can be easily manipulated with a fork in one hand. Sandwiches are also easily managed with one hand.

Elimination If the patient does not have a pedal infusion, he may be allowed out of bed to use a commode or may be wheeled to the bathroom. Generally, a bedpan is used for the first 24 hours. The nurse should ensure that the patient can balance adequately, as his balance will be altered by having one arm strapped to his side. The danger is that he may lean to his affected side, and either fall or put his weight through that arm by leaning on his elbow. After 24 hours, the patient will be able to get out of bed and walk to the bathroom with assistance. He may need help with cleaning after opening his bowels, particularly if the dominant arm is the affected one.

Activity/rest It is important that patients are encouraged to rest to promote tissue repair and healing. Although the deep, nagging arthritic pain is removed by the surgery, pain will still be experienced within the muscles and soft tissues of the shoulder. Analgesia should be given regularly as prescribed and its effectiveness monitored. It is especially important that the patient is given adequate analgesia at night to allow him to sleep, and before any nursing or physiotherapy intervention during the day.

When permitted by the surgeon, the physiotherapist will begin to mobilize the affected shoulder. Before mobilization, finger, wrist and hand movements are carried out in order to maintain normal joint range. Static exercises of the deltoid muscle are also taught while the patient is wearing the body bandage.

Following removal of the body bandage, extension exercises of the elbow and movements of the forearm are encouraged. Static shoulder exercises are reinforced with assisted shoulder movements, especially flexion with external rotation. Although the programme is individually tailored for each patient, exercises will include movement of the shoulder using the unaffected arm or pulleys to assist, finger-walking up a wall, use of a gymnastic ball, and pendulum exercises

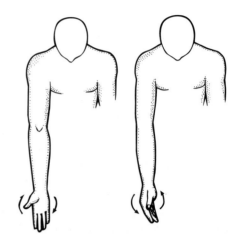

Fig. 15.11 Pendulum exercises; each arm is circled outwards, then inwards while bending at the waist.

(see Fig. 15.11). Hydrotherapy may also be encouraged if the condition of the wound allows.

When the patient's functional movements are restored, strengthening exercises are introduced. These include isolated isometric exercises for each of the deltoid muscles. Latex bands of graded strengths may also be used in dynamic exercises, especially external rotation (see Fig. 15.12). At this point the occupational therapist becomes involved to encourage the patient to follow functional exercises, such as medial and lateral rotation, so that he will be able to lift his hand to his mouth. The patient should, however, be cautioned not to lift or carry heavy objects, as these muscles have not been used fully for some time and will remain weak.

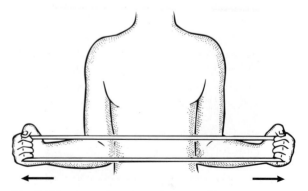

Fig. 15.12 External rotation using graded latex strip.

Solitude/social interaction This is not generally a problem for the patient who has undergone shoulder surgery. He is able to mobilize after 24 hours, and so may interact with other patients or spend time alone as he wishes.

Prevention of hazards When the patient returns from theatre, the affected shoulder is immobilized by means of a body bandage in order to allow healing of the soft tissues and prevent dislocation. By keeping the shoulder immobile, pain can also be controlled (Follman 1988). When the body bandage is removed, the arm is supported in a collar and cuff or in a broad arm sling.

A wound suction drain is in place for the first 48 hours, and the amount of drainage should be monitored hourly at first, decreasing to 4-hourly after the first 6 hours.

The physical reaction to surgical trauma results in increased permeability of the blood vessels, causing oedema of the soft tissues. As it is not possible to elevate the affected arm because it is immobilized in a body bandage, careful observation of the neurovascular status is essential. Both radial pulses should be monitored and compared to ensure equality of strength. Sensation and movement should be examined in all fingers, as should the colour and warmth of the hand. Medical advice should be sought if there is any alteration in perfusion or in the neurological status of the hand.

Assisting the patient to a sitting position helps to decrease swelling around the immediate shoulder area. However, the patient may find it difficult to maintain a sitting position and may have a tendency to slide down the bed. The resultant friction with the bed linen will cause a shearing force and may leave the patient at risk of pressure sores. Use of a 'monkey pole' and teaching the patient to lift himself by bending his knees and pushing with his feet help him to keep himself upright while in bed. As soon as he is mobile the problem will disappear as he will be able to sit out in a chair. However, he should be warned to avoid leaning on the affected arm by, for example, resting on the chair arm when sitting.

Being normal As soon as possible following surgery, the patient will wish to change into his own clothes. Baggy tops or nightdresses allow adequate room for the body bandage. Female patients may prefer to use a shawl rather than a dressing gown or cardigan in order to keep warm. When the body bandage is removed, the incision will need protection from the friction arising from the patient's clothing. Female patients will find that blouses with skirts or trousers are more convenient than dresses, as they allow easier access to the shoulder when necessary.

All patients find that their level of independence is initially reduced and that they need assistance with personal hygiene and dressing, especially if the operation has been carried out on their dominant arm. Skin care of the affected arm is important as irritation where two skin surfaces touch, such as in the axilla, may cause discomfort, particularly in hot weather. The skin should be washed and dried thoroughly by the nurse who should take care to support the affected arm. A cotton pad placed in the axilla helps to keep the skin dry, but talcum powder or deodorants should be avoided due to the proximity of the wound.

Health deviation Care of the wound ensures good healing with minimal scarring. The suction drain is removed at 48 hours, at which point the wound may be redressed if the surgeon allows the body bandage to be removed. The dressing is reduced using an aseptic technique, but subsequently should not be removed until healing is complete, unless there is evidence of infection (such as pyrexia), inflammation around the dressing or exudate onto the dressing pad. Generally, shoulder sutures are removed at between 7 and 10 days postoperatively.

In order to shorten the period of rehabilitation, patients should be active participants in their own care (Doheny & Ceccio 1988) and understand the reasons for their rehabilitation exercises. The nurse should make time to listen to their worries. Members of the patient's family should also be involved in the patient's rehabilitation, as they can encourage him to do his exercises and provide emotional support as he adjusts to his new body image. Rehabilitation following shoulder arthroplasty may take as long as a year before full function and strength are regained. Education on the time-scale of recovery ensures that the patient has realistic expectations of his progress and becomes less frustrated (see Care plan 1).

Recurrent anterior dislocation of the shoulder

This is usually the result of an initial traumatic dislocation which tears the soft tissue structures and results in an unstable joint. Repeated dislocation may then occur following minor shoulder movements. Surgery is undertaken to repair and tighten the soft tissues of the shoulder in order to increase the stability of the joint.

Specific postoperative care

Much of the general care required is as outlined for patients undergoing shoulder arthroplasty. The patient's arm is immobilized in a body bandage, which allows finger movements only. The neurovascular status of the hand must therefore be monitored carefully. A suction drain is in situ, and is removed at 24–48 hours, when drainage is minimal.

When the body bandage is removed, the arm rests in a collar and cuff. On removal of the body bandage, the axilla, arm and trunk are gently washed with minimal movement of the shoulder. Deodorant or talcum powder should not be used due to the proximity of the wound.

Care plan 1   Joan S, 68 years old; left total shoulder replacement

Problem	Aim	Nursing intervention
1. Joan has pain in her left shoulder following surgery	For Joan to say that she has no pain	Ask Joan whether she has any pain and get her to describe it by using the pain chart Observe for any non-verbal signs of pain, such as sweating, grimacing Position Joan comfortably in the bed or chair using pillows for support Offer analgesia as prescribed Ensure that nursing actions and physiotherapy follow analgesia
2. Joan cannot be fully independent while wearing a body bandage	a. Joan will be able to wash herself each day as she wishes	Assist Joan with washing the areas she cannot reach with her right arm Ensure she has all necessary articles within reach when in the bathroom
	b. Joan will be able to eat meals as she wishes	Encourage Joan to select her meals from the menu Ensure her meals are presented so that she can eat them with one hand, and that her food is cut into adequate portions Liaise with occupational therapist re: eating aids
	c. Joan will be wearing the clothes she wants to each day	Assist Joan with dressing each day, such as fastening buttons Encourage her to wear loose nightdress or blouse and skirt to allow ease of access to her shoulder Assist her to undress as she requires
3. Joan has to wear a body bandage for one week to prevent dislocation of her total shoulder replacement	For Joan to feel comfortable in the bandage and to suffer no ill effects	Check the bandage daily to ensure it remains in position Reapply the bandage if it becomes loose Check the neurovascular status of Joan's left hand for alteration Observe Joan's fingers for oedema
4. Joan has a surgical wound in her left shoulder	For Joan's wound to heal within 10 days	Observe the body bandage for any excess wound leakage Monitor exudate into the suction drain Remove drain aseptically at 48 hours Record vital signs 4-hourly and observe for pyrexia
5. Joan has reduced movement in her left shoulder following surgery	For Joan to be able to regain the use of her shoulder	Reinforce instructions from the physiotherapist about shoulder exercises Encourage Joan to practise these shoulder exercises Offer support and encouragement as to her progress

When and how quickly the patient's shoulder is mobilized are dictated by the surgeon. The patient starts with gentle assisted exercises initially and gradually increases to active and strengthening exercises over several months. He should be warned not to abduct or laterally rotate his shoulder to prevent further injury to the repaired soft tissues.

To support his shoulder at night, the patient is advised to wear a tight T-shirt. When he is lying in bed, a pillow tucked into the side under the upper arm stops it falling posteriorly. The patient should be advised to keep the arm next to the body at all times, and not to put any clothing directly onto the arm at first. Any clothes must go over the whole arm, and female patients should initially be dissuaded from wearing a bra.

Any dressings should be left intact, provided there is no exudate or inflammation around the wound. Sutures are removed at between 7 and 10 days postoperatively, when the wound is healed. Some physiotherapists now use biofeedback in order to retrain the muscles which have become used to functioning abnormally when they have allowed the shoulder to dislocate easily.

Painful arc syndrome

This syndrome is characterized by pain in the shoulder and upper arm during movement (see Fig. 15.13). There is generally little or no pain when the arm is next to the patient's side, but as he begins to lift the arm and so abduct the shoulder, pain begins and lasts until the arm is above the level of the shoulder, and then lessens again.

This syndrome can limit the patient's function; he may find himself unable to dress easily, comb his hair, or reach articles which have been placed in cupboards.

Treatment is conservative, with hydrocortisone injection and physiotherapy to the affected shoulder. While these patients are not generally admitted to hospital, the nurse may encounter this problem in patients in the community or in those who have been admitted for other reasons.

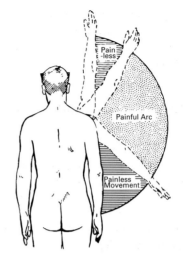

Fig. 15.13 Painful arc syndrome. (From Adams 1990, with permission.)

THE ELBOW

The elbow is a hinge joint with the movements of flexion and extension. Immediately distal to the elbow, there is a further joint between the radius and ulna which allows pronation and supination of the forearm (see Fig. 15.14).

Any loss of function at the elbow may have dramatic effects on the patient's daily life. Loss of flexion, for example, prevents him from lifting his hand to his mouth, washing his face or combing his hair. Loss of extension makes it extremely difficult for him to pick up articles from surfaces, as does loss of pronation or supination.

Many patients undergoing surgery to the elbow region experience similar problems, despite differing surgery. The following section aims to identify those problems arising from one surgical procedure, ulnar nerve transposition; other surgical interventions are then discussed.

Preoperative considerations

A full nursing assessment allows early identification of potential problems for the patient. Hand dominance should be noted; if the dominant arm is to have reduced function for a time, the patient should be encouraged to practise using the opposite hand for self-care activities. A

CORONAL SECTION OF ELBOW JOINT

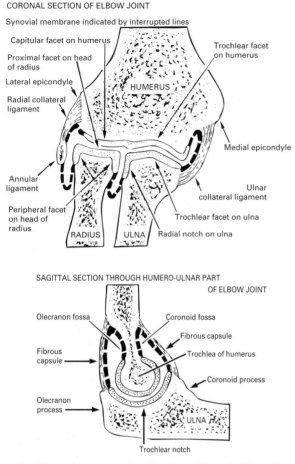

Synovial membrane indicated by interrupted lines

Capitular facet on humerus

Proximal facet on head of radius

Lateral epicondyle

Radial collateral ligament

HUMERUS

Trochlear facet on humerus

Medial epicondyle

Annular ligament

Peripheral facet on head of radius

Ulnar collateral ligament

Trochlear facet on ulna

RADIUS   ULNA   Radial notch on ulna

SAGITTAL SECTION THROUGH HUMERO-ULNAR PART OF ELBOW JOINT

Olecranon fossa

Fibrous capsule

Olecranon process

Coronoid fossa

Fibrous capsule

Trochlea of humerus

Coronoid process

ULNA

Trochlear notch

Fig. 15.14 Anatomy of the elbow joint. (From Smith et al 1983, with permission.)

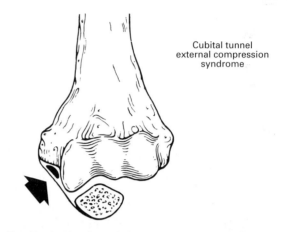

Cubital tunnel external compression syndrome

Fig. 15.15 Exposure of ulnar nerve to pressure at the elbow. (From Wadsworth 1982, with permission.)

baseline assessment of the neurovascular status of both hands allows accurate interpretation of postoperative observations.

Much of the preparation is as for shoulder surgery, and the reader is referred to the previous section for details.

Ulnar neuritis (cubital tunnel syndrome)

This condition results from damage to the ulnar nerve where it passes by the medial epicondyle of the humerus (see Fig. 15.15). The most common cause of damage to the ulnar nerve at this point is pressure, a condition which has been recognized for over a century (Wadsworth 1982);

it results in altered sensation in the little and ring fingers. It is not uncommon for the ulnar nerve to become damaged as a result of other orthopaedic procedures. Pressure may be exerted on the patient's elbow while he is undergoing a total hip replacement, due to positioning on the operating table. Equally, poor application of plaster of Paris to the arm may also compress the nerve. Any patient who has to spend time in bed is at risk of developing ulnar neuritis by taking weight on his elbows while attempting to reposition himself in bed, especially as the space in which the ulnar nerve lies is reduced when the elbow is flexed.

Many patients who have developed this syndrome require surgical transposition of the nerve away from the medial epicondyle of the humerus to lie deeper within the subcutaneous tissues. All patients returning from theatre following a procedure of more than 30 minutes' duration, especially those who have undergone hip arthroplasty, should have the sensation and movement of their little and ring fingers assessed. Any numbness or paraesthesia should be reported immediately to the medical staff. The same observations also should be carried out daily on patients who are confined to bed, and who may therefore be using their elbows to help them change their position.

Postoperative care

Much of the general postoperative care of the patient has already been decribed in the section on the shoulder, and the reader should refer back to this for details. This section will deal only with specific care.

Activity/rest   As the patient is mobile within a relatively short period of time postoperatively, he is able to decide on his own periods of rest and activity. However, he should be encouraged to take adequate rest to allow the tissues to heal and repair. Analgesia should be given regularly, as prescribed, and its effectiveness monitored. It is especially important that the patient is given adequate analgesia at night to ensure that he sleeps, and also before any nursing or other intervention such as physiotherapy during the day.

Immediately on return from theatre, the patient begins exercising the fingers of the affected arm. Shoulder and wrist movements are also carried out to maintain the normal joint range. Movements of the elbow commence at the surgeon's discretion, following reduction of the theatre dressing at 24–48 hours postoperatively. These are minimal at first until healing is established.

Prevention of hazards   On return from theatre, the patient's elbow is supported in a wool and crêpe bandage dressing. A small suction drain may be in place; this is removed at 24–48 hours when drainage is minimal. During the initial postoperative period the elbow is not moved, to allow healing of the soft tissues to commence.

As with any other surgery, there is increased permeability of the local blood vessels as a direct result of the procedure, and so there is a risk of oedema. The patient's arm may be elevated in a roller towel or supported on pillows, with the nurse ensuring that the hand and wrist are higher than the elbow to encourage lymphatic drainage. When the patient is mobile around the ward his arm will be supported in a broad arm sling.

Careful observation of the colour and warmth of the hand should be carried out to ensure that there is adequate perfusion. The neurological status of the hand also must be assessed and compared to its status preoperatively. Full movement and sensation are unlikely to return immediately to the little and ring fingers, and may take some months to do so.

Being normal   As soon as possible following surgery, the patient should be encouraged to get up and change into his own nightclothes, preferably with loose sleeves to fit over the dressing. Patients find it easier to dress if they put their affected arm into the sleeve first, before the unaffected arm. Most patients find that their level of independence is reduced due to the limited use of their affected arm. They may need help with personal hygiene and dressing, particularly with small tasks such as combing their hair or fastening buttons, and especially if their dominant arm is affected.

Health deviation   Good wound care ensures optimum healing with minimum scarring. When requested to do so by the surgeon, the nurse should remove the theatre dressing using an aseptic technique and protect the wound with a light dressing, which should not subsequently be removed until healing is complete at 7–10 days postoperatively.

The physiotherapist supervises the exercise programme for the patient's elbow, and this should be reinforced by the nurse. The patient should be made aware that recovery of sensation and movement in the affected fingers may take as long as 6 months to a year, especially if the nerve was severely compressed (see Care plan 2).

Total elbow replacement

Arthroplasty of the elbow is less developed than hip or knee arthroplasty. However, it is performed in centres around the country and as knowledge advances its use will increase. A growing number of designs of elbow prostheses have been developed since the first one by Boerema and De Waard in 1942 (Swanson & Herndon 1982) (see Fig. 15.16).

The problems experienced by a patient following this procedure are similar to those of any patient who has an immobilized elbow, and the

Care plan 2 Peter E, 47 years old; ulnar nerve decompression

Problem	Aim	Nursing intervention
1. Peter has pain in his elbow following surgery	For Peter to say that he has no pain	Ask Peter whether he has any pain and ask him to score it on his pain chart Position Peter comfortably in the bed or chair using pillows for support Ensure his arm is well elevated in a roller towel or sling Offer analgesia as prescribed Ensure that nursing actions occur after analgesia has been given
2. Peter has loss of independence due to restriction of use of his arm	For Peter to be able to maintain his self-care activities	Ensure Peter has any articles he needs within reach of his unaffected arm Assist him with dressing as he requires, such as fastening buttons Ensure his food is presented to be eaten with one hand
3. Peter has a surgical wound in his elbow	For Peter's wound to be healed within 10 days	Observe dressing for any exudate Monitor drainage into wound drain Remove drain aseptically at 48 hours Monitor neurovascular status of Peter's hand following surgery
4. Peter has limited function of his arm following surgery	For Peter to regain full use of his arm	Reinforce elbow exercises as taught by physiotherapist Offer Peter analgesia prior to physiotherapy Ensure all other joints of his arm are put through a normal range of movement twice per day

reader is referred to the previous discussion of care following ulnar nerve transposition. The elbow is completely immobilized in a padded plaster of Paris backslab at 90° flexion for approximately 5 days, according to the surgeon's

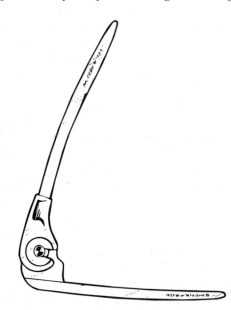

Fig. 15.16 Stanmore total elbow replacement. (From Wadsworth 1982, with permission.)

instructions. A suction drain is also in place for the first 48 hours.

In order to reduce postoperative oedema, the patient's arm is elevated in a roller towel, and supported by a broad arm sling when mobile. Because of the risk of oedema at the elbow, the nurse should undertake careful observation of the patient's hand to monitor the neurovascular status, observing especially for any signs of compression of the ulnar nerve, as discussed previously.

Rehabilitation and recovery following elbow arthroplasty may be prolonged, as many of these patients, especially those patients with rheumatoid arthritis, have disruption of the surrounding soft tissues due to their diseased elbow. They may remain dependent on others for some of their self-care needs for several weeks, and require sympathetic and tactful nursing interventions to maintain their level of morale. Many of their rehabilitation exercises are aimed at carrying out functional activities, such as increasing their elbow flexion in order to be able to lift their hands to their mouths. It should be remembered, however, that the primary reason for replacing the elbow joint is relief of pain, and patients should be advised that they are unlikely to regain a full range of elbow movements.

THE WRIST

As with the elbow, the wrist contains two joints. The joint between the radius and carpal bones allows the movements of flexion, extension, abduction and adduction. Proximal to this is a joint between the radius and ulna which allows pronation and supination of the forearm.

Although such a variety of movements is possible at the wrist, immobilization may not affect the patient's function radically, provided that there is good movement in the elbow and hand.

Carpal tunnel syndrome

This condition results from compression of the median nerve at the wrist as it passes, with the flexor tendons, beneath a band of fascia known as the flexor retinaculum (see Fig. 15.17). Although the cause of this is usually idiopathic, any disorder which reduces space at the wrist may predispose a patient to this syndrome; for example, rheumatoid arthritis, Colles' fracture and hand oedema in pregnancy.

Carpal tunnel syndrome may affect one or both hands and can be relatively disabling in its severe forms. Mild forms result in altered sensations, such as numbness or tingling, in the palmar side of the thumb, index, middle and ring fingers. In more severe forms motor function may also be disturbed with, for example, loss of grip. Functionally this can be very limiting for patients, especially when the dominant hand is affected, as all fine and small movements of the fingers may be reduced or lost.

Although non-invasive treatments, such as a local steroid injection, may be tried initially, patients who are admitted to hospital will undergo surgical decompression of the carpal tunnel.

Preoperative considerations

These are as for any patient undergoing surgery to the arm and the reader is referred to the previous sections on the shoulder and elbow.

Postoperative care

Water/food The patient will be able to eat and drink when he is fully conscious after the anaesthetic. All items should be placed within easy reach of the unaffected arm to allow maximum independence. However, if both wrists have been operated upon, the patient will need assistance with drinking as he will be unable to hold a cup himself, or to manipulate cutlery, until the dressings have been reduced.

Elimination As soon as he is fully conscious, the patient will be able to walk to the bathroom to use the toilet. Assistance with removal of clothing and cleaning after opening his bowels is needed by the patient who has had bilateral surgery. Help may also be required by the patient whose dominant hand is affected. If the patient wears a plastic glove over the dressing he will be able to clean himself without soiling or contaminating the wound dressing.

Activity/rest The patient may find it difficult to sleep at night with his arm elevated, as this limits the number of positions in which he can sleep. This is especially true for those patients who have had bilateral surgery, as they will be able to sleep only on their backs initially, with both hands elevated. It is therefore essential that they have adequate analgesia, and that the nurse takes time to help them settle into a position where they feel able to sleep.

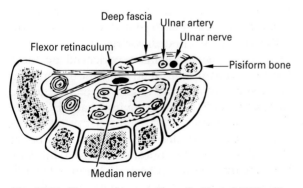

Fig. 15.17 The carpal tunnel. (From Smith et al 1983, with permission.)

Prevention of hazards On his return from theatre, the patient's wrist is immobilized in a wool and crêpe bandage dressing, which may encase most of the hand apart from the fingers. This dressing is generally reduced at 24–48 hours postoperatively, prior to the patient's discharge, to allow greater movement of the hand.

Following surgery, the increased permeability of the blood vessels predisposes the patient to the risk of oedema. Therefore, his hand should be elevated overnight to aid lymphatic drainage (see Fig. 15.18). The neurovascular status of the fingers also should be monitored as previously outlined in the general principles of care.

Being normal As soon as possible following surgery the patient should be encouraged to get up. Patients who have undergone bilateral surgery will have to accept that initially they will be dependent on others for what may seem basic activities:

- When eating and drinking they will be unable to hold cups and utensils easily.
- When dressing they will be unable to fasten their clothing.
- For personal hygiene they will initially be unable to get their hands wet.

The patient may find difficulty in adjusting to these limitations after what may seem 'minor' surgery, and the nurse should show tact and understanding when providing assistance.

Health deviation The patient needs to be made aware that the altered sensations of his

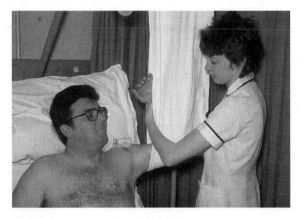

Fig. 15.18 Elevation in roller towel.

hand will not resolve immediately after surgery. The longer the nerve has been compressed the longer it will take to recover, and it may be up to 6 months before full sensation is restored in the affected hand.

The patient should be taught the principles of good wound care so that he can be self-reliant at home. A supply of plastic gloves will allow him to be independent in everyday activities, such as personal cleaning following elimination. His affected arm should be elevated in a high arm sling for the first few days, and both the patient and his relatives should be taught adequately about its application so that it is worn correctly. At night he should be advised to sleep with his hand resting on a pillow, to keep it higher than his elbow. The patient who has had bilateral surgery will be unable to have both arms elevated in slings, and so should be advised about keeping his arms elevated when sitting, by resting them on a cushion or pillow (see Care plan 3).

Wrist arthrodesis

This is generally performed for severe osteoarthritis of the wrist, to relieve pain and provide maximum function. Careful preparation of the patient is necessary preoperatively to ensure that he has adequate hand function postoperatively. Close liaison with the occupational therapist is necessary to assess the patient's ability to carry out self-care activities. A light-weight wrist splint is worn by the patient; this immobilizes the wrist joint and allows him to assess the potential value of an arthrodesis (see Fig. 15.19). In some cases the patient may prefer to continue wearing the splint if it provides sufficient pain relief, rather than undergo surgery.

Many of the problems experienced by these patients are common to any patient undergoing wrist surgery, and the reader is referred to the discussion of care following carpal tunnel decompression.

Assistance is needed with self-care activities at first, as the affected arm cannot be used. Initially, the patient's wrist is completely immobilized in a plaster of Paris backslab, which will be extended to a full cast several days postoperatively

Care plan 3 Julie B, 34 years old; bilateral carpal tunnel decompression

Problem	Aim	Nursing intervention
1. Julie has loss of independence following surgery	a. For Julie to be able to wash each day as she wishes	Assist Julie with washing until dressings to her hands are reduced Once dressings are reduced, protect wounds with plastic gloves so Julie can wash herself Ensure she has all necessary articles within reach when washing
	b. For Julie to be able to dress as she wishes	Assist Julie with dressing each day Once dressings are reduced, assist with small tasks such as buttons, as required
2. Julie is at risk of developing hand oedema	For Julie's hands to remain unoedematous	Elevate both arms in roller towels Show Julie how to elevate her hands using pillows when sitting in a chair Monitor neurovascular status of her hands Ensure Julie understands the reasons for elevating her hands
3. Julie has continued paraesthesia following surgery	For Julie to accept that this will resolve eventually	Monitor neurovascular status to record resolution of altered sensations Explain to Julie that this is not uncommon and will resolve with time

when the initial oedema has subsided. The patient needs to be instructed in the care of his plaster cast prior to discharge home, including such advice as:

- Do not get it wet.
- Do not expose it to direct heat.
- Maintain hand elevation.

The patient's arm should be elevated in a roller towel to minimize postoperative oedema and kept in a high arm sling when he is mobile. He and his relatives should know how to apply the sling and be aware of the importance of maintaining a full range of movement in the other joints of the arm.

Wrist orthoses and splints

Splints may be dynamic or static; that is, they are used either to aid movement or to support and immobilize. Others may be used only at night to rest joints in a good position (see Fig. 15.20).

Regardless of the reasons for their application, there are common considerations to be noted for all patients who need to wear hand splints. The splint should fit well and not impinge on joints other than the one for which it is designed; for example, there should be full movement at the metacarpophalangeal joints when a wrist splint is worn.

The patient should be taught how to put the splint on and when to use it, and given advice

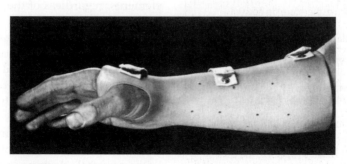

Fig. 15.19 Cylindrical wrist splint. (From Adams 1990, with permission.)

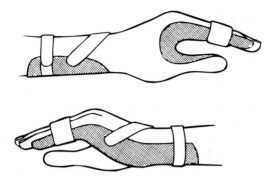

Fig. 15.20 Resting splint.

about its care. Initially it should be worn for short periods of about half an hour, after which the skin should be checked for any signs of redness, oedema, increased pain or altered sensation, such as numbness. Straps should fasten tightly enough to hold the wrist in a good position in the splint without pinching. Provided that the skin condition remains satisfactory, the amount of time that the splint is worn can be increased to raise the patient's level of tolerance.

Most splints are now made from thermoplastics and as such are heat-sensitive. Patients should therefore be advised on how to care for the splint (see Fig. 15.21).

THE HAND AND FINGERS

Much of everyday life depends on the use of the hand (see Fig. 15.22), and Crawford Adams (1981) comments that, due to the practical and economic consequences of any loss of hand func-

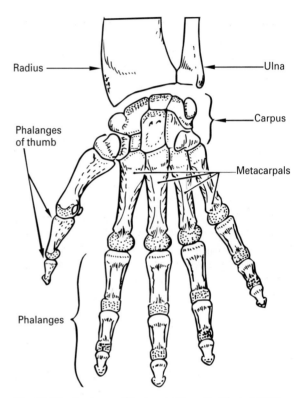

Fig. 15.22 Anatomy of the hand. (From Smith et al 1983, with permission.)

tion, hand surgery is now becoming a distinct and separate branch of orthopaedics. The main emphasis in treating any disorder of the hand must be on restoration of function. The joints of the hand tolerate immobilization poorly and quickly become stiff, so any approach must include early mobilization.

The care required by patients undergoing surgery to the hand will contain many common elements, regardless of the nature of the surgery undertaken.

Eating and drinking Patients will need assistance with the preparation of food, although independence in eating and drinking can often be preserved with the use of aids, such as large-handled cutlery for patients with impaired grip, or the use of non-slip mats and plate guards for patients eating with one hand.

Elimination The patient may require help with personal cleaning following elimination.

CARE OF YOUR SPLINT
Your splint is heat sensitive, therefore do not:
   leave it on a radiator
   leave it in direct sunlight (e.g. in a car)
   place it in hot water
   dry it using a hair dryer
To clean your splint:
   wash in lukewarm soapy water
   tough stains may be removed with nail polish
   remover
Always dry your splint thoroughly before wearing

Fig. 15.21 Instructions to patients regarding the care of splints.

Toilet tissue is very flimsy and difficult to handle without fine grip. Equally, fastening or un-fastening zips and buttons may be awkward. Many patients find it acutely embarrassing to have to ask for help, and it is often more tactful to offer assistance than to wait until the patient has to ask.

Activity/rest   Sleep may often be disturbed for one of two reasons. First, pain in the hand may be severe and the nurse should try and relieve this using non-pharmacological methods such as heat or ice and elevation of the affected hand. If these are not successful, suitable analgesia should be given. Second, elevation of the hand may impair the patient's ability to sleep. Every assistance should be given to the patient to help him find a position which is comfortable.

Hand exercises are commenced by the physiotherapist as soon after surgery as possible, in order to prevent joint stiffness and restore function to the affected area of the hand. Sometimes the treatment continues for several months to gain maximum benefit; this should be explained to the patient at the outset so that he has realistic expectations.

Prevention of hazards   As with any other surgery to the upper limb, there is a risk of oedema developing postoperatively. All jewellery, including rings, should be removed preoperatively. After surgery the hand is elevated, initially in a roller towel and subsequently in a sling when the patient is mobile. By careful observation of the neurovascular status of the hand the nurse is able to check for any inadvertent trauma during surgery and detect any compression from oedema as early as possible.

Health deviation   Many patients find it difficult to accept their reduced level of independence as a result of what they perceive to be 'minor' surgery. Elderly people, in particular, may find their level of functioning severely reduced by having one hand immobile. It may be that, due to shorter hospital admissions, they require assistance at home when initially discharged, and it is valuable for the nurse to work in conjunction with the occupational therapist in assessing the patient's ability to cope with his activities of living.

Dupuytren's contracture

This condition occurs as a result of thickening and the formation of nodules within the palmar fascia or aponeurosis, which cause it to shorten (see Fig. 15.23). Eventually joint contractures occur with the fingers being pulled down into the palm. Although most commonly occurring in the hand, Dupuytren's contracture may also present on the sole of the foot.

Treatment is surgical, involving the excision of the contracted areas of fascia. Postoperatively, the patient's hand is enclosed in a wool and crêpe dressing. High elevation is necessary, as the palm is a highly vascular area and there is a considerable risk of bleeding or oedema. Careful observation of the neurovascular status of the fingers is therefore vital.

Wound care is a major part of the nursing care for this group of patients. Haematomas are not uncommon due to the vascularity of the affected area. The skin of the palm contracts when healing and, without careful attention, this may cancel out any surgical benefits. For this reason, the

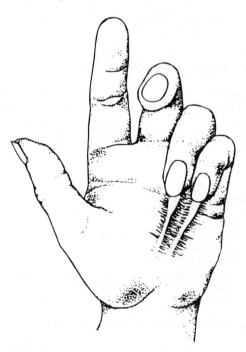

Fig. 15.23   Dupuytren's contracture. (From American Society for Surgery of the Hand 1983).

incision is Z-shaped to minimize any further contractures. The fingers are also kept at a slight stretch to reduce contracture, and so the wound is under some tension. A strictly aseptic technique is vital, and careful observation of the wound edges is needed to monitor for any necrosis.

Many of these patients are now discharged home after 2–3 days, and are then cared for as outpatients. They should be instructed in strict hand hygiene, and told to avoid wetting their wounds until they are healed. Sutures are generally removed at 7–10 days postoperatively, depending on the rate of healing in the palm.

In order to maintain the fingers in as straight a position as possible, the patient may return from theatre with a volar (dorsal) splint on his hand, similar to a night resting splint (Fig. 15.20). However, some surgeons are now beginning to use a backsplint with a bar over the affected fingers to hold them straight as pulling is more effective than pushing, and the fingers may tend to push out of a volar splint. The use of splints will vary according to the surgeon; some will not use one at all, others will want the patient to wear one for up to 6 months. If a splint is used, the patient should be told how to care for it, as outlined in Figure 15.21.

Rehabilitation may take some months, and the patient should be made aware of this. Massage of the scar with oils will help to keep it supple while the finger joints are reaching their maximum extension. Some units may also use silicone hand baths in order to oxygenate the wound edges and promote healing, although the evidence for the value of their use is by no means conclusive.

REFERENCES

American Society for Surgery of the Hand 1983 The hand: examination and diagnosis, 2nd edn. Churchill Livingstone, Edinburgh

Boore J 1978 Prescription for recovery. Royal College of Nursing, London

Crawford Adams J 1990 Outline of orthopaedics, 11th edn. Churchill Livingstone, Edinburgh

David J 1986 Wound management. Martin Dunitz, London

Diers D 1981 Clinical and political issues in nursing practice. In: Hockey L (ed) Recent advances in nursing: current issues in nursing. Churchill Livingstone, Edinburgh

Doheny M O, Ceccio C M 1988 Total shoulder replacement: preparing patients for discharge. Orthopaedic Nursing 7(3): 13–20

Follman D 1988 Nursing care concerns in total shoulder replacement. Orthopaedic Nursing 7(3): 29–31

Footner A 1987 Orthopaedic nursing. Bailliere Tindall, London

Hayward J 1975 Information: a prescription against pain. Royal College of Nursing, London

McCaffery M L 1979 Nursing management of the patient with pain, 2nd edn. Lippincott, Philadelphia

Orem D 1980 Nursing concepts of practice. McGraw-Hill, New York

Rogers R, Salvage J 1988 Nurses at risk: a guide to health and safety at work. Heinemann, London

Royal College of Nursing 1990 Standards of care for orthopaedic nursing. RCN, London

Smith J W, Murphy T R, Blair J S G, Lowe K G 1983 Regional anatomy illustrated. Churchill Livingstone, Edinburgh

Swanson A B, Herndon J H 1982 Surgery of arthritis. In: Wadsworth T G (ed) The elbow. Churchill Livingstone, Edinburgh

Wadsworth T G (ed) 1982 The elbow. Churchill Livingstone, Edinburgh

Walsh M, Judd M 1989 Long term immobility and self care: the Orem approach. Nursing Standard 3(41): 34–36

FURTHER READING

Aggleton P, Chalmers H 1986 Nursing models and the nursing process. MacMillan, Basingstoke

Crawford Adams J 1990 Outline of orthopaedics, 11th edn. Churchill Livingstone, Edinburgh

Footner A 1987 Orthopaedic nursing. Bailliere Tindall, London

Kessel L, Bayley I 1986 Clinical disorders of the shoulder, 2nd edn. Churchill Livingstone, Edinburgh

Lamb D W, Hooper G 1984 Hand conditions. Churchill Livingstone, Edinburgh

Royal College of Nursing 1990 Standards of care: orthopaedic nursing. RCN, London

Wadsworth T G (ed) 1982 The elbow. Churchill Livingstone, Edinburgh

16

Spinal problems

Jacqueline Scott

INTRODUCTION

The first part of this chapter looks at the medical causes of low back pain, its prevalence and its cost in terms of medical care and number of working days lost. The incidence and causes of low back pain among nurses are then examined in more detail. This leads on to a discussion of the application of ergonomics to improving nurses' working conditions and the importance of the Health and Safety at Work Act.

The second part of the chapter discusses the 'sick role' and its relationship to the individual's health beliefs. The principles involved in the nursing care of the patient with spinal problems are described, identifying the rehabilitative phase.

The chapter does not cover the nursing of spinal-injured patients or children with conditions such as scoliosis. The approach of this chapter is very much one of prevention through individuals taking responsibility for their own health maintenance.

INCIDENCE OF BACK PAIN

Back pain is one of the most common medical symptoms experienced by the British population. It is also one of the least understood.

The causes of low back pain, as suggested by the Arthritis and Rheumatism Council (Papageorgiou & Rigby 1990), vary with age. Disc disorders, back strain and trauma are the commonest causes in the younger age groups (especially males under 45 years) and disc degeneration is more common in those aged over 45 years (Kelsey & White 1980, OHE 1985, Wood & Badley 1987).

Radiographic investigation will be required to help establish the cause of the pain. X-rays may reveal the presence of degenerative changes in the vertebrae such as osteophyte formation or bone thickening, which will cause narrowing of the nerve root access. Other abnormalities may indicate malalignment of vertebrae or deformities. However, radiographs may not reveal any obvious abnormality despite the intense clinical indication of pain.

Further radiographic examination may include ultrasound scanning and computerized axial tomography (CAT or CT scanning), which is a series of pictures taken as a cross-section of the spine (or other region of the body) and adjacent tissues at any given point. CT scanning uses low-dose radiation. MRI (magnetic resonance imaging) is extremely useful in the diagnosis of spinal problems due to the magnetic resonance's ability to expose fluid-retaining areas such as intervertebral discs. A series of pictures are produced using a sensor from a powerful magnetic field which measures the 'movement' of atomic protons within the anatomical structure. Images can be created onto radiographic film either as an anatomical or pathological representation. Contraindications to MRI include the presence of a pacemaker or any other metal implant, such as metal clips, a prosthetic cardiac valve, or a metal prosthesis such as a hip replacement or Harrington rod.

Osteoarthritis of the spine increases with age. Each year, one in 22 persons (4.5%) of all ages is diagnosed by their general practitioner as having low back pain; this incidence rises to one in five (6.6%) for those aged 45–64 years. This represents approximately 2.25 million persons consulting their general practitioners annually in the UK because of problems with back pain (OHE 1985).

General practitioner consultation and referral rates of patients with low back pain are listed in Figure 16.1 (OHE 1985). Proportionally, more males are admitted to hospital than females; half of these are aged between 25 and 44 years and a further third between 45 and 64 years (DHSS

General practitioner consultations	2 250 000
	1 : 4 population
General practitioner referrals (outpatient)	350 000
Hospital inpatients (average 12 days) ♀ > ♂	65 000
Surgical intervention (prolapsed intervertebral disc or laminectomy)	10 800 inpatient
	1 : 6 population

Fig. 16.1 Back pain statistics (Office of Health Economics 1985).

1982, OHE 1985, Wood & Badley 1987). Further, it is suggested that, despite the fact that approximately one in six of these patients undergo surgery (Halliwell 1988), just under one-third fail to be rehabilitated.

SOCIOECONOMIC COST OF BACK PAIN

The social and economic cost of low back pain on the individual's life is impossible to measure. The impact of low back pain on the National Health Service (NHS) and national economy can, however, be estimated. The cost to the NHS in terms of general practice, hospital and community service and drugs for this condition accounted for 1.15% of NHS expenditure during 1982 (OHE 1985).

Further, the Office of Health Economics (1985), in their survey on back pain, estimated that back pain and associated disorders such as neck pain and ankylosing spondylitis account for a loss of over 33 million working days, i.e. 9.2% of all working days lost through certificated incapacity in 1982, 14 days being the calculated mean for time off work. On any one day, some 10 000 people have been incapacitated by low back pain for 6 months.

Unrecorded sickness and reduced work effectiveness cannot be measured efficiently and monitored, nor can the costs of the chronic back pain sufferers' decisions to use alternative or complementary therapies and medicines. The above figures, therefore, are an underestimation of the financially draining effect that low back pain has on the community as a whole.

CAUSES OF LOW BACK PAIN

The majority of individuals suffering from low back pain who visit their general practitioners will have either an inflammatory or mechanical spinal disturbance. However, it is important to remember that pain is a symptom and the source of the problems may arise from many other factors. Therefore, the cause of low back pain must be clearly identified (see Fig. 16.2).

Incidence of back pain in nurses

The high incidence of back pain within the nursing population is the result of a combination of moderate dynamic spinal stress and high static stress; most episodes of both occur over a short period during the working day. Observations of posture on the ward established that nurses spend one-third of their day (i.e. 1.6–2 hours/day) in forward flexion (Stubbs & Buckle 1983).

The most frequent reasons for lifting patients (Bell 1979) were:

- Lifting on and off chairs (8–9%)
- Lifting on and off toilets (8–9%)
- Repositioning in chairs or beds (8–9%)
- Lifting in and out of bed (9–10%)
- Lifting in and out of baths (10–11%).

Nurses, in particular, experience a great deal of low back pain. This is usually assumed to be from abuse of the spine caused by lifting and transferring patients and also from adopting a harmful posture (i.e. forward flexion) when caring for bedridden patients. This is particularly so in Denmark (Kaur & Pederson 1986), the USA (Owen & Damron 1984, Harber et al 1985) and the UK (Cust et al 1972, Stubbs & Buckle 1984, Raistric 1981).

The environmental factors that can give rise to back pain in nurses have been identified in four broad areas;

1. Failure by nursing management to appreciate that problems can arise in moving patients
2. Inefficient training and improperly supervised practice
3. Lack of understanding of how to use strength efficiently

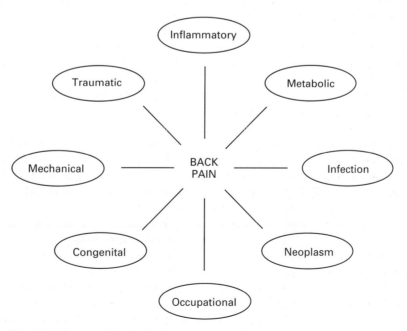

Fig. 16.2 Causes of low back pain.

4. Inefficient systems of work which disregard individual capabilities, limitations and resistance to change.

Ergonomic studies have been used to try and improve these conditions (Simpson 1984).

Ergonomics

Ergonomics has been defined as the scientific study of the relationship between man and his working environment (Murrell 1965).

Troup et al (1987) identified three main possible causes of the high injury rate for nurses within the clinical area:

1. The design of ward furniture and the ward environment has evolved without much regard for the problems of patient handling.

2. In the absence of ergonomic principles, the standards of training in the safe handling of patients have been universally low.

3. Nurses do not complain about their working environment.

The term 'environment' is taken to cover not only the surroundings in which nurses may work, but also the equipment, the method of work and the organization of their work, either as individuals or within a working team of nurses. It must be remembered also that there are other factors affecting the individual apart from the working environment which will have an effect on expected outcome and efficiency; these include personality, work, family and community.

Ergonomics aims to accommodate the demands of the individual's work within his limitations and capabilities. The classical ergonomic approach is to find out how a machine or situation can be modified most easily to suit the worker. It is, therefore, important to identify the duty demands of an individual's employment, to indicate both knowledge of the tasks for which individuals are suited and those for which machines are better employed, and also the cost/value of acquisition and selection training (Singleton 1972) (see Fig. 16.3).

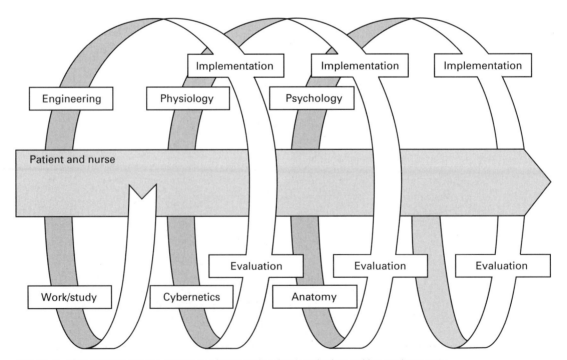

Fig. 16.3 Ergonomics: relation between science and technology in the working environment.

Reducing back problems

Factors which indicate that the design of the working environment is inadequate may include an increased accident rate, poor morale, high absenteeism, complaints of undue fatigue, unspecified illness and poor service quality. A design which is ergonomically satisfactory should offer a safe and satisfying place in which to work and also be labour-efficient.

A simple ergonomic action plan to review nurses' handling and lifting of patients in the clinical area is illustrated in Figure 16.4.

Health and safety

The purpose of the Health and Safety at Work Act (1974) is to provide the legislative framework to promote, stimulate and encourage high standards of health and safety at work (HSC 1991). A health authority has a statutory duty to ensure that staff who are involved in handling or lifting patients are not exposed to working practices or risks which are likely to result in injury (Fig. 16.5).

The lifting of Crown Immunity protection and the directive from the Commission of the European Communities (1990) further highlight the responsibilities of employers to safeguard their staff. The Commission proposed that the following measures be taken where there is a risk of back injury for workers:

- Pre-employment 'back' screening
- Safety precautions such as safety training programmes for all staff, not just new employees
- The management of the back and of back pain at work.

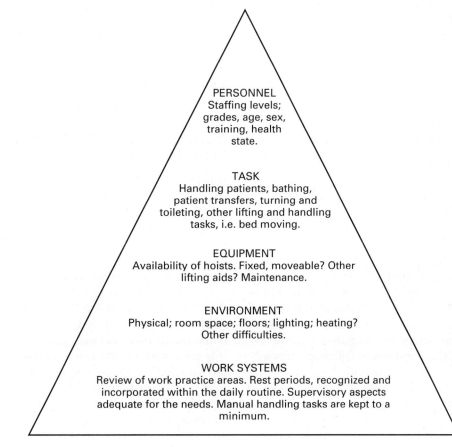

Fig. 16.4 Ergonomic action plan (adapted from Simpson 1984).

DUTIES TO EMPLOYEES

The general duties of employers to their employees are set down in Section 2 of the Act.

1. It shall be the duty of every employer to ensure, so far as is reasonably practicable, the health, safety and welfare at work of all his employees.

2. Without prejudice to the generality of the above, the matter to which that duty extends include in particular:
   a. the provision and maintenance of plant and systems of work that are, so far as is reasonably practicable, safe and without risks to health.
   b. arrangements for ensuring, so far as reasonably practicable, safety and absence of risks to health in connection with the use, handling, storage and transport of articles and substances.
   c. the provision of such information, instruction, training and supervision as are necessary to ensure, so far as is reasonably practicable, the health and safety at work of all his employees.
   d. so far as is reasonably practicable as regards any place of work under the employer's control, the maintenance of it in a condition that is safe and without risks to health and the provision and maintenance of means of access to and egress from it that are safe and without such risks.
   e. the provision and maintenance of a working environment for his employees that is, so far as is reasonably practicable, safe, without risks to health and adequate as regards facilities and arrangements for their welfare at work.

3. Except in such cases as may be prescribed, it shall be the duty of every employer to prepare and as often as may be appropriate revise a written statement of his general policy with respect to the health and safety at work of his employees and the organization and arrangements for the time being in force for carrying out that policy, and to bring the statement and any revision of it to the notice of all his employees.

Fig. 16.5 Health and Safety at Work Act 1974.

The Health and Safety Executive (1990) guidelines emphasize:

- Safe systems at work
- Appropriate and adequate equipment
- Training in the use of equipment in appropriate situations.

The framework directive initiated from the European Commision and made under Article 118A of the Treaty of Rome mirrors the Health and Safety at Work Act 1972 by establishing the broad general duties of employees and employers in all working activities.

Implementation of the directive in all European Community Member States at the end of 1992 places the primary responsibility for ensuring health and safety on employers; however, the impact of the regulations will vary depending on the extent of existing law.

More than a quarter of the accidents reported each year to the enforcing authorities are associated with the manual handling of loads. Strains and sprains, particularly of the back, are the injuries most commonly reported; however, amputations, fractures, cuts and bruises are also reported.

NURSING PATIENTS WITH SPINAL PROBLEMS

Adults are autonomous, independent and responsible for their own health. The professional relationship between the nurse and the patient is seen as one of equality, where the responsibility for the patient's health is seen as a priority and one in which the nurse may assist the patient in the pursuit of optimum wellness.

It is important to remember that individuals with back pain who are treated are not always in an acute phase of their illness. If the patient is unable to meet his own self-care needs, then it is necessary for the nurse to ensure that they are satisfied. A positive approach with constant reassurance is essential.

A distinct role of nursing is to help patients towards optimum wellness and, by so doing, to enable individuals to manage changes in their health.

Compliance

It is important that all persons suffering from spinal problems comply with their prescribed treatment in order to achieve a successful outcome. Compliance is a necessary prerequisite for achieving and maintaining the desired level of wellness identified by the individual. Compliance to prescribed therapy may include adhering to medications such as anti-inflammatory drugs, and treatment routines such as strict bedrest and traction or daily hydrotherapy. It should be remembered, however, that the patient's perceived view of his illness, such as duration, severity and knowledge of his back problem, will affect his degree of compliance.

Becker's (1976) health belief model is a guide to identifying factors that enhance or hinder compliant behaviour and a move towards optimum wellness. It acknowledges the concept of the perceived value of an outcome and the individual's expectation that a given action will result in a positive outcome. Becker's model has three main components:

1. Readiness and motivation to take action to comply with the therapeutic regimen.

2. An evaluation of the benefits of the action and the barriers to action. Benefits for a patient with a prolapsed intravertebral disc could be perceived as reduced pain when sitting and standing. Barriers may be that family, job commitments and finance inhibit adequate 'space' for management.

3. A cue to action, either internally or externally, must be present to trigger advocated action. The cue may be pain or a life-threatening situation. The patient, however, must perceive that compliance will reduce the threat.

Disc lesions

The lumbar and cervical regions are the most common areas for spinal problems to develop.

Identification of the specific region is made by clinical examination in conjunction with the patient's medical history; this examination includes radiological investigations such as a myelogram, radiculogram or discogram to confirm the diagnosis.

The causes of spinal problems have been identified in Figure 16.2. However, the events leading to a rupture or prolapse of an intervertebral disc are cumulative and uncertain. Rupture of the annulus fibrosus and the posterior ligament allows the protrusion of the nucleus pulposus – i.e. a prolapsed intervertebral disc (Fig. 16.6). With a small protrusion, the bulge will impinge on the posterior longitudinal ligament and cause pain in the back.

The effects of a prolapsed intervertebral disc include pain felt in the area of nerve distribution, commonly the sciatic nerve. Consequently, the

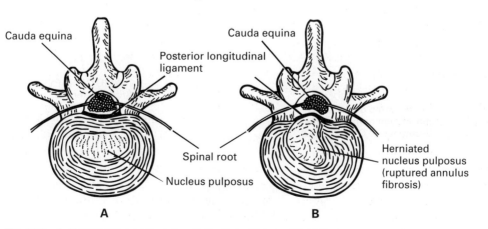

Fig. 16.6 A. Normal intervertebral disc; B. Prolapsed intervertebral disc.

pain is characteristically in the buttocks radiating to the thigh, calf and toes. However, it is important to note that pain also may be due to a compressed nerve, muscle spasm and oedema. This pain may affect one or both legs and straight leg raising will often exacerbate the pain. Muscle weakness and sensory loss in the area of the nerve distribution also may occur.

Conservative nursing management

All individuals who have spinal problems such as disc lesions will be treated in a conservative manner initially, in the hope that such measures and a re-education programme on walking and lifting will be enough to control the patient's back pain problem.

Conservative nursing management includes bedrest, relief of pain and rehabilitation (Fig. 16.7). The length of conservative treatment varies from person to person depending on the assessment of the individual's needs. Generally,

most individuals recover after approximately 14 days of bedrest when they are given relaxants, non-steroidal anti-inflammatory drugs and/or analgesics. These may include diclofenac sodium (Voltarol), diazepam (Valium) and buprenorphine (Temgesic).

A firm base mattress is essential. Many individuals may prefer to maintain bedrest at home provided there is support from family, friends and community services. Bedrest is generally described as lying in bed, with one pillow under the head, for 23 hours a day for at least 10–14 days, during which an allowance of 1 hour per day is made for hygiene and toilet purposes only. However, bedrest at home is not always feasible, as distraction from the daily routine of the home may hinder recovery and encourage premature mobilization, thus creating an opportunity for relapse. There are those individuals who for various reasons, such as having a young family, may respond more effectively to support and care as an inpatient.

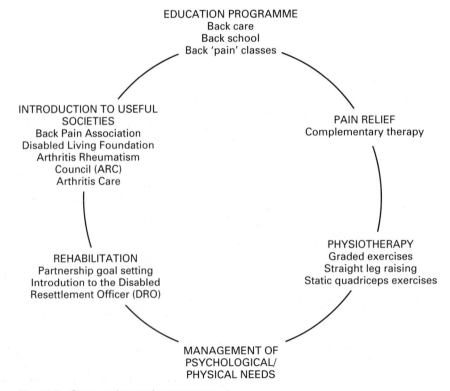

Fig. 16.7 Conservative nursing management.

Traction – either bilateral extensions, Bucks traction or pelvic corset traction – may be used in addition to total bedrest and helps to reduce muscle spasms of the lumbosacral region (Fig. 16.8); however, the benefits of traction are now being questioned.

The patient must lie supine with one pillow under the head for support and must be encouraged to do lower limb exercises regularly (Fig. 16.9). These would include 'static quad' exercises, which encourage quadriceps muscle tone and are essential if the patient is to have a rapid

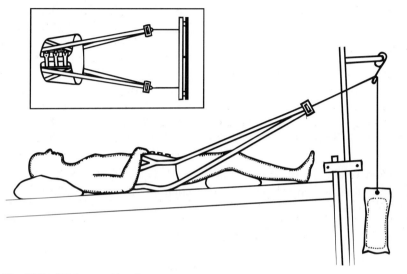

Fig. 16.8 Pelvic corset traction.

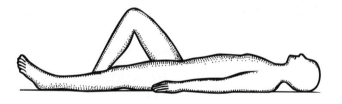

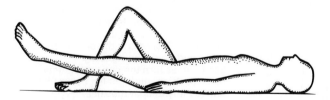

STRAIGHT LEG RAISING (SLR)
With legs resting on bed, one knee bent, one leg extended

On extended leg:
Toes pointing upright, tighten thigh muscle; raise leg off bed (5"-6"); hold for count of 10—increasing to 15 when able, leg down and rest, alternate legs

FOOT PUMPS
Lying or sitting down with legs out straight, push your toes away from you until your calf muscles tighten; relax both feet; pull your toes towards you until you feel your calf muscles tighten; relax and repeat as often as you can throughout the day

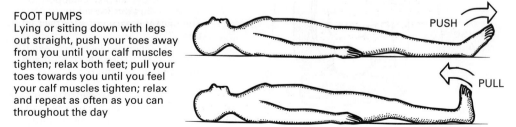

PUSH

PULL

Fig. 16.9 Caption see overleaf.

STATIC QUADRICEPS EXERCISE

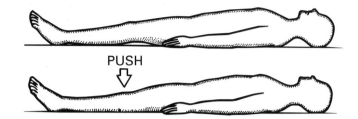

PUSH

Legs extended, toes relaxed

With alternate legs: tighten thigh muscles and
push knee into the mattress;
relax; repeat as often as
you can throughout the day

Fig. 16.9 Lower limb exercises and static quadriceps exercise.

and safe mobilization when his back pain has abated. Plantar- and dorsiflexion exercises encourage calf muscle activity and reduce some of the risks of complications of bedrest such as deep vein thrombosis (see Ch. 5).

A physiotherapist is involved with the nurse in each patient's assessment and plan of care. Together they teach and encourage the patient to carry out the exercises mentioned above, as well as exercises to alleviate further problems such as pulmonary embolism. While on bedrest the patient is encouraged to roll over from side to side on his back as if he were a 'log', therefore avoiding any twisting movements when changing position; such twisting could result in more pain and discomfort. Figure 16.10 outlines the process of 'log rolling'.

The nursing care of patients in traction is

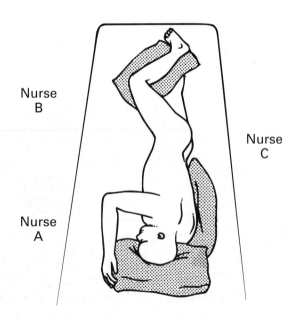

Nurse B

Nurse C

Nurse A

Explain the procedure to the patient.
Reassure.
The patient is lying supine.
Remove the pillows supporting the feet under the legs.
Two nurses stand on the left side of the bed. Nurse A at the head of the patient puts her arm around the shoulders, so the forearm supports along the back, and Nurse B supports the base of the spine and holds the right leg.
Both nurses turn the patient together towards them, the right leg being lifted and slightly bent at the knee.
Nurse C provides pillow support for the spine, behind the patient.
The patient is asked to relax back into this pillow.
A further pillow is placed between the legs in order to provide comfort and support between the knees.

This procedure is explained using three nurses and turning the patient onto his LEFT SIDE, reverse for RIGHT SIDE.

Fig. 16.10 Log rolling.

covered in Chapter 6. Once a period of rest, in some cases 4–6 weeks, has allowed the symptoms to abate, the patient may gradually begin to mobilize.

Some people respond well to lumbar corsets (Fig. 16.11) for support and may continue to wear the corset for many months after the acute phase. However, there are many who are not offered lumbar support corsets; this may be due to the identification on initial medical assessment of the need for immediate surgery due to acute pain and/or the presence of disabling features such as a limp and an inability to carry on with reasonable daily activities. Alternatively, many surgeons prefer not to prescribe the corset at all, preferring physiotherapy, exercises and surgery.

As part of the conservative management, whether the patient is an inpatient or outpatient, a re-education programme including back care and simple exercises should be discussed and demonstrated in the rehabilitative phase.

A stiff spine with weak supporting muscles is not able to respond well to the additional stress that may be imposed on it by different or sudden awkward movement. It is, therefore, important and necessary that movement is included in the maintenance of a healthy spine. In order to improve spinal mobility and strengthen the muscles which control movement and posture of the spine, gentle exercises such as abdominal strengthening exercises and spinal mobilizing and stretching exercises should be encouraged. Some of these will be performed in a horizontal position whereas others, such as back and hip extensor strengthening exercises, will require the patient to be upright.

No exercise that causes pain which continues after the exercise is completed should be repeated. However, the spine may be stiff and some discomfort may be expected while stretching.

The individual should be instructed in labour-saving, 'back-saving' techniques. Alternative, physically more efficient ways of tackling any situation can minimize the spinal stress and therefore cause less pain. Altering or redesigning the working environment may minimize postural stress on the spine; measures may include choosing the correct chair for the desk, using a foot stool when sitting and adjusting the height of the working surface.

Advice should be given to avoid prolonged bending and stooping by kneeling or by using a long-handled implement which can be provided by the practice nurse or hospital unit.

Heavy loads are a hazard. Patients should be advised never to lift a load without adequate preparation for the task, and never to twist the body while lifting.

Despite a re-education programme on back care, symptoms often recur. In the acute phase, it is quite likely that the patient will be faced with the prospect of surgical intervention.

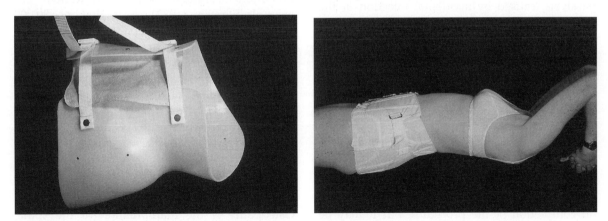

Fig. 16.11   Lumbar corsets. (From Institute of Orthopaedics, Royal National Orthopaedic Hospital, with permission.)

SURGERY FOR BACK PROBLEMS

There are many surgical procedures which may be offered to the patient; the choice is based on the clinical assessment in conjunction with the patient's need to be mobile as soon as possible. Surgical procedures for back pain include chemonucleolysis, percutaneous discectomy, and laminectomy and discectomy.

Chemonucleolysis

Chemonucleolysis is a method often chosen because it provides relief of symptoms without operative excision of the disc, thus allowing early mobilization. It is a procedure whereby a surgeon, who must hold a special licence to practice this technique, injects an enzyme, chymopapain, into the nucleus pulposus of one or more intervertebral discs. This action causes the chemical decompression (shrinking) of the chondromucoprotein within the nucleus, thus reducing the fluid pressure, with subsequent release of pressure on the surrounding structures. A discogram is performed prior to this injection to confirm the diagnosis of a disc protrusion, and also to enable correct placement of the injecting needle. The risk of anaphylaxis is high, so the patient is given a prophylactic dose of hydrocortisone 100 mg i.m. The procedure may be performed under sedation or general anaesthetic. However, due to the risk of anaphylaxis, an anaesthetist should always be in attendance. A further risk attached to this procedure is paralysis, caused by accidental injection of the enzyme into the lumber theca. Paralysis below the level of injection will cause paraplegia.

The amount of chymopapain injected varies from 0.8 to 1 ml per disc. The activity of the enzyme is instant, and it may not be withdrawn once instilled.

Recovery from this procedure may not be immediate; latent pain and stiffness may continue for some weeks, possibly months. In some cases, the discomfort may seem greater initially, due to intrusion of muscle and nerve fibres at the site of puncture. A pressure bandage is applied on completion of the procedure but it may be removed at any stage provided the puncture site is clean and dry. Postoperatively, the patient may be as mobile as he feels able. A care plan for the nursing management of a patient after chymopapain injection is set out in Table 16.1.

Percutaneous discectomy

A percutaneous discectomy is performed to release a nerve root which is being compressed, causing a neurological deficit and painful symptoms such as sciatica.

Laminectomy and discectomy

A laminectomy and discectomy is carried out if symptoms become intolerable for the individual and conservative measures have been unsatisfactory. The lamina lying over the involved nerve root and the underlying ligamentum flavum are excised. The nerve root is then gently retracted and the herniated nucleus pulposus is removed. The amount of pain following this procedure is variable, and specific to each individual. The responsibility of the nurse is to provide therapeutic caring which includes touch, massage, empathy and relaxation, and management of physical needs such as the effective control of pain.

COMPLEMENTARY THERAPIES

Many people who are seeking relief from back pain do not choose orthodox or traditional methods of treatment; however, the total number of people who consult complementary practitioners annually is not fully known. For example, Stanway (1982) reports that over 80 000 visited the outpatient department of the six homeopathic hospitals run by the NHS in 1982; furthermore, many people treat themselves.

The principle manipulative therapies used in treating the joints of the spine are osteopathy, chiropractic and reflexology. Osteopathy and chiropractic are used more specifically for spinal problems and are described briefly (Inglis & West 1983).

Osteopathy

Osteopathy is the manipulation of the spine, which concentrates specifically on a particular

Table 16.1 Care plan for the management of a patient before and after chemonucleolysis

Patient's problem/need	Expected outcome for patient	Action	Date
1. Informed decision about whether to have procedure under sedation or general anaesthetic	Safe preparation of patient for chymopapain injection procedure	Ensure 'informed' consent is obtained (Tait 1989)	
2. Comfort and position	Patient will feel comfortable and safe post-chemonucleolysis procedure	*After sedation* Nurse patient in any position patient desires Patient is able to lie in semirecumbent position; if comfortable, patient may sit up *After general anaesthetic* Nurse patient in lateral position or supine until patient recovers from anaesthetic Patient's legs elevated on pillows if desired as this reduces lumbar lordosis when lying supine Patient should be encouraged to turn frequently from side to side to back to reduce pressure on the skin Log rolling (Fig. 16.10) is the most comfortable method (taught to the patient preprocedure)	
3. Anxiety regarding risks of procedure, i.e. anaphylactic shock, paraplegia	Patient will feel safe and informed about procedure and experience no excessive anxiety	Identify cause of anxieties by interviewing patient and providing opportunity for him to ask questions Provide information about preprocedure preparation, transfer to and from theatre, what to expect postprocedure (Hayward 1975, Boore 1978)	
4. Pain due to prolapsed disc	Relief of pain/discomfort controlled to a level acceptable to the patient	Assess degree of discomfort by verbal/non-verbal communication (Hayward 1975). Administer appropriate prescribed pain-relieving agents, i.e. anti-inflammatory drugs, antispasmodics, analgesics or alternative therapy (McCafferey 1983, Sofaer 1983) Position and support patient comfortably	
5. Loss of independence	Retain as much independence as possible during hospitalization	Provide opportunity for patients to retain independence by helping themselves as much as possible Encourage active participation All aspects of life are affected by this admission as described in Figure 16.3	
6. Potential shock	Early recognition of abnormal signs	Observe and record blood pressure and pulse; be aware of signs of shock – hypovolaemic or anaphylactic – and report	
7. Potential problem of altered neurovascular status (particularly the lower limbs)	Early recognition of abnormal signs	Observe and record neurovascular status – i.e. colour, warmth, movement, sensation – and report	
8. Wound management	Promote healing and prevent infection	Pressure bandage applied over puncture site initially Can be removed at any time provided that a haematoma has not developed	
9. Potential inability to eliminate urine and/or faeces normally	No discomfort from urinary retention or bowel disturbance	Ensure privacy Encourage fluid/high fibre intake Use slipper bedpan/bottle as appropriate	
10. Unable to maintain personal hygiene	Provide independence for the patient during his 24-hour bedrest so that he can deal with personal hygiene	Assist patient with his personal hygiene and offer advice upon discharge	

Table 16.1 (*contd*)

Patient's problem/need	Expected outcome for patient	Action	Date
11. Restricted mobility for 24 hours	Prevent complications of immobility	Encourage patient to perform exercise, i.e deep breathing, straight leg raising, static quadriceps exercises After 24 hours bedrest, patient to mobilize gradually, walking with a straight back	
12. Further anxiety of recurring back pain	Prevent recurrence of back pain	Arrange outpatient appointment for 2 weeks after discharge Continue education programme while patient is in hospital, i.e. how to bend down, how to lift and carry heavy weights Reinforce 'back-saving' exercises at back school Encourage good posture Encourage personal action plan	

vertebra. The technique involves locking the vertebra on either side of the joint, then using the movement of the patient's body to provide momentum to apply a corrective thrust.

Chiropractic

Chiropractors use a slightly different manipulative method aimed at specific joints. They combine many related therapies such as massage, aromatherapy, reflexology, Alexander technique, acupuncture, herbalism, homeopathy and applied kinesiology.

These therapies are not readily available within the NHS. However, a general practitioner may refer a patient to a medical practitioner with osteopathic or chiropractic qualifications.

REHABILITATION

The goals of rehabilitation include the prevention of further disability, maintenance of remaining abilities and restoration of as much function as possible in activities of daily living and in social roles.

Rehabilitation nursing also involves advising and teaching the patients and their families to adapt to familiar or new lifestyles, so that realistic goals are set to enable individuals to reach their maximum potential.

Educating the individual

The concept of using education in the treatment of people with back problems is not new. The aim is to increase the patient's ability to take care of his back by informing him of what is known about his condition, in order to facilitate self-management.

Most 'back schools' function as multidisciplinary programmes and run effectively as an outpatient educational resource. However, they are not available in every district general hospital. The schools usually run programmes with 2-hour sessions weekly over 6 weeks. Prior to the commencement of the programme each person is reassessed and has the opportunity to discuss any further problems relating to his case.

Although content varies from school to school, the main focus is on self-management. Introductory aspects of basic anatomy are explained providing a platform for understanding the mechanics of the human frame and body movement. Ergonomic counselling and the instruction of useful muscle strengthening exercises such as extension and isometric abdominal exercises are provided. Lifting and carrying techniques are taught and practised in a practical manner, ensuring that bending occurs at the knees and not the back. Advice on pain and stress management, and relaxation techniques such as the Alexander technique are also included.

CONCLUSION

Nursing practice in relation to low back problems is based on an accurate knowledge of the problem causing the patient discomfort. The incidence of back pain is high, and nurses themselves are prone to the development of this condition because of the physical demands of their employment. Nursing involves helping patients to achieve optimum wellness, and nurses have a valuable role to play in the achievement and maintenance of a healthy spine.

REFERENCES

Becker M H 1976 Sociobehavioural determinants of compliance. In: Fitzgerald Miller J (ed) 1983 Coping with chronic illness. F A Davis, USA

Bell F 1979 Hospital ward patient lifting tasks. Ergonomics 22(11): 1257–1273

Boore J 1978 Prescription for recovery. RCN, London

Commission of the European Communities 1990 Amended proposal for a council directive on the minimum health and safety requirements for handling heavy loads where there is a risk of back injury for workers. Presented by the Commissioner under article 149–3 of the Treaty, 25 April Brussels

Cust G, Pearson J C G, Muir A 1972 The prevalence of low back pain in nurses. International Nursing Review 19: 169–179

Department of Health and Social Security Office of Population Census and Surverys (OPCS) 1982 Hospital in-patient enquiry. HMSO, London

Halliwell R S 1988 Some current areas of interest in back pain research. Rheumatology in Practice 6: 21–4

Harber P, Billet E, Gutowski M, Soohoo K, Lew M, Roman A 1985 Occupational low-back pain in hospital nurses. Journal of Occupational Medicine 17: 518–524

Hayward J 1975 Information: a prescription against pain. RCN, London

Health & Safety Commission 1991 Proposals for health and safety (general provisions consultative document) regulations and approved code of practice. Health and Safety Executive. HMSO

Health and Safety at Work Act 1974 HMSO

Inglis B, West R 1983 The alternative health guide. London

Kaur B, Pederson H 1986 Mind your backs! Nursing Times 82(16): 45–47

Kelsey J L, White A A 1980 Epidemiology and impact of low back pain. Spine 5(2): 133–142

McCafferey M 1983 Nursing the patient in pain. Harper & Row, London

Murrell K F H 1965 Man in his working environment. Thanet, London

Office of Health Economics 1985 Back pain. White Crescent, London

Owen B D, Damron C F 1984 Personal characteristics and back injury among hospital nursing personnel. Research in Nursing and Health 7: 305–313

Papageorgiou A, Rigby A 1990 Review of UK data on the rheumatic diseases. Arthritis and Rheumatism Council for Research, Manchester

Pheasant S R 1984 Anthropometrics: an introduction for schools and colleges. Royal Free Hospital School of Medicine, London

Raistrick A 1981 Nurses with back pain – can the problem be prevented? Nursing Times 77(20): 853–856

Simpson G 1984 Ergonomic problems and solutions. In: Brotherwood J (ed) Occupational aspects of back disorders. Society of Occupational Medicine

Singleton W T 1972 Introduction to ergonomics. WHO, Geneva

Sofaer B 1983 Pain relief – the core of nursing practice. Nursing Times 79(47): 38–42

Stanway A 1982 Alternative medicine. Penguin, Harmondsworth

Stubbs D A, Buckle P W 1984 The epidemiology of back pain in nurses. Nursing 2: 935–938

Tait A 1989 Informed consent. Nursing Standard 3: 55

Troup J D G, Martin J W, Lloyd D C 1987 The handling of patients – a guide for nurses, 2nd edn. Back Pain Association, RCN, London

Wood P H N, Badley E M 1980 Back pain in the community. In: Grahame R (ed) Clinics in rheumatic diseases, vol 6, no 1. Pitman, London, Ch. 1 p 3–16

Wood P H N, Badley E M 1987 Epidemiology of back pain. In: Jayson M I V (ed) The lumbar spine and back pain, 3rd edn. London, Ch. 1 p 1 15

17

The amputee

Sarah Wallis

The aim of this chapter is to identify problems specific to amputee patients and to improve awareness of the specialized nursing care required.

Amputation evokes a multitude of individual responses. Like bereavement, it has physical and psychological repercussions for the individual, and can cause deep emotional stress and an inability to cope with daily life. Routinely, the nurse observes denial, shock, fear and anger, grief for loss of the body part, worry about the loss of mobility and fear of pain or lack of healing. Anxiety, depressive reactions, identified body image concerns, stress, isolation and negative emotions have all been documented as psychosocial consequences of amputation (Weinstein 1985) (Fig. 17.1). As reactions to amputation are bio-psycho-social in nature, nursing care should reflect this.

THE STRUCTURE OF NURSING CARE

The nursing care that the patient requires needs to be individualized, knowledgeable, empathetic and holistic. Indeed, caring for the amputee patient requires tremendous skill and expertise from the nurse. At present many individuals following amputation are nursed on different wards by nurses with variable expertise and knowledge. Clinical nurse specialists or link nurses were suggested as early as 1986 (Potterton) as the ideal, meeting the patient preoperatively and following through to discharge and commu-

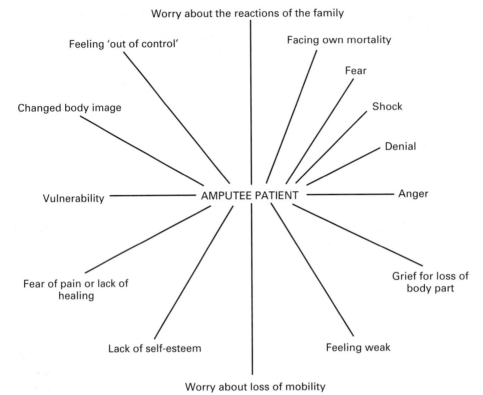

Fig. 17.1   Physical and psychological responses to amputation.

nity care. The nurse would be able to act as a resource facilitating care for the patient's social, psychological, and physical problems as they arise. However, most districts do not have such a post and care is given to the best of the nurse's ability.

The nurse–patient relationship

Virginia Henderson (1966) identifies the unique role of the nurse. However, her definition concentrates on the skills of nursing and does not take full account of the nurse's feelings. McFarlane (1976) identified the two compoments of caring as activities and feelings. Nurses need to examine carefully their own feelings – for example fear, embarrassment, revulsion and despair – when caring for amputee patients. They should analyse their feelings and become aware of their attitudes, values and beliefs about amputation and amputee patients (see Fig. 17.2).

This can be done by giving nurses the opportunity to discuss their feelings towards amputation in ward meetings, within primary nurse teams and at appraisal or performance reviews. Talking to patients who have accepted their loss can be very helpful, giving nurses a useful insight into patients' emotional reactions generated by amputation and how nurses can help. Due to swift turnover of staff in many areas this analysis of nurses' attitudes, values and beliefs needs to be frequent, and many wards do have a meeting every month facilitated by an experienced nurse specialist.

The nurse's awareness and understanding of her own thoughts and feelings helps her build a nurse–patient relationship firmly based on trust, mutual respect and honesty. How can the nurse who has not explored her own feelings about amputation, or who holds attitudes, values and beliefs that are potentially harmful, hope to treat the patient with honesty and respect?

Values may be:	An affective disposition towards a person, object or idea. They give direction to life.
Attitudes may be:	A disposition or feeling towards a person, object or idea.
Beliefs may be:	A special class of attitudes in which the cognitive component is based more on faith than fact.

Fig. 17.2 Statements regarding attitudes, values and beliefs.

Initially, the nurse may feel, from her perspective, that she would 'rather die than have an amputation' or alternatively 'not know what the fuss is about, the patient is much better off without his limb anyway'. Her feelings are very likely to influence her approach to her nursing care. Misplaced sympathy or inadequate control of feelings can generate patient dependence and negative emotion – all potentially harmful to patient recovery.

Setting goals with the patient

Goals used to plan achievable nursing care can promote a positive feeling of progression; this positive approach is of the utmost importance to the amputee patient. The nurse and patient together can easily plan these goals, and can structure them by identifying subject, behaviour, condition and criteria (McFarlane & Castledine 1982), for example:

Subject – Mr Smith
Behaviour – to walk
Condition – with his crutches and prosthesis on his affected limb
Criteria – with one nurse to the table for meals by (date)

If one page of nursing documentation is given to one problem, over time the patient and nurse can see improvement. Progression determined by achievement of goals is easily visible.

However, the nursing process will not function without some underlying theoretical or conceptual framework (Campbell & Walker 1989).

In the next section Orem's model of nursing will be used (see Chs 11 and 16).

Orem's model of nursing

Amputee patients need to feel in control of their care and Orem's model (1985) allows the patient to do this while he is being given health care and treatment. The structure of assessment as detailed in Figure 17.3 is particularly applicable when used to identify patient problems. Deviations from normal health are assessed and any behavioural patient problems arising as a result of medical intervention are observed. Grief for loss of the body part could be one such problem manifesting as anger, denial or shock.

Nurses should give information and appropriate support and assistance to the patient, enabling him to participate in his own care and so contribute to the maintenance of his own health. Orem's (1985) model acts as an ideal tool for nurses to use when devising care for their patients undergoing amputation, with the emphasis on self-care, patient participation and education.

Patients' reactions to amputation

An amputation is a stressful event for the patient, whose reactions differ depending on the reasons for and significance of the amputation. Limb loss results in a myriad of responses dependent upon the patient's personality, developmental stage, life experiences and the significance of the loss of a limb. For example,

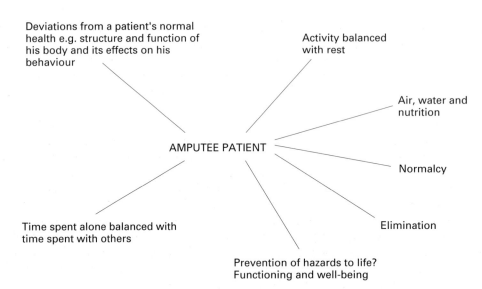

Deviations from a patient's normal health e.g. structure and function of his body and its effects on his behaviour

Activity balanced with rest

Air, water and nutrition

AMPUTEE PATIENT

Normalcy

Time spent alone balanced with time spent with others

Elimination

Prevention of hazards to life? Functioning and well-being

Fig. 17.3 Assessment structure using Orem's (1985) model.

traumatic amputation or amputation to save or prolong life allows little time for preparation: the patient and his family are expected to adjust quickly. However, for the patient who has a long-term disability or a painful, immobile, useless limb, surgery is usually scheduled. The patient is, in general, not only physically ready for amputation, but relieved and eager to get on with life. If the patient has been suffering from long-term ill health, he may have had time to adjust to the reality of amputation, but be physically or psychologically unable or unwilling to take on this 'challenge'.

The nurse must be careful not to generalize at this stage, as the reaction the patient has is not dependent upon any one factor but on a combination of factors.

Site of amputation

In many cases the level of amputation is determined by the patient's disease and its state of advancement. The site of the amputation also affects the patient's psychological reactions to surgery, in addition to the degree of disability with which he has to cope (Fig. 17.4). Thus, the nurse needs to know not only the reason for the amputation but also where the amputation site will be to be prepared for the patient's emotional reactions and physical incapabilities. For exam-

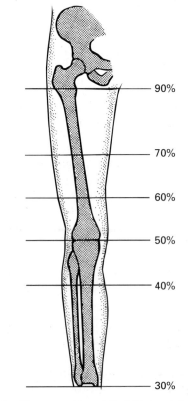

90%

70%

60%

50%

40%

30%

Fig. 17.4 The percentage of disability in relation to amputation level.

ple, the patient who has a mid-thigh amputation to prolong his life would be expected to have more problems with acceptance and disability than a patient who has had some toes amputated because of a congenital abnormality. However, these examples are over-simplifications. Care must be individualized using a nursing model, and as such the assessment could reveal that the patient with a mid-thigh amputation is very positive. He may have a very supportive family, a loving relationship with his partner, be financially secure with an optimistic, open personality and a good past experience of hospital and medical interventions. The patient who has had his toes amputated may feel quite alone, and his relationship with his partner may be strained; in fact, he may not be visited at all. He may be a lonely, introverted person who finds it difficult to talk to people, and he may never have been in hospital before and so find it very disconcerting. This patient is more likely to experience problems after amputation than the patient described first.

Preparation of the patient for amputation

Prior to surgery the patient may have additional problems which are specifically associated with the amputation and of which the nurse must take account. These are:

1. Normalcy – acceptance of the amputation; the breaking of bad news
2. Prevention of hazards to life, functioning and well being – stress and its effect on the patient about to undergo amputation; why is the reduction of stress important?; preparation of the limb for surgery
3. Deviation from the patient's normal health, structure and function – phantom limb pain – preparation of the patient.

These problems are discussed below within the framework of Orem's model of nursing.

Normalcy: acceptance of the amputation

Orem (1985) describes normalcy as having four different aspects. One of these is the individual maintaining a realistic self-concept and actively trying to develop as a human being. The others are: the individual looking after his own body to promote optimum function; being aware of any deviations from his norm; and acting on that awareness. All these aspects will be affected if the patient undergoes amputation.

The first step to be taken when preparing the patient for amputation is to inform him of the operation. This is an area that doctors and nurses find difficult. Moos (1986) identified the nurse's role when helping patients adapt to a life crisis: 'Caregivers need to be conversant with knowledge of coping tasks and skills and to be sensitive to people's emotional reactions and needs. Coupled with their own empathy and understanding of crisis situations this information can help them diffuse the negative impact of life's crisis and nurture the potential for growth intrinsic in such situations'.

There are several factors which need to be remembered when informing patients that they are to have an amputation. One is to accept that bad news is bad news however it is broken. Another is to realize that the key to breaking it is to give the information slowly at the patient's pace (Maguire & Faulkner 1988).

Assessment

Assessment of the patient should be made when the nurse knows that the patient is to have an amputation. Although doctors make the decision as to when the amputation is necessary, the experienced nurse has usually known for some time that it is unavoidable. As the patient needs time to adjust to the fact that the operation is necessary, he should be prepared for the surgery as soon as possible. The nurse can introduce the idea gradually in a positive way, by perhaps using other patients who have progressed well as examples, or including amputation as an option when explaining the different types of surgical intervention available for the patient's condition. Although amputation is an ever-present fear in many patients' minds, they often 'block it out' and do not perceive it as a reality because they do not want to do so. Gentle introduction of the subject by the nurse, when she suspects that it is a possibility, can lengthen the time available for the patient to accept it. Initially the level of the patient's knowledge and understanding is assessed to detect and correct any deficits. Asking questions to determine this is helpful. For example:

'How do you feel your wound is healing?'
'How does your pain feel now?'
'What do you think is going to happen to you now?'
'Have the doctors said anything to you about more surgery?'

When preparing the patient for surgery, the patient's present body image has to change in order that he can accept the now altered perception which results in recognition of and adaptation to amputation (Novotny 1986).

Body image disturbances occur when the patient cannot accept the changes and clings to old images which may be inconsistent with reality. Often these difficulties are related to societal values which emphasize vitality and physical fitness and consequently view amputation as a failure. The nurse needs to assess this area, taking into consideration the attitudes of the patient's family and friends. For example, the family could place much importance on the patient's sporting accomplishments in the past and their negative feelings about amputation could reinforce the patient's own feelings of failure. The nurse in her assessment could identify any problems by asking questions such as:

'What sport were you playing before this happened?'
'Did you get any benefits out of playing sport?'
'Did your friends play sport as well?'

Feelings can then be communicated which enable the nurse to devise strategies to alleviate the problem and encourage adoption of different, more realistic goals in a positive way.

Once amputation has been decided upon by the medical and nursing staff, the patient needs to be informed. It is hoped that patient prepara-tion will have gradually changed the patient's perception of the problem. Maguire and Faulkner (1988) proposed some strategies for breaking bad news that are detailed in Figure 17.5.

Inclusion of the patient's partner or relatives, at their request, is important as it allows them to voice fears and concerns, receive support and obtain answers to questions. It also increases the network of available support for the patient, who will need understanding, encouragement and empathy.

Evaluation

The patient's evaluation of goals achieved is an excellent way of assessing the effectiveness of care given. Transition stages in coping are identified in Figure 17.6, and Moos (1986) has identified the adaptive tasks necessary for coping with a life crisis (Fig. 17.7). Both of these diagrams are worth remembering, as they show how the process of acceptance can be broken down into stages, making it easier for patients and nurses to set realistic achievable goals which can then help to identify patient progression in an area that has tended to be ignored in the past.

Prevention of hazards to life, functioning and well-being: stress and its effect on the patient about to undergo amputation

Orem (1985) describes the prevention of hazards as contributing to the maintenance of human integrity and thus to the promotion of human functioning. Prolonged stress has been shown to induce illness and jeopardize body functioning (Feist & Brannon 1988). A parallel has been drawn between the loss of a limb and the loss of a spouse (Parkes 1986); by using the social readjustment scale (Holmes & Rahe 1967) (Fig. 17.8) it is clear that amputation, with a score of 400 or more, is a very stressful event. This supports Weinstein's (1985) identification of stress as a major factor arising from the threat of amputation.

Hans Selye (1956) suggests that individuals adapt to stress in the way outlined in his 'general

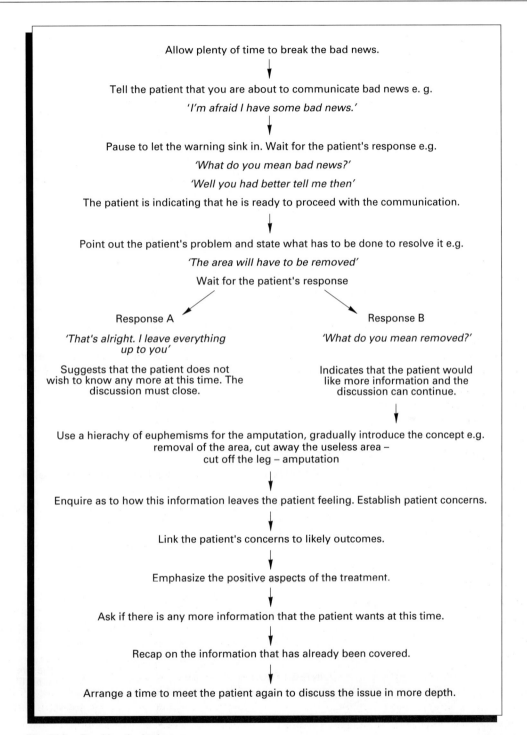

Fig. 17.5 Breaking the bad news.

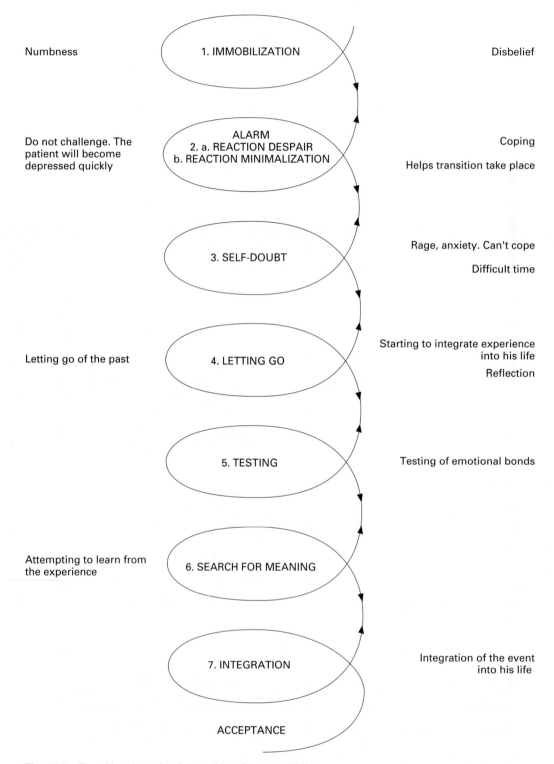

Numbness

1. IMMOBILIZATION

Disbelief

Do not challenge. The patient will become depressed quickly

ALARM
2. a. REACTION DESPAIR
b. REACTION MINIMALIZATION

Coping

Helps transition take place

3. SELF-DOUBT

Rage, anxiety. Can't cope

Difficult time

Letting go of the past

4. LETTING GO

Starting to integrate experience into his life

Reflection

5. TESTING

Testing of emotional bonds

Attempting to learn from the experience

6. SEARCH FOR MEANING

7. INTEGRATION

Integration of the event into his life

ACCEPTANCE

Fig. 17.6 Transitions in coping (adapted from Hopson 1981).

1. Establish the meaning and significance of the situation
2. Confront reality
3. Sustain relationships with family and friends
4. Maintain a reasonable emotional balance
5. Preserve a satisfactory self-image

Fig. 17.7   Adaptive tasks necessary to cope with life crisis.

LIFE EVENT	VALUE	SCORE	LIFE EVENT	VALUE	SCORE
Death of spouse	100	☐	Son or daughter leaving home	29	☐
Divorce	73	☐	Trouble with in-laws	29	☐
Marital separation	65	☐	Outstanding personal achievement	28	☐
Jail term	63	☐	Spouse begins or stops work	26	☐
Death of a close family member	63	☐	Begin or end school	26	☐
Personal injury or illness	53	☐	Change in living condition	25	☐
Marriage	50	☐	Revision of personal habits	24	☐
Fired at work	47	☐	Trouble with boss	23	☐
Marital reconcilation	45	☐	Change in work hours or conditions	20	☐
Retirement	45	☐	Change in residence	20	☐
Change in health of family member	44	☐	Change in schools	20	☐
Pregnancy	40	☐	Change in recreation	19	☐
Sex difficulties	39	☐	Change in church activities	19	☐
Gain of new family member	39	☐	Change in social activities	18	☐
Business adjustment	39	☐	Mortgage or loan less than one year's net salary	17	☐
Change in financial state	38	☐			
Death of a close friend	37	☐	Change in sleeping habits	16	☐
Change to different line of work	36	☐	Change in number of family get-togethers	15	☐
Change in number of arguments with spouse	35	☐	Change in eating habits	15	☐
Mortgage over one year's net salary	31	☐	Holiday	13	☐
Foreclosure of mortgage or loan	30	☐	Christmas	12	☐
Change in responsibilities at work	29	☐	Minor violations of the law	11	☐

Enter your total here _____

Under 150: If your score is less than 150 units, you have a 30% chance of a serious change in your health within the next year.
150–300: Up to 300 units, you have a 50% chance of suffering stress-related illness.
Over 300: If you score more than 300, you stand an 80% chance of getting sick if you don't take some preventative action.

Note that the ratings only apply to stresses that you have undergone over the last 24 months.

Fig. 17.8   Social readjustment scale. (From Holmes & Rahe 1967.)

adaptation syndrome'. After the initial alarm re-action and the stage of resistance, adaptation is achieved. During the adaptation period, the indi-vidual's ability to react to an additional stressor is greatly diminished. There are two important factors for the nurse to remember at this stage. First, the amputee patient may have suffered ill health through diabetes, peripheral vascular disease, failed surgery or chronic pain for some time and may be already a stressed individual; with exposure to an additional stressor such as amputation, adaptation will be lengthy and difficult. Second, if the individual maintains a stressed state for an extended period of time (for example, when he has difficulty in accepting the loss of amputation), the body can rapidly become exhausted. It is practically impossible for the patient then to withstand another stressor. Problems can occur as a direct result of these additional stressors, such as wound in-fection, hypertension, lethargy and weakness, leading to a lack of motivation, depression and even exacerbation of the medical condition that necessitated the amputation (Atkinson et al 1987).

Preoperatively, stress reduction is an impor-tant part of the nurse's role. She must provide strategies that help the patient adapt to his changing circumstances, causing him as little additional stress as possible.

Assessment

The individual's feelings of stress before being informed of the amputation are compared to his feelings after being told. If these have increased, care is planned and given accordingly. A ques-tion that the nurse can ask to ascertain the degree of stress is: 'How do you feel now compared with before you knew that you were having an amputation?' The patient will often then identify his own degree of adaptation for the nurse. For example: 'I used to feel in control, now I feel so helpless', or 'I used to feel calm, but now I feel jumpy and anxious'. Nurses also need to observe the patient's mood and signs of stress, as the patient's verbal responses may not accurately reflect his feelings. Monitoring the vital signs

is another indication; tachycardia, hypertension and hyperventilation are all indicative of stress (Feist & Brannon 1988). Mood and emotion can be detected by the nurse looking at and listening to her patient as well as by asking questions.

Planning and intervention

The patient's problem will dictate whether the nurse's role should be wholly or partially com-pensatory or educative and supportive. What-ever role the nurse undertakes, she should always aim to help the patient feel in control of his care, as this will help to relieve his anxiety and stress (Wilson-Barnett & Batehup 1988).

Patients undergoing amputation often feel vulnerable. Vulnerability exists when insuffi-cient resources create a potentially threatening or harmful situation (Feist & Brannon 1988). Very often the amputee patient only requires knowledge and support to make him feel in con-trol, alleviate his anxiety and reduce his vulner-ability. Nurses should always be ready to give information on request, and any care planned should be with the patient's knowledge and, wherever possible, participation.

The nurse should respond to and encourage the patient who is about to undergo an amputa-tion to release his emotions. Culturally, this may be an unfamiliar concept both to the nurse and patient, but unexpressed emotion can manifest itself in many ways, all potentially harmful to the patient. Physical tension and emotional prob-lems can be avoided if emotion is released at this stage (Burnard 1988). Reich (1976) suggests that the release of repressed emotion can lead to the person feeling healthier physically, as well as emotionally more stable and secure.

The nurse, in her assessment, may detect the patient's degree of physical tension by his complaints of tension or pain in the shoulders or upper trunk. A person who cannot cope with his unexpressed sorrow will often experience tension in his stomach.

However, it is often not easy for the nurse to allow patients to freely express their emotions. Socially the nurse's reflex is to rush in and 'reassure' the emotional patient to stop him getting too upset; it is as if the patient's emotions stir up the nurse's own unexpressed emotions and make her unhappy (Burnard 1988). Burnard (1988) suggests that after the expression of emotion the patient needs time to reflect on the situation. Often the patient gains much comfort from a nurse sitting quietly by his side while he thinks the situation through.

Implementation of the care planned and the release of tension are aided by a sympathetic environment with a degree of privacy and quiet. Light touch can also often promote and encourage emotional release (Montague 1978, Heron 1973); where appropriate, nurses can convey their comfort and empathy through touch.

Evaluation

Realistic goals set individually with each patient should lead to a patient prepared for surgery who is as relaxed as he can be, feeling supported and comforted by relatives and nurses and in control of his care.

Nurses who deal with the emotional release of others frequently must take time to explore their own emotions. If the nurse carries around much unexpressed emotion herself, she will become distressed by others' emotional release. She might then avoid the latter situation by indirectly disallowing the patient's expression of feelings, for example by saying: 'Dry your tears now, it's not good to get too upset'. 'You really must not get so angry, it upsets your family'. Confidential support groups can encourage nurses to talk through their feelings and gain support from their colleagues (Burnard 1988). This self-development is the first stage in preparing the nurse to help others express their emotions. If a more detailed or in-depth knowledge is needed by the nurse, or if she feels reluctant or unsure about when to intervene, then more knowledge and skills in the form of a counselling course could be of value (see Figs 17.6 and 17.7).

Preparation of the limb for surgery

Nurses are often confused as to how much they should prepare a limb for amputation. The pa-tient who is in pain will not tolerate shaving or cleansing of the limb preoperatively. However, patients such as those requiring amputation of a deformed limb can be prepared in this way.

Preparation of the operation site has been found to affect the incidence of infection. One study found the lowest incidence of infection (0.9%) in patients who were not shaved or clipped preoperatively. Infection rates increased depending on the method of hair removal: 1.4% with the use of an electric razor, 1.7% if the operation site was clipped and 2.5% if manual shaving was carried out (Wysocki 1989). In trials that compared shaving with the use of depilatory creams, the creams were found to be more comfortable for the patient but made no difference to the postoperative infection rates (Winfield 1986). However, if removal of hair is essential then it should be done as near to the time of surgery as possible as this will reduce the risk of infection. The utmost care must be taken not to break the skin in any way as this would increase the risk of infection.

Skin cleansing to reduce skin flora preoperatively may be necessary and should be done according to the surgeon's preference. However, if the patient is in pain then this should be performed in theatre.

Assessment

The nurse observes the limb the evening or morning before the amputation. She assesses the patient's pain and mobility and plans the intervention accordingly. The surgeon's wishes are noted, and if they cannot be followed then this is documented in the patient's notes.

Evaluation

Measuring evaluation against infection rates is difficult as many patients who have an amputation are at risk of delayed wound healing just from the nature of their condition. If care has been successful, then:

1. Patients should show that they have understood the care that they have received and the rationale behind that care.

2. Patients should not have experienced any pain as a result of any preoperative preparation.

3. The infection rates on the ward or department among the amputee patients should not rise.

Deviations from the patient's normal health, structure and function

Phantom limb sensation is an extremely common occurrence, affecting 84–100% of all amputee patients (Wall et al 1985, Herbener 1988). Phantom limb pain affects 35% of all patients almost immediately postoperatively and 5–10% suffer from it chronically (Herbener 1988). Because most patients are going to experience some sensation postoperatively, the nurse should prepare all her patients so that they know what to expect. By providing this information the nurse will help to lower their level of anxiety and thus their potential for pain. To feel that his limb is still present may make the uninformed patient question his own sanity; elderly patients can feel particularly fearful of appearing foolish and may not report their limb sensations.

Assessment

It is essential that the nurse, when preparing the patient preoperatively, allows him enough time to absorb the relevant information, but does not start preparing him too soon while he is still adjusting to the news of the amputation.

Planning and intervention

The nurse should limit the type of information she gives the patient to facts, in particular how the sensations will affect him. Phantom limb sensations can be described as tingling, numbness, itching, warmth, coldness, heaviness or tightness, and they are most commonly felt in the distal part of the limb. The nurse should concentrate on describing the sensations rather than the pain, but if the patient enquires directly about it she must on no account avoid the issue.

The patient will retain more information if it is given in short sessions on several occasions rather than for one long period. At the beginning of each session, the nurse should encourage the patient to give feedback on the information that he has remembered. The use of a visual aid (Fig. 17.9) is helpful and encourages memory retention. The nurse should also be aware that information sessions could increase the patient's anxiety or stress if not supported with reassurances such as:

- The sensations are felt by most amputee patients and it is less common to feel actual pain.
- The sensations can come very quickly after the operation and patients may feel them immediately.
- The sensations gradually recede when mobilization with a prosthesis commences (Herbener 1988, Ceccio & Horosz 1988).

Preoperatively, the patient will be anxious and generally will not want a detailed explanation of phantom pain.

1. Sensations are more commonly felt in the part of the amputated limb furthest away from you.

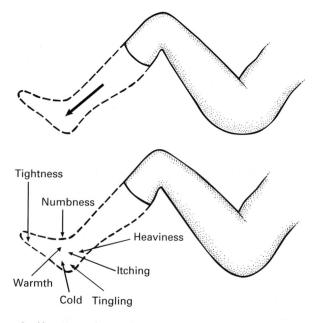

2. How your phantom limb might feel to you.

Fig. 17.9 Visual teaching aid used when preparing the patient prior to amputation about phantom limb sensations.

Evaluation

Evaluation is provided by the patient's feedback from the information-giving session. This indicates the patient's level of understanding and thus the effectiveness of intervention.

Multidisciplinary team

Before surgery the nurse needs to ensure that the patient, wherever possible, is known and has been seen by other members of the multidisciplinary team. The physiotherapist should see the patient preoperatively to show him the exercises necessary for strengthening the sound limbs. The affected limb muscles above the lines of expected surgery are also strengthened. The patient with a lower limb amputation should practise walking with crutches, and the effect of amputation on balance should be explained to him.

If at all possible, the patient should go to the artificial limb centre to meet the prosthetist and see some examples of prostheses. However, it is important for the nurse to assess whether the patient is ready for this, i.e. whether he would welcome the visit or find it overwhelming and upsetting.

The occupational therapist should be contacted to make an assessment of the patient's needs after discharge and to liaise with social services, if appropriate, for home alterations.

The social worker may need to be informed if the patient requires financial and family support whilst in hospital and on discharge.

SPECIFIC POSTOPERATIVE NURSING CARE OF THE PATIENT FOLLOWING AMPUTATION

After surgery the patient has several problems specific to recovery from amputation. These may be summarized as follows.

Deviations from the patient's normal health

Fear of pain has been found to be one of the major concerns of amputee patients (Weinstein 1985). This fear can cause anxiety and sleeplessness and thus result in further pain (Spencer 1989). Forced immobilization due to unrelieved pain could lead to reduced lung ventilation, ineffective cough and poor limb movements (Goodwin 1986).

As described in the preoperative care of the amputee patient, phantom limb pain and sensations are common postoperatively. Phantom limb pain is more likely to develop in the patient whose limb was painful prior to surgery, and the higher the amputation the more likely the patient is to experience it (Herbener 1998). Different types of phantom limb pain are described in Figure 17.10. The onset is variable but is usually soon after amputation.

Muscle tension can exacerbate pain around the stump site, and in such a case relaxation is of more value to the patient than painkillers. Deep breathing is one form of relaxation that can decrease the sympathetic nervous activity as well as improve lung ventilation and decrease the need for narcotic analgesia. The patient also feels in control, so his anxiety is reduced (Spencer 1989).

Other methods of non-analgesic pain relief include heat, distraction, position change, massage and the use of transcutaneous nerve stimulation (Gartside 1986). The use of heat aids muscle

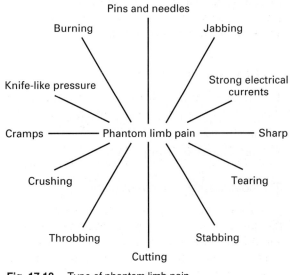

Fig. 17.10 Type of phantom limb pain.

relaxation and enhances circulation, facilitating the resolution of oedema. The provision of routine comfort measures and diversional activities refocus the patient's attention, and promote relaxation, and may enhance coping abilities.

Elevation of the stump or the end of the bed, or the use of a sling for the upper arm amputee, lessens oedema formation by enhancing venous return, reduces muscle fatigue and skin/tissue pressure and so reduces pain.

Gentle massage of the stump, often performed by the patient, enhances circulation and reduces muscle tension, and is also useful in the relief of phantom limb sensations and pain.

In addition to reducing anxiety levels, patient-controlled analgesia administration prevents fluctuations in pain and associated muscle tension and spasms (Doenges 1989). Thus, self-medication with supervision from the nursing staff is to be recommended for patients with chronic stump pain.

Evaluation can be carried out by observing the drug charts to ascertain how much and how frequently analgesia is administered. The level of pain also can be calculated from the scale of the transcutaneous nerve stimulation machine; the lower the number on the scale the less pain the patient is experiencing.

Prevention of hazards to life, functioning and well-being

Nursing care of the stump involves the following:

1. Awareness of the potential risk of haemorrhage
2. Specific care of the wound
3. Awareness of the potential risk of joint contractures
4. Maintenance of stump shape.

The potential risk of haemorrhage

Amputation can cause a haemorrhage postoperatively. The operation necessitates the complete severence of bone, muscles, skin, blood vessels and nerves: bleeding from severed arteries and veins is relatively common.

A primary haemorrhage occurs at the time of surgery, and haemostasis is achieved with the use of diathermy and ligation of the larger vessels.

A reactionary haemorrhage occurs within the first 24 hours after surgery and can be venous or arterial; it is caused by a vessel being inadequately sealed or by a ligature becoming dislodged.

Amputee patients who have conditions preoperatively and postoperatively that contribute to delayed wound healing are susceptible to secondary haemorrhage; for example, diabetics. Secondary haemorrhage occurs approximately 10 days after surgery and is associated with wound infection. It may involve an artery and may lead to sudden collapse or even exsanguination (Blake 1989).

Patients should be monitored for reactionary bleeding during the first 24 hours postoperatively. Nurses' awareness of the risk of secondary haemorrhage will make them alert to any patient complaints of pain or change of condition in the initial 10 days postoperatively. Blood pressure and pulse are monitored to ascertain if there is any loss of circulating blood volume.

Skin colour and temperature also indicate blood loss. The peripheral vessels vasoconstrict, which causes the skin to become pale and cool. It may also feel clammy due to the activity of the sympathetic nervous system.

Frequent observation of the dressings and wound drains for the amounts and characteristics of the drainage is necessary. Dark red oozing is indicative of venous bleeding; arterial loss is bright red. While the patient is in bed in the immediate postoperative period, the area around the stump, particularly between the legs and behind the small of the back for above-knee amputees and underneath the shoulders for above-elbow cases, should be observed for the pooling of blood.

Some bleeding is expected after amputation, but bright red bleeding is a serious problem and would possibly necessitate ligation of the artery. If this does occur, the medical staff should be informed as for an emergency. Pressure is applied to the stump wound or nearest pressure point, and the foot of the bed raised. Some hospitals stipulate that a tourniquet should be used in such situations, and one is kept for this purpose in the vicinity of the patient postoperatively.

Specific care of the wound

Problems associated with wound healing are outlined in Figure 17.11 The following factors can delay wound healing and increase the risk of infection:

- Age is significant, as 60% of all amputee patients are over the age of 60 years (Footner 1987).
- Essential organs function less well in older people, and they have nutritional deficiencies which may delay healing.
- Prolonged stress results in the production of cortisol which has been implicated in delayed wound healing (Cooper & Schumann 1979). The instability of blood pressure, metabolic rate and heart rate as a result of stress can also be detrimental to recovery and wound healing.
- Bereavement and grief for the loss of a limb are additional stressors which act to suppress the individual's immune response contributing to a delay in wound healing (Parkes & Weiss 1983).
- Patients who have had an amputation because of diabetes are five times more likely to develop wound infection than those without diabetes (Wilson-Barnett & Batehup 1988).

- Radiation therapy, if the patient received it prior to surgery, damages tissue. Infection is a common problem among such patients, as is poor wound healing.
- Steroid therapy will suppress the repair process if administered within 2–3 days of surgery.
- Chemotherapy can cause an increased rate of wound dehiscence and wound infection; this is worse if therapy is given near to the time of the operation.
- Peripheral vascular disease, which is the most common reason for amputation (Footner 1987), causes tissue hypoxia, thus seriously affecting the process of wound healing (Torrance 1986).
- Amputee patients often feel too ill preoperatively to take an adequate diet: this again is likely to delay wound healing.
- Haemorrhage resulting in hypovolaemia causes underperfusion of the edges of the wound, which may lead to underperfusion of the wound after restoration of blood volume; this would seriously affect wound healing.
- Haematoma can also result in a delay in wound healing (Ceccio & Horosz 1988).

The nurse's role in the specific care of wounds is to minimize the risks of delayed wound healing for the patient by devising a suitable care plan.

Assessment of the patient on admission should alert the nurse to any nutritional deficiencies and the patient's experience of pain and stress. Documentation of the wound's appear-

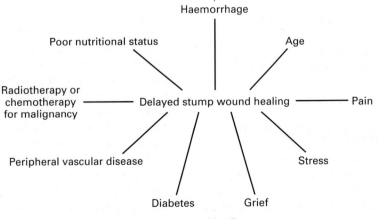

Fig. 17.11   Factors that delay stump wound healing.

ance is essential to ensure continuity of care. Selection of the wound dressing is dependent on the wound assessment and not on the particular preference of the nurse or surgeon. Morison (1987) has written extensively on this subject, discussing and describing the process of wound assessment and the selection of appropriate cleansing solutions and dressings.

There are several factors of which the nurse should be aware when planning this care:

1. Use an aseptic technique when changing dressings; this minimizes the opportunity for the introduction of bacteria.
2. Inspect dressings and the wound, noting characteristics of drainage. Early detection of developing infection provides the opportunity for timely intervention and the prevention of more serious complications such as osteomyelitis.
3. Maintain patency and routinely empty wound drainage. This promotes wound healing and reduces the risk of infection.
4. Expose the limb to air; wash it with mild soap and water after dressings have been discontinued. This maintains cleanliness and increases the resilience of tender or fragile skin.
5. Monitor vital signs such as pyrexia and tachycardia as they may indicate a developing infection.
6. Refer the patient to the dietician:
   a. if his nutritional intake has been impaired for more than 1 week prior to surgery
   b. if he has had inadequate feeding for 5 days or more after surgery
   c. if he has fasted prior to and after surgery. The earlier the nurse refers the patient the better will be the patient's response to treatment.

The potential risk of joint contractures

Joint contractures are a potential problem because the combined effects of the weight of the limb and the antagonistic quality of muscle tension which have kept the limb in its normal position have disappeared with amputation. The stump has nothing to keep it straight and in alignment.

Fixed flexion deformities of joints such as the knee and elbow are common, as are abduction contractures at the hip and shoulder. These contractures occur rapidly after surgery and have been reported as developing after 36 hours of immobility (Judd 1989). It is important to prevent them because they are painful, unsightly and inhibit the fitting and use of the prosthesis.

The nurse needs to assess the patient's general condition to see whether he can move his own limbs. Wherever possible, he should be encouraged to do this.

The nurse should also assess whether the patient needs to have the rationale for this nursing care explained. If joint contractures are seen to be developing, then the physiotherapist and the doctors should be alerted.

Joint contractures are prevented by:

- correct positioning
- exercise: passive, assisted or active
- early weight-bearing.

Correct positioning of the stump is essential from the immediate postoperative period. The stump is placed flat on the bed and never flexed over a pillow. Muscle spasms may make it difficult to keep the stump flat on the bed, but by handling the stump firmly and gently (preferably done by the patient) and using gentle pressure, the stump can be placed firmly back on the bed.

To prevent abduction contractures, amputation stumps of the lower limb are placed near the sound limb in anatomical alignment.

Lying prone for the prevention of hip flexion contractures is not always necessary (Fig. 17.12) and many patients cannot tolerate it. However, if they lie completely flat with a pillow underneath the sacrum and gentle pressure is applied down on the top of the stump, this will serve to strengthen extension muscles and prevent fixed flexion deformities of the hip (Fig. 17.13).

Exercises for the affected as well as the unaffected limbs begin early on in the postoperative period. The physiotherapist should be contacted to explain the specific movements to both nurse and patient.

Early ambulation, i.e. the movement of the

No pillows or *one* pillow

Nurse call bell placed within patient's reach

Head turned to sound side

Arms positioned wherever comfortable for patient

Patient wearing a watch to time period prone

Both hips completely flat on bed

Stump lying flat (with knee straight if b/k) *no pillow*

Remaining leg supported on a pillow to prevent toes from digging into bed

Footboard and bedclothes turned right back out of the way

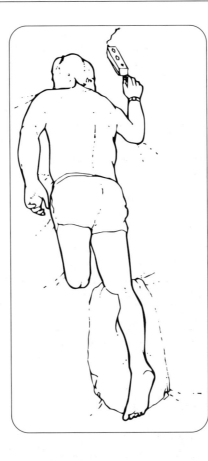

POINTS TO REMEMBER
1. To roll prone, the patient must turn towards the sound side, the nurse ensuring that the stump is lowered gently.
2. Initially the patient lies prone for about 10 minutes.
3. The patient should then build up to lying prone for ½ hour three times a day

Fig. 17.12 Patient lying prone; b/k, below knee. (From Engstrom & Van de Ven 1993, with permission.)

Gentle pressure by nurse or patient to extend the hip

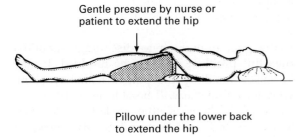

Pillow under the lower back to extend the hip

Fig. 17.13 Position of the patient with pillows to aid extension of the hip.

patient from bed to chair, is encouraged from the first day postoperatively. However, below-knee amputees must be aware of the risk of hanging the stump over the end of their chairs: the stump should be supported on a stool. This prevents excessive oedema formation, aids venous return and prevents fixed flexion deformities that are all exacerbated by inadequate support of the stump.

Evaluation

Evaluation is achieved by observation of the limb, reports of joint stiffness or pain, and ultimately the correct fitting of the prosthesis.

Maintenance of stump shape

The ideal shape for a stump is conical, to facilitate fitting the prosthesis. There are many ways of ensuring that the stump shape is maintained, two of these being by use of plaster of Paris and by fitting a prosthesis immediately after the operation. However, by far the most common is stump bandaging (Fig. 17.14). If performed by an experienced nurse, stump bandaging is very effective in maintaining stump shape. Unfortunately, it is not unusual for the amputee patient to be nursed by inexperienced nurses who apply the stump bandage either much too tightly or ineffectively (Fig. 17.15). In both instances it is better for the patient to have no bandage at all. Incorrectly applied stump bandages which constrict a vulnerable stump can result in ischaemia of the surrounding tissues, leading to wound breakdown and infection and thus prolonging the patient's stay in hospital.

Once the wound is healed a stump sock is a good alternative to stump bandaging. It is easy to apply, both for nurses and patients, and gives continuous pressure over the stump, encouraging a conical shape.

The stump is observed initially half-hourly postoperatively, gradually reducing to 4-hourly as the patient's condition dictates. The nurse assesses:

- The patient's pain
- The patient's skin condition
- The extent of oedema and its effect on the neurovascular status of the stump
- The patient's complaints of pain, cold, excessive heat or numbness.

The effectiveness of the stump sock or bandaging is assessed by judging its effects on the above factors.

The stump sock or bandage is applied immediately postoperatively as oedema can occur rapidly (Doenges 1989). Routine stump care, for example inspection of the skin area and thorough cleansing and drying, provides an opportunity to check for any complications. Once the stump has been inspected the support is reapplied immediately.

Patients can be encouraged to provide as much self-care as possible. In this way the nurse can help the patient adapt to his new situation.

Activity and rest

Chapters 5 and 6 discuss the necessary balance between activity and rest. However, for the purposes of this section, the focus will be on activity and how the nurse facilitates it.

Amputee patients cite problems with mobility as their second major concern after pain (Ceccio & Horosz 1988); they have to adapt to a permanent change and learn new ways of moving around. The level of mobility aimed for is decided on an individual basis, the nurse ensuring that the patient has the knowledge and capabilities to cope with his disability.

How soon an amputee starts mobilizing will depend on his physical and mental fitness but should not be delayed, in order to avoid the complications that can arise from immobility. Mobility also increases the patient's motivation and encourages a healthier mental state.

The patient's ability to mobilize is affected by several factors:

- pain
- effects of anaesthesia
- strength
- motivation
- knowledge.

If the pain is enough to discourage mobility, then this problem needs to be resolved. It may be exacerbated by the patient's anxiety about whether or not he will be able to mobilize. To assess the extent of this anxiety, scales (see Teasdale 1987) can be used by the nurse to ascertain the level of pain he is experiencing.

Motivation, or lack of it, can be a result of

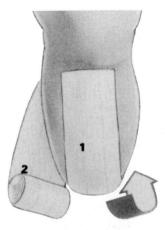

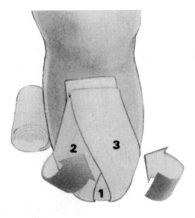

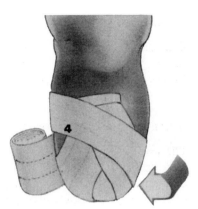

1 Commence bandaging just below the patella and cover the distal end of the stump, (turn 1), by taking the bandage to just below the popliteal space. Fold the bandage and bring back to the outside of the stump (turn 2).

2 Return to the starting point and fold the bandage taking it to the inside of the distal end of the stump (turn 3). It is now taken behind to the upper part of the stump on the medial side.

3 Bring the bandage diagonally across the front of the stump (turn 4) to partially cover turn 3 and around the back to the medial side at the distal end.

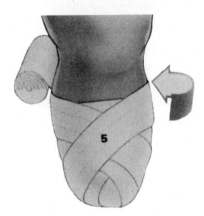

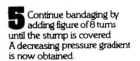

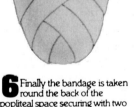

4 Figures of 8 are now commenced by passing the bandage diagonally over the front of the stump (turn 5), around the back and returning diagonally to the base of the stump.

5 Continue bandaging by adding figure of 8 turns until the stump is covered A decreasing pressure gradient is now obtained.

6 Finally the bandage is taken round the back of the popliteal space securing with two turns above the knee, ensuring the joint is left free.

Fig. 17.14   Stump bandaging technique for a below-knee amputation. The bandage used in this illustration is 'Elset-S' (courtesy of Seton Products). (From Powell 1986, with permission.)

the patient's level of acceptance of his loss. The patient who has not yet achieved acceptance will be less keen to commence mobilizing; he will spend time dwelling on the loss, trying to come to terms with it and begrudging the reminders that mobilization brings of his disability.

Knowledge alleviates anxiety. If the patient does not know how to move, he will worry about it and be reluctant to try.

Figure 17.16 outlines a suggested mobility plan. Both nurse and patient decide on the plan: the goals are identified by a cross. For example,

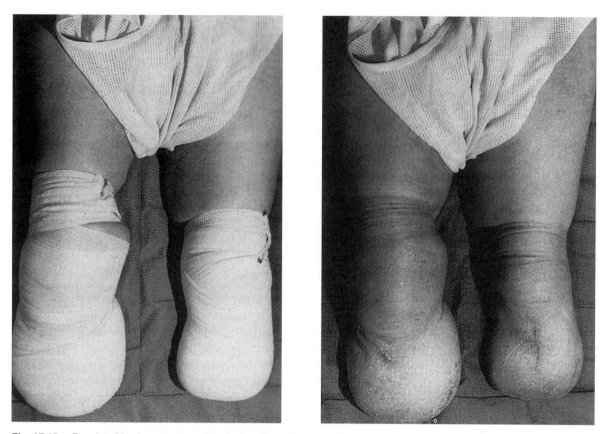

Fig. 17.15 Results of inadequate stump bandaging. (From Engstrom & Van de Ven 1993, with permission.)

in this plan the patient's goal is to stand with a frame by day 4 post-amputation. The plan encourages individualized care as the crosses are positioned in accordance with the patient's needs and abilities. The physiotherapist could also be included to help the patient and nurse to set realistic, achievable goals. Patients following amputation will become demoralized and depressed if they do not achieve set targets.

Bereavement and loss

Adjustment to amputation can continue for a long time after discharge and will affect the patient and his family, who are important for the emotional, physical, spiritual and cultural support they give to the amputee (Craig et al 1988).

Nurses can assist new amputees to become aware of their capabilities, and work with patients and families to ensure that no artificial limitations are imposed. Often the family's response is to do much that the amputee could do himself. Over-protection not only increases his anxiety and sense of insecurity, but also decreases his initiative, independence and sense of self-worth because very little is expected of him (Novotny 1987).

The nurse can assess the family for its level of support. A family with a large support network can 'spread the load' in terms of the care. Each family member supports the other who in turn supports the patient. The smaller family, with perhaps only one or two members, may need additional support to fulfil this role while the patient is in hospital and after discharge.

It is important for the nurse to identify the patient's level of acceptance so that she can plan strategies to encourage acceptance (Figs 17.6 and 17.7).

Postoperative days

Mobility	1	2	3	4	5	6	7	8	9	10	11	12	13	14	15	16	17	18	19	20	21	22	COMMENTS
1. Lying flat twice a day with pillow under sacrum.		✕																			✕		
2. Bed to chair, twice a day, gradually increasing to four times a day.			✕						✕														
3. Transferring independently from bed to chair.						✕															✕		
4. Chair only. To bed to lie flat twice a day.								✕													✕		
5. Standing with a frame learning to get one's balance.			✕					✕															
6. Hopping with a frame around the bed.								✕	✕														
7. Hopping with a frame to the bathroom independently.									✕												✕		
8. Gym to walk on the parallel bars.			✕																		✕		

Fig. 17.16 A suggested plan of mobility progress. Goals marked with a cross.

Parkes (1986) identifies five bereavement reactions that the amputee patient is likely to experience:

1. A process of realization, i.e. from denial or avoidance to recognition of the loss towards acceptance
2. An alarm reaction: anxiety, restlessness and the physiological signs of fear or stress
3. Mourning for lost intactness: yearning for wholeness and full mobility
4. Anger and guilt directed towards those who are intact; anger towards those who prematurely pressurize the patient to accept his loss
5. Feelings of internal loss or mutilation.

The patient who is finding it difficult to accept his situation is more likely to need his family's support on discharge. The nurse must ensure that the patient's family understands the amputee's feelings and know ways to support him as constructively as possible (Craig et al 1988).

Once the patient's primary carer in the family has been identified, regular meetings with that individual should be arranged to discuss progress and feelings generated by the amputation and its aftercare. The patient should be included in these discussions unless he states otherwise.

A resource manual to inform families of available community services upon discharge is helpful and should be given to the patient and members of his family as soon after the operation as possible. Once the nurse has assessed how supportive the family is as a unit she can plan whether and how often she needs to meet family members.

Changes in feelings of sexuality following amputation

Disruptions to an individual's sexuality are common in patients following amputation. Physiological problems can arise – for example, in patients who suffer from peripheral vascular disease which can inhibit penile erection. Anaemia as a result of surgery causes tiredness and lethargy. Drugs such as analgesics, antiemetics and antihypertensives can interfere with sexual function (Hine & Daines 1987).

Environmental factors within the hospital can contribute to sexual dysfunction. It is difficult to ensure privacy in hospital, which can be a worry for patients and their partners who need to have time together to talk over the more intimate details of their lives. Physical expression of emotion is discouraged by the hospital environment and, at times, by the hospital staff, leading to frustration and anxiety (Judd 1989). The feelings generated by amputation can exacerbate any existing problems or create new ones in a previously stable relationship.

A deteriorating self-esteem and a distorted body image can both be a result of amputation and can have disastrous effects on the patient's sexual feelings and performance. For example, the patient or his partner may believe that disabled people are not meant to be sexual. Amputee patients generally view their bodies in a negative way, feeling guilty that they cannot be attractive to their partners, whose reassurances are viewed as pity. They can easily plummet into a depression and be overwhelmed by feelings of inadequacy while the partner can feel helpless and frustrated.

Assessment of this private aspect of the patient's life needs to be conducted sensitively. Inclusion of the subject by the nurse when she is involved in a family discussion could provide her with the opportunity to talk to both partners together; or the subject could be introduced along with other aspects of care as a natural part of the patient's life. In doing this the nurse gives the patient permission to discuss any problems.

The role of the nurse is to assist patients in their understanding of sexuality so that patient and partner will be able to assume responsibility for their own sexuality under the most helpful circumstances (Hine & Daines 1987).

The patient may require information on any constraints on his sexual activity. Once the stump has healed, sexual intercourse can be resumed in whatever position is comfortable. If the patient has sexual difficulties as a result of his medical condition or medication, then referral to the medical staff should be considered.

If the patient is finding it difficult to accept his amputation he will be more likely to experience sexual problems. Some of these are complex and beyond the skills of most nurses to resolve; referral to a sexual counsellor must be considered.

Evaluation can only be achieved if the nurse asks the patient and his partner about the success of the intervention and compares this information with the goals set. Too often this is an area of care ignored by nurses and addressed only when the patient 'plucks up courage' to ask advice. It is hoped that this will change as nurses become more aware of the degree to which amputee patients are susceptible to sexual problems.

CONCLUSION

After surgery and during rehabilitation, the nurse needs to ensure that all members of the multidisciplinary team provide the care the amputee patient needs to help him recover from this radical surgery and live as independently as possible.

As a result of the amputation, the individual's status changes, at least temporarily, from active independence to disabled dependence. The aim of this chapter is to provide the nurse with the information she needs to help the amputee patient accept his disability, gradually acknowledge his loss and utilize his remaining potential to become a productive and self-reliant individual.

As the date of discharge approaches, the patient may find it reassuring to have the addresses of people or groups to contact in the community who can give him some support. It should be possible to obtain these local addresses from the Social Work department in the hospital.

Useful national addresses are listed below:

National Association for Limbless Disabled
134 Martindale Road, Hounslow, Middlesex
TW4 7NQ
Tel: 081 572 5337

Royal Association for Disability and Rehabilitation
25 Mortimer Street, London W1N 8AB
Tel: 071 637 5400

Disabled Living Foundation
380–384 Harrow Road, London W9 2HV
Tel: 081 289 6111.

REFERENCES

Atkinson R L, Atkinson R C, Smith E E, Hilgard E R, 1987 Introduction to psychology, 9th edn. Harcourt, Brace & Jovanovich, New York

Blake C 1989 Care of the patient requiring surgical intervention. In: Hinchliffe S M, Norman S E, Schober J E (eds) Nursing practice and health care. Edward Arnold, London

Burnard P 1988 Coping with other peoples emotions. Professional Nurse 4(1): 11–14

Campbell S M, Walker J M 1989 Pain assessment, nursing models and the nursing process. Recent Advances in Nursing 24: 47–61

Ceccio C M, Horosz J E 1988 Teaching the elderly amputee to meet the world. Registered Nurse Sept: 70–76

Cooper D M, Schumann D 1979 Post surgical nursing intervention as an adjunct to wound healing. Nursing Clinics of North America 11(4): 713–725

Craig M C, Copes W S, Champion H R 1988 Psychosocial considerations in trauma care. Critical Care Nursing Quarterly 11(2): 51–58

Doenges M E 1989 Nursing care plans. Guidelines for planning patient care, 2nd edn. F A Davis, Philadelphia

Engstrom B, Van de Ven C 1993 Physiotherapy for amputees, 2nd edn. Churchill Livingstone, Edinburgh

Feist J, Brannon L 1988 Health Psychology. Wadsworth, Belmont, California

Footner A 1987 Orthopaedic nursing. Heinemann Nursing, Oxford

Gartside G 1986 Alternative methods of pain relief. Nursing (London) 3(11): 405–407

Goodwin J 1986 Post operative pain: is it being adequately managed? Medical Dialogue. 104 A

Henderson V 1966 The nature of nursing: a definition and its implications for practice, research and education. Macmillan, New York

Herbener D 1988 The phantom limb phenomenon. Physicians Assistant 12(7): 57–66

Heron J 1973 Co counsellors teacher's manual. Human potential research project. University of Surrey, Guildford

Hinchliffe S M, Norman S E, Schober J E 1989 Nursing practice and health care. Edward Arnold, London

Hine J, Daines B 1987 Sexuality and the renal patient. Nursing Times 83(20): 35–36

Holmes T H, Rahe R H 1967 Journal of Psychosomatic Research 11: 212–218

Hopson B 1981 Response to papers by Schlossberg, Branner and Abrego. Counselling Psychology 9(36): 39

Judd M 1989 Mobility patient problems and nursing care. Heinemann Nursing, Oxford

Maguire P, Faulkner A 1988 Communicate with cancer patients: in handling bad news and difficult questions. British Medical Journal 8 Oct: 907–908

McFarlane J K 1976 A charter for caring. Journal of Advanced Nursing 1: 187–196

McFarlane F, Castledine G 1982 A guide to the practice of nursing using the nursing process. C V Mosby, London

Montague A 1978 Touching: the human significance of the skin. Harper & Row, New York

Moos R H 1986 Coping with life crisis. An integrated approach. Plenum, New York

Morison M J 1987 Wound assessment. Professional Nurse 2(10): 315–317

Novotny M P 1986 Body image changed in amputee children. Journal of Association of Paediatric Oncology Nurses 3(2): 8–13

Orem D E 1985 Nursing: concepts for practice, 3rd edn. McGraw Hill, New York

Parkes C M Weiss R S 1983 Recovery from bereavement. Basic Books, New York

Parkes C M 1986 Bereavement. Studies of grief in adult life. Penguin, Harmondsworth

Potterton D 1986 The avoidable disability. Nursing Times 83(13): 18–19

Powell M 1986 Orthopaedic nursing and rehabilitation, 9th edn. Churchill Livingstone, Edinburgh

Reich W 1976 Character analysis. Simon & Schuster, New York

Selye H 1956 The stress of life. McGraw Hill, New York

Spencer K E 1989 Post operative pain: the alternatives to analgesia. Professional Nurse 4(10): 479–480

Teasdale K 1987 Giving reassurance to anxious patients. Professional Nurse 2(4): 112–113

Torrance C 1986 The physiology of wound healing. Nursing (London) 3(5): 162–168

Wall R, Novotny J P, MacNamara T E 1985 Does pre amputation pain influence phantom limb pain in cancer patients? South Medical Journal 78(1): 34–36

Weinstein C L 1985 Assertiveness, anxiety and interpersonal discomfort among amputees: implications for assertiveness training. Archives of Physical Medicine and Rehabilitation 66: 687–689

Wilson-Barnett J, Batehup L 1988 Patient problems. A research base for Nursing Care. Scutari, London

Winfield V 1986 Too close a shave. Nursing Times 82(24): 64–66

Wysocki A B 1989 Surgical wound healing American Operating Room Nursing Journal 49(2): 502–518

Glossary

Abscess – Local collection of pus

Achlorhydria – Absence of hydrochloric acid in the stomach

Amyloidosis – Accumulation of abnormal protein in various tissues of the body

Antibody (immunoglobulin) – specific protein produced by the immune system in response to invasion by a specific antigen

Antigen – Any foreign substance stimulating the body's immune system to respond by producing specific antibodies. Bacterial cells, pollen grains, foreign cells from tissue grafts and transplants all operate as antigens

Arthralgia – Pain in a joint

Arthroplasty – Refashioning of a joint

Atelectasis – Shrunken and airless state of the lungs due to failure of expansion or resorption of air from the alveoli

Bactericide – A physical or chemical agent able to destroy vegetative bacteria

Chemotaxis – Attraction of white cells by chemicals

Chondroblast – Cartilage-secreting cell

Cushingoid – The characteristic round face of Cushing's syndrome

Diapedesis – A property of neutrophils, allowing them to leave the capillaries and enter the tissues by squeezing through narrow slits between neighbouring capillary endothelial cells

Dyspareunia – Painful sexual intercourse

Electromyography – Recording of the electrical currents generated by muscular activity

Endogenous – Originating or produced within an organism, or from some part of it

Exogenous – Originating or produced outside the organism

Fibroblast – Cell present in connective tissue which responds to tissue damage by synthesizing collagen fibres necessary for repair; when fibroblasts are inactive they are often described as fibrocytes

Fomite – Object able to carry infection from one person to another, contributing to cross-infection, e.g. bedpans, urinals, blankets etc.

Gangrene – Tissue necrosis on which the infective activity of bacteria belonging to the clostridium group is imposed

Gram-positive bacteria – Many bacteria contain chemicals in their cell walls allowing them to take up the blue or purple colour of a laboratory dye, Gram's stain, widely used in identification and diagnosis, e.g. *Staphylococcus*. Gram-negative bacteria retain the red colour of a counterstain and are thus distinguishable, e.g. *Proteus, Klebsiella, Pseudomonas, E. coli*

Hyperaemia – Initial response of the tissues to damage during acute inflammation. Vasoconstriction causes whitening of the tissue followed by a dull red flare as vasodilation causes increased vascular supply

Inflammation – Non-specific protective response of living tissues to any kind of trauma, e.g. excess heat or cold, radiation, chemicals, bacteria

Kinins – A group of biologically active proteins released during the inflammatory response. The best known is bradykinin, which produces extravascular smooth muscle contraction, vasodilation, increased capillary permeability and pain in response to noxious stimuli. It may chemotactically attract white cells active in the inflammatory response

Leucopenia – Abnormal reduction in the number of white cells in the blood

Lymphopenia – Reduction of the number of lymphocytes in the blood

Neutropenia – Abnormally small number of neutrophils in the blood

Opportunist – Microorganism of low-grade pathogenicity able to invade the tissues and cause development of clinical infection in a severely debilitated patient. Opportunists do not infect healthy individuals

Osteo – Referring to bone

Osteomyelitis – Infection of bone; may be acute or chronic

Osteophytes – Bony outgrowths

Osteosclerosis – Thickening of bone

Pathogenicity – Ability to produce disease

Phagocytosis – A process by which bacteria are engulfed by white cells (mainly neutrophils and macrophages) and actively destroyed by the action of hydrolytic enzymes

Pyogenic – Ability of a bacterium to induce pus

formation. Pyogenic infections are usually acute

Sequestrum – Necrotic, non-viable bone

Sinus – Long tortuous track discharging pus and wound exudate from a chronic focus of infection deep in the tissues onto an external or internal body surface

Suppuration – Pus formation; pus is a mixture of dead cells, including neutrophils, bacteria and debris contaminating a wound

Thomas' sign – Test for fixed flexion deformity of the hip. Lying supine, the patient can compensate for a fixed flexion deformity of a hip by arching the lumbar spine. If the other hip is then passively flexed to its fullest range, the spine will flatten. Any attempt to flex it further will cause the affected hip to flex, revealing the deformity

Tophi – Gritty concretion due to gout, found most commonly on the edge of the auricle of the ear or in the joints

Totipotency – Ability of cells to undergo mitosis and regenerate

Toxin – Poison produced by bacteria, usually contributing to the specific signs and symptoms of the infection. Toxins have a damaging effect on the host and contribute to virulence; i.e. a species able to produce very potent toxins will be highly virulent

Trendelenburg sign – Test for instability of hip joint (weakened glutei). The patient stands on one leg, unsupported. The test is positive if the crease of the opposite buttock falls (the pelvis tilts down) and negative if it rises (pelvis tilts upwards)

Index